PROGRESS IN CLINICAL AND BIOLOGICAL RESEARCH

RECENT TITLES

Vol 50: **Rights and Responsibilities in Modern Medicine: The Second Volume in a Series on Ethics, Humanism, and Medicine,** Marc D. Basson, *Editor*

Vol 51: **The Function of Red Blood Cells: Erythrocyte Pathobiology,** Donald F. H. Wallach, *Editor*

Vol 52: **Conduction Velocity Distributions: A Population Approach to Electrophysiology of Nerve,** Leslie J. Dorfman, Kenneth L. Cummins, and Larry J. Leifer, *Editors*

Vol 53: **Cancer Among Black Populations,** Curtis Mettlin and Gerald P. Murphy, *Editors*

Vol 54: **Connective Tissue Research: Chemistry, Biology, and Physiology,** Zdenek Deyl and Milan Adam, *Editors*

Vol 55: **The Red Cell: Fifth Ann Arbor Conference,** George J. Brewer, *Editor*

Vol 56: **Erythrocyte Membranes 2: Recent Clinical and Experimental Advances,** Walter C. Kruckeberg, John W. Eaton, and George J. Brewer, *Editors*

Vol 57: **Progress in Cancer Control,** Curtis Mettlin and Gerald P. Murphy, *Editors*

Vol 58: **The Lymphocyte,** Kenneth W. Sell and William V. Miller, *Editors*

Vol 59: **Eleventh International Congress of Anatomy,** Enrique Acosta Vidrio, *Editor-in-Chief.* Published in 3 volumes: Part A: **Glial and Neuronal Cell Biology,** Sergey Fedoroff, *Editor* Part B: **Advances in the Morphology of Cells and Tissues,** Miguel A. Galina, *Editor* Part C: **Biological Rhythms in Structure and Function,** Heinz von Mayersbach, Lawrence E. Scheving, and John E. Pauly, *Editors*

Vol 60: **Advances in Hemoglobin Analysis,** Samir M. Hanash and George J. Brewer, *Editors*

Vol 61: **Nutrition and Child Health: Perspectives for the 1980s,** Reginald C. Tsang and Buford Lee Nichols, Jr., *Editors*

Vol 62: **Pathophysiological Effects of Endotoxins at the Cellular Level,** Jeannine A. Majde and Robert J. Person, *Editors*

Vol 63: **Membrane Transport and Neuroreceptors,** Dale Oxender, Arthur Blume, Ivan Diamond, and C. Fred Fox, *Editors*

Vol 64: **Bacteriophage Assembly,** Michael S. DuBow, *Editor*

Vol 65: **Apheresis: Development, Applications, and Collection Procedures,** C. Harold Mielke, Jr., *Editor*

Vol 66: **Control of Cellular Division and Development,** Dennis Cunningham, Eugene Goldwasser, James Watson, and C. Fred Fox, *Editors.* Published in 2 Volumes.

Vol 67: **Nutrition in the 1980s: Constraints on Our Knowledge,** Nancy Selvey and Philip L. White, *Editors*

Vol 68: **The Role of Peptides and Amino Acids as Neurotransmitters,** J. Barry Lombardini and Alexander D. Kenny, *Editors*

Vol 69: **Twin Research 3, Proceedings of the Third International Congress on Twin Studies,** Luigi Gedda, Paolo Parisi, and Walter E. Nance, *Editors.* Published in 3 volumes: Part A: **Twin Biology and Multiple Pregnancy** Part B: **Intelligence, Personality, and Development** Part C: **Epidemiological and Clinical Studies**

Vol 70: **Reproductive Immunology,** Norbert Gleicher, *Editor*

Vol 71: **Psychopharmacology of Clonidine,** Harbans Lal and Stuart Fielding, *Editors*

Vol 72: **Hemophilia and Hemostasis,** Doris Ménaché, D. MacN. Surgenor, and

See pages following the index for previous titles in this series.

Harlan D. Anderson, *Editors*

Vol 73: **Membrane Biophysics: Structure and Function in Epithelia,** Mumtaz A. Dinno and Arthur B. Callahan, *Editors*

Vol 74: **Physiopathology of Endocrine Diseases and Mechanisms of Hormone Action,** Roberto J. Soto, Alejandro De Nicola, and Jorge Blaquier, *Editors*

Vol 75: **The Prostatic Cell: Structure and Function,** Gerald P. Murphy, Avery A. Sandberg, and James P. Karr, *Editors.* Published in 2 volumes: Part A: **Morphologic, Secretory, and Biochemical Aspects** Part B: **Prolactin, Carcinogenesis, and Clinical Aspects**

Vol 76: **Troubling Problems in Medical Ethics: The Third Volume in a Series on Ethics, Humanism, and Medicine,** Marc D. Basson, Rachel E. Lipson, and Doreen L. Ganos, *Editors*

Vol 77: **Nutrition in Health and Disease and International Development: Symposia From the XII International Congress of Nutrition,** Alfred E. Harper and George K. Davis, *Editors*

Vol 78: **Female Incontinence,** Norman R. Zinner and Arthur M. Sterling, *Editors*

Vol 79: **Proteins in the Nervous System: Structure and Function,** Bernard Haber, Jose Regino Perez-Polo, and Joe Dan Coulter *Editors*

Vol 80: **Mechanism and Control of Ciliary Movement,** Charles J. Brokaw and Pedro Verdugo, *Editors*

Vol 81: **Physiology and Biology of Horseshoe Crabs: Studies on Normal and Environmentally Stressed Animals,** Joseph Bonaventura, Celia Bonaventura, and Shirley Tesh, *Editors*

Vol 82: **Clinical, Structural, and Biochemical Advances in Hereditary Eye Disorders,** Donna L. Daentl, *Editor*

Vol 83: **Issues in Cancer Screening and Communications,** Curtis Mettlin and Gerald P. Murphy, *Editors*

Vol 84: **Progress in Dermatoglyphic Research,** Christos S. Bartsocas, *Editor*

Vol 85: **Embryonic Development,** Max M. Burger and Rudolf Weber, *Editors.* Published in 2 volumes: Part A: **Genetic Aspects** Part B: **Cellular Aspects**

Vol 86: **The Interaction of Acoustical and Electromagnetic Fields With Biological Systems,** Shiro Takashima and Elliot Postow, *Editors*

Vol 87: **Physiopathology of Hypophysial Disturbances and Diseases of Reproduction,** Alejandro De Nicola, Jorge Blaquier, and Roberto J. Soto, *Editors*

Vol 88: **Cytapheresis and Plasma Exchange: Clinical Indications,** W.R. Vogler, *Editor*

Vol 89: **Interaction of Platelets and Tumor Cells,** G.A. Jamieson, *Editor;* Alice R. Scipio, *Assistant Editor*

Vol 90: **Beta-Carbolines and Tetrahydroisoquinolines,** Floyd Bloom, Jack Barchas, Merton Sandler, and Earl Usdin, *Organizers*

Vol 91: **Membranes in Growth and Development,** Joseph F. Hoffman, Gerhard H. Giebisch, and Liana Bolis, *Editors*

Vol 92: **The Pineal and Its Hormones,** Russel J. Reiter, *Editor*

Vol 93: **Endotoxins and Their Detection With the Limulus Amebocyte Lysate Test,** Stanley W. Watson, Jack Levin, and Thomas J. Novitsky, *Editors*

Vol 94: **Animal Models of Inherited Diseases,** Robert J. Desnick, Donald F. Patterson, and Dante G. Scarpelli, *Editors*

Vol 95: **Gaucher Disease: A Century of Delineation and Research,** Robert J. Desnick, Shimon Gatt, and Gregory A. Grabowski, *Editors*

Vol 96: **Mechanisms of Speciation,** Claudio Barigozzi, *Editor*

Vol 97: **Membranes and Genetic Disease,** John R. Sheppard, V. Elving Anderson, and John W. Eaton, *Editors*

Vol 98: **Advances in the Pathophysiology, Diagnosis, and Treatment of Sickle Cell Disease,** Roland B. Scott, *Editor*

Vol 99: **Osteosarcoma: New Trends in Diagnosis and Treatment,** Alexander Katznelson and Jacobo Nerubay, *Editors*

Vol 100: **Renal Tumors: Proceedings of the First International Symposium on Kidney Tumors,** René Küss, Gerald P. Murphy, Saad Khoury, and James P. Karr, *Editors*

RENAL TUMORS

Proceedings of the
First International Symposium
on Kidney Tumors

RENAL TUMORS
Proceedings of the First International Symposium on Kidney Tumors

Paris, France
November 1981

Editors

RENÉ KÜSS, MD
Professor of Urology
Chief of Urology Clinic
Hôpital de la Pitié
Paris, France

GERALD P. MURPHY, MD, DSc
Institute Director
Roswell Park Memorial Institute
Buffalo, New York, USA

SAAD KHOURY, MD
Professor of Urology
Hôpital de la Pitié
Paris, France

JAMES P. KARR, PhD
Experimental Surgery Department
Roswell Park Memorial Institute
Buffalo, New York, USA

ALAN R. LISS, INC. • NEW YORK

Address all Inquiries to the Publisher
Alan R. Liss, Inc., 150 Fifth Avenue, New York, NY 10011

Library of Congress Cataloging in Publication Data

International Symposium on Kidney Tumors (1st:
  1981: Paris, France)
  Renal tumors.

    Includes bibliographies and index.
    1. Kidneys—Tumors—Congresses. I. Küss, René
Robert. II. Title. [DNLM: 1. Kidney neoplasms—
Congresses. WI PR668E v. 100/WJ 358 I59 1981r]
RC280.K5148   1981   616.99′461   82-14008
ISBN 0-8451-0100-5

Contents

Contributors . . . . **xiii**

Welcome and Introduction
René Küss . . . . **xxi**

NEPHROBLASTOMA (WILMS' TUMOR)

Histopathological Aspects of Renal Tumors in Children
J. Bruce Beckwith **1**

An Experimental Wilms' Tumor
Gerald P. Murphy **15**

Wilms' Tumor: Genetic Aspects and Etiology
G.J. D'Angio and A.E. Evans **43**

Evaluation of Nephroblastomas
Sylvia Neuenschwander, Jean Philippe Montagne, and
Clément Fauré **59**

Computerized Tomography and Nephroblastomas
Dominique Couanet, Anne Geoffray, Francoise Le Bras,
Jean Daniel Piekarski, Daniel Vanel, and Jacques Masselot **67**

**Evaluation of Unusual Nephroblastomas and Differential
Diagnosis**
Jean Philippe Montagne, Sylvia Neuenschwander, and
Clément Fauré **71**

Preoperative Diagnosis of Wilms' Tumor
Denys Pellerin **83**

Surgery of Wilms' Tumor
Denys Pellerin **85**

**TMM Description and Staging of Wilms' Tumors. Prognostic
Factors**
Jean Lemerle **91**

**Radiation Therapy of Wilms' Tumor. Methods and Immediate
Complications**
Pierre Bey **97**

**Chemotherapy in Wilms' Tumor — Indications and Early Side
Effects**
Annie Boilletot **111**

Complications and Sequelae of the Treatment of Wilms' Tumor
Jean Lemerle **119**

Wilms' Tumor Updated: Evolution of Ideas and Trends
G.J. D'Angio and A.E. Evans **123**

Preoperative Chemotherapy in Wilms' Tumour. Results of
Clinical Trials and Studies on Nephroblastomas Conducted by
the International Society of Paediatric Oncology (SIOP)
J. de Kraker, P.A. Voûte, J. Lemerle, M.-F. Tournade, and
H.J.M. Perry 131

Wilms' Tumor: Histologic Grading as a Prognostic Factor in
Tumors Beyond 10 cm in Diameter
Julio Pow-Sang, Graciela Ramírez, and Víctor Benavente 145

Surgical Aspects of Simultaneous Bilateral Wilms' Tumors
M. Gruner, B. Chaouachi, and M. Bitker 155

Late-Recurring Wilms' Tumors
N. Clausen 165

The Treatment of Wilms' Tumor in 1982. The Status of the Art
Jean Lemerle 167

KIDNEY TUMORS IN ADULTS

Murine Renal Cell Carcinoma: A Suitable Human Model
Gerald P. Murphy 175

The Clinical Significance of NMRI Nu/Nu Mice Tumor Model
Ullrich Otto and Hartwig Huland 207

Evaluation of Effective Vinblastine–Sulfate Dosage in Different
Renal Cell Carcinomas After Transplantation to the Nu/Nu Mice
U. Otto, H. Huland, and H. Klosterhalfen 209

Receptor Profiles in Renal Cell Carcinoma
James P. Karr, Sarah Schneider, Hanna Rosenthal,
Avery A. Sandberg, and Gerald P. Murphy 211

Steroid Receptors in Kidney Tumours
R. Ghanadian, G. Auf, G. Williams, and A.P.M. Coleman 245

Aetiology of Renal Cancer
Michele Pavone-Macaluso, Giovanni B. Ingargiola, and
Marcello Lamartina 255

Clinically Unrecognized Renal Cell Carcinoma. An Autopsy
Study
Sverker Hellsten, Thorbjörn Berge, Folke Linell, and Lennart Wehlin 273

Paraneoplastic Syndromes: Introduction
Geoffrey D. Chisholm 277

Fever in Adult Renal Cancer
L. Friocourt, J. Jouquan, S. Khoury, R. Richard, G. Chomette, and
P. Godeau 283

Hypercalcaemia
Geoffrey D. Chisholm 293

The Nonmetastatic Hepatic Dysfunction Syndrome Associated
With Renal Cell Carcinoma (Hypernephroma): Stauffer's
Syndrome
Kamal A. Hanash 301

Metastatic Renal Cell Adenocarcinoma
Wafic S. Tabbara, Amira M. Mehio, and George P. Aftimos 317

Clinical Signs in Renal Neoplasia. A Comparison of Two Series of Three Hundred Cases
A. Haertig and R. Küss 337

Positive and Differential Diagnosis, and Diagnostic Pitfalls of Malignant Tumors: I.V.P.
J. Grellet 341

Nephrotomography in Patients With Renal Carcinoma
Karen Damgaard and Flemming Lund 345

Arteriography and Cancer of the Kidney
C. Bollack and J.J. Wenger 349

How Does Ultrasound Show Renal Cancer, Diagnostic Difficulties and Reliability
M. Ch. Plainfosse and S. Merran 369

Computed Tomography in the Diagnosis and Evaluation of Renal Cell Carcinoma
François Richard, Saad Khoury, and René Küss 377

Computed Tomography Detection of Inferior Vena Cava Obstruction in Renal Cancers
L.M. Rognon and Ch. Caron-Poitreau 399

Local Recurrence After Nephrectomy for Renal Cancer: CT Recognition
Roger A. Parienty, Janine Pradel, François Richard, and Saad Khoury 409

Does Percutaneous Puncture Still Have a Role to Play in the Diagnosis of Renal Tumors
Adolphe Steg 417

Cytologic Diagnosis of Renal Cell Carcinoma
Sixten Franzén and Eva Brehmer-Andersson 425

Diagnostic Value of Lipid Content in Cyst Fluid
S. Pettersson, H. Kleist, O. Jonsson, S. Lundstam, J. Nauclér, and A.E. Nilson 433

Is Explorative Lumbotomy Still Indicated as a Means of Diagnosing a Kidney Tumor?
G. Arvis 435

Renal Tumour Syndrome: Hierarchy of Investigations
J. Auvert, C.C. Abbou, and V. Lavarenne 437

Staging of Renal Cell Carcinoma
Charles J. Robson 439

The Natural History of Renal Cell Carcinoma
Charles J. Robson 447

Thoracophrenolaparotomy
W. Grégoir 453

Lumbar Flank Approach
Saad Khoury 457

The Abdominal Approach in Kidney Tumors of the Adult
Herbert Brendler 461

**The Anterior Transabdominal Transversal Sub-Costal Approach
for Removal of Renal Cancer**
B. Dufour and Ch. Choquenet 465

The Choice of Surgical Incision
Philip H. Smith and David F. Green 471

**Results of Radical Nephrectomy Without Lymphadenectomy in
Renal Cell Carcinoma**
C. Chatelain 475

**Results of Radical Thoraco-Abdominal Nephrectomy in the
Treatment of Renal Cell Carcinoma**
Charles J. Robson 481

**Comparative Study of Actuarial Survival Rates in Stage II and III
Renal Cell Carcinomas Managed by Radical Nephrectomy Alone
or Associated With Formal Retroperitoneal Lymph Node
Dissection**
A. Gilloz and J. Tostain 489

**Should Lymphadenectomy be Associated to Radical
Nephrectomy in Renal Cell Carcinoma?**
C. Chatelain 493

**Locally Extensive Renal Cell Carcinoma — Current Surgical
Management of Invasion of Vena Cava, Liver, or Bowel**
Ruben F. Gittes 497

Bench Surgery in Renal Tumors
Ruben F. Gittes 509

Conservative Surgery in Renal Cell Carcinoma
René Küss 519

**Renal Cell Carcinoma Extending Into the Inferior Vena Cava.
Technical Problems**
J. Cinqualbre, J.M. Py, and C. Bollack 529

Is Radical Nephrectomy Useful When Metastases Are Present?
C. Chatelain 533

The Treatment of Metastasis From Renal Cell Carcinoma
Saad Khoury 541

**Tumor Recurrence in the Renal Fossa and/or the Abdominal
Wall After Radical Nephrectomy for Renal Cell Carcinoma**
Aurelio C. Uson 549

**Reflections on the Treatment of Transitional-Cell Tumours of the
Upper Urinary Tract**
Etienne Mazeman 561

**Autotransplantation With Direct Pyelovesical Anastomosis in
Renal Pelvic and Ureteric Tumours. A New Approach**
S. Pettersson, H. Brynger, Ch. Henriksson, S. Johansson,
A.E. Nilson, and T. Ranch 569

Renal Angiomyolipoma
Alain Jardin 573

The Transplanted Kidney as a Vector of Malignant Cells
P. Frantz, C. Chatelain, J. Poisson, J. Luciani, C. Jacobs, and R. Küss 581

Renal Oncocytoma (Pathology, Preoperative Diagnosis, Therapy)
H.D. Lehmann and M.H. Blessing 589

Needle Tract Seeding Following Puncture of Renal Oncocytoma
J. Auvert, C.C. Abbou, and V. Lavarenne 597

Natural History of Renal Cell Carcinoma Left in Place
G. Vallancien, Djedje Madi, F. Richard, and R. Küss 599

Improvements of the Renal Tumor Embolization Technique
Ph. Curet 601

**The Indications of Embolisation in Renal Tumor: What Remains
to Be Said?**
M. Le Guillou and J.J. Merland 603

Pre- and Postoperative Radiotherapy, Influence on Prognosis
Lennart Andersson and Folke Edsmyr 609

Kidney Carcinoma: Is Preoperative Radiotherapy of any Value?
L. Boccon Gibod, G. Benoit, F. Eschwege, and A. Steg 617

Hormonal Therapy of Renal Cell Carcinoma (RCC)
Ulrico Bracci, Franco DiSilverio, and Giuseppe Concolino 623

Treatment of Advanced Renal Cell Carcinoma
Jean B. deKernion and Arie Lindner 641

**Combined Chemotherapy and Radiotherapy in Metastatic Renal
Carcinoma**
Lennart Andersson and Folke Edsmyr 661

Methyl-GAG in Advanced Renal Cell Carcinoma
J.A. Child 663

Chemotherapy of Renal Tumours. Personal Experience
C. Jacquillat, G. Auclerc, M.F. Auclerc, N. Chamsedine, J. Mara,
and M. Weil 669

Thermomagnetic Surgery for Renal Cancer
Robert W. Rand, Harold D. Snow, and W. Jann Brown 673

Index 687

Contributors

C.C. Abbou, Service d'Urologie, Hôpital Henri Mondor, 94010 Creteil, Cedex, France **[437, 597]**

George P. Aftimos, Pathology Department, St. Joseph University Medical School, Hotel Dieu de France and Barbir Medical Center, Beirut, Lebanon **[317]**

Lennart Andersson, Department of Urology and Radiumhemmet, Karolinska sjukhuset, Stockholm, Sweden **[609, 661]**

G. Arvis, Department of Urology, Hôpital Saint-Antoine, 75012 Paris, France **[435]**

G. Auclerc, Medical Oncology Service, Hôpital de la Salpétrierè, Paris, France **[669]**

M.F. Auclerc, Medical Oncology Service, Hôpital de la Salpétrierè, Paris, France **[669]**

G. Auf, Royal Postgraduate Medical School, Hammersmith Hospital, London W.12 OHS, England **[245]**

J. Auvert, Service d'Urologie, Hôpital Henri Mondor, 94010 Creteil, Cedex, France **[437, 597]**

E. Baum, Children's Memorial Hospital, Chicago, Illinois, USA **[43, 123]**

J. Bruce Beckwith, Children's Orthopedic Hospital and Medical Center, PO Box C-5371, Seattle, Washington, 98105, USA **[1, 43, 123]**

Víctor Benavente, Instituto Nacional Enfermedades Neoplásicas, Av. Alfonso Ugarte 825, Lima 1, Peru **[145]**

G. Benoit, Clinique Urologique de l'Hôpital Cochin 75014, Department de Radiation, Service de Telecobaltherapie, Institut Gustave Roussy, 94800 Villejuif, France **[617]**

Thorbjörn Berge, Department of Pathology, Malmö General Hospital, S-214 01 Malmö, Sweden **[273]**

Pierre Bey, Department of Radiotherapy, Centre Alexis Vautrin, 54511 Vandoeuvres Les Nancy, France **[97]**

M. Bitker, Hôpital Trousseau, Paris, France **[155]**

M.H. Blessing, Departments of Urology and Surgical Pathology, Hospitals of the City of Cologne, Cologne, RFA, France **[589]**

L. Boccon Gibod, Clinique Urologique de l'Hôpital Cochin 75014, Department de Radiation, Service de Telecobaltherapie, Institut Gustave Roussy, 94800 Villejuif, France **[617]**

Annie Boilletot, Service des Maladies du Sang, Hôpital de Hautepierre, Strasbourg, France **[111]**

The number in brackets following each contributor's affiliation is the number of the first page of that contributor's article.

C. Bollack, Department of Urology, Hôpital Central, 67005 Cedex Strasbourg, France **[349, 529]**

Ulrico Bracci, University of Rome, 00161 Rome, Italy **[623]**

Eva Brehmer-Andersson, Departments of Cytology and Pathology, Karolinska sjukhuset, Stockholm, Sweden **[425]**

Herbert Brendler, Department of Urology, Mount Sinai Medical Center, New York, New York, USA **[461]**

Norman Breslow, Fred Hutchinson Cancer Research Center, Seattle, Washington, USA **[43, 123]**

W. Jann Brown, Department of Pathology, UCLA School of Medicine, Los Angeles, California, USA **[673]**

H. Brynger, Sahlgrenska sjukhuset, University of Göteborg, S-413 45 Göteborg, Sweden **[569]**

Ch. Caron-Poitreau, C.H.U. Angers, 49040 Angers, Cedex, France **[399]**

N. Chamsedine, Medical Oncology Service, Hôpital de la Salpétrierè, Paris, France **[669]**

B. Chaouachi, Hôpital Trousseau, Paris, France **[155]**

C. Chatelain, Hôpital de la Pitié, Paris, France **[475, 493, 533, 581]**

J.A. Child, The General Infirmary at Leeds, Leeds LS1 3EX, England **[663]**

Geoffrey D. Chisholm, University Department of Surgery/Urology, Western General Hospital, Edinburgh, Scotland **[277, 293]**

G. Chomette, Service de Médecine Interne, Hôpital de la Pitié, Paris, France **[283]**

Ch. Choquenet, Service d'Urologie, Hôpital Necker, Paris, France **[465]**

J. Cinqualbre, Department of Urology, Hôpital Central 67005. Cedex. Strasbourg, France **[529]**

N. Clausen, University Clinic of Paediatrics, Rigshospitalet, Copenhagen, Denmark **[165]**

A.P.M. Coleman, Royal Postgraduate Medical School, Hammersmith Hospital, London W.12 OHS, England **[245]**

Giuseppe Concolino, University of Rome, 00161, Rome, Italy **[623]**

Dominique Couanet, Institut Gustave Roussy, 94805 Villejuif Cedex, France **[67]**

Ph. Curet, Department of Radiology, Hôpital de la Pitié, 83 Bld de l'hôpital, 75013 Paris, France **[601]**

Karen Damgaard, University of Copenhagen Medical School, Copenhagen, Denmark **[345]**

G.J. D'Angio, Children's Hospital Cancer Research Center, Philadelphia, Pennsylvania, USA **[43, 123]**

Jean B. deKernion, Department of Urologic Oncology, UCLA School of Medicine, Los Angeles, California 90024, USA **[641]**

J. de Kraker, Department of Pediatric Oncology, Institut Gustave Roussy, Villejuif, France **[131]**

Alfred de Lorimier, University of California, San Francisco, California, USA **[43, 123]**

Franco DiSilverio, University of Rome, 00161 Rome, Italy **[623]**

B. Dufour, Service d'Urologie, Hôpital Necker, Paris, France **[465]**

Folke Edsmyr, Department of Urology and Radiumhemmet, Karolinska sjukhuset, Stockholm, Sweden **[609, 661]**

F. Eschwege, Clinique Urologique de l'Hôpital Cochin 75014, Department de Radiation, Service de Telecobaltherapie, Institut Gustave Roussy, 94800 Villejuif, France **[617]**

A.E. Evans, Children's Hospital Cancer Research Center, Philadelphia, Pennsylvania, USA **[43, 123]**

Clément Fauré, Hôpital Trousseau, 75571 Paris, Cedex 12, France **[59, 71]**

Donald Fernbach, Baylor College of Medicine, Houston, Texas, USA **[43, 123]**

P. Frantz, Hôpital de la Pitié, Paris, France **[581]**

Sixten Franzén, Departments of Cytology and Pathology, Karolinska sjukhuset, Stockholm, Sweden **[425]**

L. Friocourt, Service de Médecine Interne, Hôpital de la Pitié, Paris, France **[283]**

Anne Geoffray, Institut Gustave Roussy, 94805 Villejuif Cedex, France **[67]**

R. Ghanadian, Royal Postgraduate Medical School, Hammersmith Hospital, London W.12 OHS, England **[245]**

A. Gilloz, Department of Urology, University of Saint-Etienne, Hôpital Bellevue, 42100 Saint-Etienne, France **[489]**

Ruben F. Gittes, Department of Urological Surgery, Harvard Medical School, Boston, Massachusetts 02115, USA **[497, 509]**

P. Godeau, Service de Médecine Interne, Hôpital de la Pitié, Paris, France **[283]**

David F. Green, Department of Urology, St. James's University Hospital, Leeds, and the University of Leeds, England **[471]**

W. Grégoir, University of Brussels, Department of Urology, Brugmann Hospital, Brussels, Belgium **[453]**

J. Grellet, Department of Radiology, Hôpital de la Pitié, 83 Bld de l'hôpital, 75013, Paris, France **[341]**

M. Gruner, Hôpital Trousseau, Paris, France **[155]**

A. Haertig, Clinique Urologique, Hôpital de la Pitié, Paris, France **[337]**

Kamal Hanash, Department of Surgery, King Faisal Specialist Hospital and Research Centre, Riyadh, Kingdom of Saudi Arabia **[301]**

Sverker Hellsten, Department of Urology, Malmö General Hospital, S-214 01 Malmö, Sweden **[273]**

Ch. Henriksson, Sahlgrenska sjukhuset, University of Göteborg, S-413 45 Göteborg, Sweden **[569]**

Ellen Hrabovsky, West Virginia University, Morgantown, West Virginia, USA **[43, 123]**

Hartwig Huland, Wissenschaftlicher Assistent, Oberarzt Urologische Klinik der Universität Hamburg, 2000 Hamburg 20, West Germany **[207, 209]**

Giovanni B. Ingargiola, Institute of Urology, University of Palermo, Palermo, Italy **[255]**

C. Jacobs, Hôpital de la Pitié, Paris, France **[581]**

C. Jacquillat, Medical Oncology Service, Hôpital de la Salpétrierè, Paris, France **[669]**

Alain Jardin, Department of Urology, Clinique Urologique de la Pitié, Paris, France **[573]**

S. Johansson, Sahlgrenska sjukhuset, University of Göteborg, S-413 45 Göteborg, Sweden **[569]**

Barbara Jones, West Virginia University, Morgantown, West Virginia, USA **[43, 123]**

O. Jonsson, Sahlgrenska sjukhuset, University of Göteborg, S-413 45 Göteborg, Sweden **[433]**

J. Jouquan, Service de Médecine Interne, Hôpital de la Pitié, Paris, France **[283]**

James P. Karr, Roswell Park Memorial Institute, Buffalo, New York 14263, USA **[211]**

P. Kelalis, Mayo Clinic, Rochester, Minnesota, USA **[43, 123]**

Saad Khoury, Clinique Urologique, Hópital de la Pitié, Paris, France **[283, 377, 409, 457, 541]**

H. Kleist, Sahlgrenska sjukhuset, University of Göteborg, S-413 45 Göteborg, Sweden **[433]**

H. Klosterhalfen, Department of Urology, University of Hamburg, West Germany **[209]**

R. Küss, Clinique Urologique, Hôpital de la Pitié, Paris, France **[xxi, 337, 377, 519, 581, 599]**

Marcello Lamartina, Institute of Urology, University of Palermo, Palermo, Italy **[255]**

V. Lavarenne, Service d'Urologie, Hôpital Henri Mondor, 94010 Creteil, Cedex, France **[437, 597]**

Françoise Le Bras, Institut Gustave Roussy, 94805 Villejuif Cedex, France **[67]**

M. LeGuillou, Bordeaux, Paris Lariboisiere, France **[603]**

H.D. Lehmann, Departments of Urology and Surgical Pathology, Hospitals of the city of Cologne, Cologne, RFA, France **[589]**

Jean Lemerle, Department of Pediatrics, Institut Gustave Roussy, 94800 Villejuif, France **[91, 119, 131, 167]**

Arie Lindner, UCLA School of Medicine, Los Angeles, California 90024, USA **[641]**

Folke Linell, Department of Pathology, Malmö General Hospital, S-214 01 Malmö, Sweden **[273]**

J. Luciani, Hôpital de la Pitié, Paris, France **[581]**

Flemming Lund, University of Copenhagen Medical School, Copenhagen, Denmark **[345]**

S. Lundstam, Sahlgrenska sjukhuset, University of Göteborg, S-413 45 Göteborg, Sweden **[433]**

Djedje Madi, Clinique Urologique, Hôpital de la Pitié, Paris, France **[599]**

J. Mara, Medical Oncology Service, Hôpital de la Salpétrierè, Paris, France **[669]**

Jacques Masselot, Institut Gustave Roussy, 94805 Villejuif Cedex, France **[67]**

Etienne Mazeman, Department of Urology, Centre Hospitalier, Lille, France **[561]**

Amira M. Mehio, Pathology Department, St. Joseph University Medical School, Hotel Dieu de France and Barbir Medical Center, Beirut, Lebanon **[317]**

J.J. Merland, Bordeaux, Paris Lariboisiere, France **[603]**

S. Merran, Central Radiology, Hôpital Broussais 96, Paris 75 674, France **[369]**

Jean Philippe Montagne, Hôpital Trousseau, 75571 Paris, Cedex 12, France **[59, 71]**

Gerald P. Murphy, Roswell Park Memorial Institute, Buffalo, New York 14263, USA **[15, 175, 211]**

J. Nauclér, Sahlgrenska sjukhuset, University of Göteborg, S-413 45 Göteborg, Sweden **[433]**

Sylvia Neuenschwander, Hôpital Trousseau, 75571 Paris, Cedex 12, France **[59, 71]**

A.E. Nilson, Sahlgrenska sjukhuset, University of Göteborg, S-413 45 Göteborg, Sweden **[433, 569]**

H.B. Othersen, Jr., Medical University Hospital, Charleston, South Carolina, USA **[43, 123]**

Ullrich Otto, Wissenschaftlicher Assistent, Oberarzt Urologische Klinik der Universität Hamburg, 2000 Hamburg 20, West Germany **[207, 209]**

Roger A. Parienty, Scanner Hartmann Inter-Cliniques, 92200. Neuilly sur Seine, France **[409]**

Michele Pavone-Macaluso, Institute of Urology, University of Palermo, Palermo, Italy **[255]**

Denys Pellerin, Department of Pediatric Surgery, Hôpital des Enfants Malades, Paris, France **[83, 85]**

H.J.M. Perry, Department of Pediatric Oncology, Institut Gustave Roussy, Villejuif, France **[131]**

S. Pettersson, Sahlgrenska sjukhuset, University of Göteborg, S-413 45 Götebrog, Sweden **[433, 569]**

Jean Daniel Piekarski, Institut Gustav Roussy, 94805 Villejuif Cedex, France **[67]**

M. Ch. Plainfosse, Central Radiology, Hôpital Broussais 96, Paris 75 674, France **[369]**

J. Poisson, Hôpital de la Pitié, Paris, France **[581]**

Julio Pow-Sang, Instituto Nacional Enfermedades Neoplásicas, Av. Alfonso Ugarte 825, Lima 1, Peru **[145]**

Janine Pradel, Scanner Hartmann Inter-Cliniques, 92200 Neuilly sur Seine, France **[409]**

J.M. Py, Department of Urology, Hôpital Central, 67005 Cedex Strasbourg, France **[529]**

Graciela Ramírez, Instituto Nacional Enfermedades Neoplásicas, Av. Alfonso Ugarte 825, Lima 1, Peru **[145]**

T. Ranch, Sahlgrenska sjukhuset, University of Göteborg, S-413 45 Göteborg, Sweden **[569]**

Robert W. Rand, Department of Surgery, UCLA School of Medicine, Los Angeles, California, USA **[673]**

François Richard, Clinique Urologique, Hôpital de la Pitié, Paris, France **[377, 409, 599]**

R. Richard, Service de Médecine Interne, Hôpital de la Pitié, Paris, France **[283]**

Charles J. Robson, Division of Urology, University of Toronto, Toronto, Ontario, Canada **[439, 447, 481]**

L.M. Rognon, C.H.U. Angers, 49040 Angers, Cedex, France **[399]**

Hanna Rosenthal, Roswell Park Memorial Institute, Buffalo, New York 14263, USA **[211]**

Avery A. Sandberg, Roswell Park Memorial Institute, Buffalo, New York 14263, USA **[211]**

Sarah Schneider, Roswell Park Memorial Institute, Buffalo, New York 14263, USA **[211]**

Philip H. Smith, Department of Urology, St. James's University Hospital, Leeds, England **[471]**

Harold D. Snow, The Leo G. Rigler Center for Radiological Sciences, UCLA Center for the Health Sciences, Los Angeles, California, USA **[673]**

Adolphe Steg, Department of Urology, Hôpital Cochin 75014 Paris, France **[417, 617]**

Wafic S. Tabbara, Pathology Department, St. Joseph University Medical School, Hotel Dieu de France and Barbir Medical Center, Beirut, Lebanon **[317]**

Melvin Tefft, Rhode Island Hospital, Providence Rhode Island, USA **[43, 123]**

Patrick Thomas, Washington University, St. Louis, Missouri, USA **[43, 123]**

J. Tostain, Department of Urology, University of Saint-Etienne, Hôpital Bellevue, 42100 Saint-Etienne, France **[489]**

M.F. Tournade, Department of Pediatric Oncology, Institut Gustave Roussy, Villejuif, France **[131]**

Aurelio C. Uson, Department of Urología, Hospital Clínico de San Carlos, Faculty of Med., Complutensis University, Madrid, Spain [549]

G. Vallancien, Clinique Urologique, Hôpital de la Pitié, Paris, France [599]

Daniel Vanel, Institut Gustave Roussy, 94805 Villejuif Cedex, France [67]

P.A. Voûte, Department of Pediatric Oncology, Institut Gustave Roussy, Villejuif, France [131]

Lennart Wehlin, Department of Diagnostic Radiology, Malmö General Hospital, S-214 01 Malmö, Sweden [273]

M. Weil, Medical Oncology Service, Hôpital de la Salpétrierè, Paris, France [669]

J.J. Wenger, Hôpital Central, 67005 Cedex, Strasbourg, France [349]

G. Williams, Royal Postgraduate Medical School, Hammersmith Hospital, London W.12 OHS, England [245]

Welcome and Introduction

We welcome you to this international symposium on kidney tumors which follows last year's conference on prostatic cancer and precedes that of next year on tumors of the bladder. In uniting the foremost specialists from various disciplines here, it is our intention naturally to assess the present state of knowledge, but also to profit from the international nature of the meeting by attempting to simplify and standardize the anatomical and clinical classifications which are still subject to considerable variation. In doing this, we hope to obtain a more objective approach to the results obtained from different treatments.

In the field of renal cancer, everyone recognizes the distinction between tumors in children and those in adults. Such a distinction is reinforced at present by the difference in the effects of treatment. However, in adults it is much more difficult, given the immense variety in microscopic appearances of the lesion, to achieve an understanding of prognosis simply by anatomical and pathological studies. This diversity can explain the variation in the natural history of the disease and it is unusual in several ways. There is the possibility of surgical enucleation of tumors because of the cleavage plane separating it from the renal parenchyma. Is this a defense mechanism for the tumor against the host, or vice versa? Again there is the hormonal nature of the lesions probably deriving from the paraneoplastic syndrome which often accompanies and may sometimes reveal the lesion.

Knowing that in some cases it is a centimeter which determines whether a tumor is benign or malignant, one must understand that the neoplasm has not begun in the formed organ, but is at the stage of embryonic nephrogenesis (dysembryoplasia). This view brings together the concept of renal cancer in the adult and in the child, where no environmental aetiological factor has as yet been identified. Faced with all the uncertainties of cancer research in general, it is reassuring to know that in the field of renal neoplasia considerable progress has been made in the last decade.

Chemotherapy has transformed the prognosis in nephroblastoma in children. This is an important example which underlines the importance of a multi-discipline approach, i.e. surgery, radiotherapy and chemotherapy all combined in the treatment of cancer.

There has also been great progress in the field of surgery in the assessment and treatment of neoplasms in the adult. For example, surgery can become more extensive with tumor embolisation or more conservative, reminding one of the idea of "out of body" surgery.

Great interest has also been focused on new methods, the advantages of which are enhanced when certain biological markers are also evaluated. These advances now allow one to consider treating a latent cancer in its early stage, thus conferring to adults with such tumors the very favorable prognosis which is afforded to children with renal tumors.

Please forgive me for continuing this slightly long-winded introduction before getting to the proper subject matter. Let me extend my thanks to all those who helped in the preparation of this meeting and in particular to Dr. Gerald P. Murphy and to all those who have agreed to participate in this symposium, which, I feel certain, will not be disappointing.

Professor René Küss

NEPHROBLASTOMA (WILMS' TUMOR)

Renal Tumors: Proceedings of the First International Symposium on
Kidney Tumors, pages 1–14
© 1982 Alan R. Liss, Inc., 150 Fifth Avenue, New York, NY 10011

HISTOPATHOLOGICAL ASPECTS OF RENAL TUMORS IN CHILDREN

J. Bruce Beckwith, M.D.

Director of Laboratories
Children's Orthopedic Hospital and Medical Center
P. O. Box C-5371
Seattle, Washington, USA 98105

Primary tumors of the kidney in infancy and childhood
are relatively uncommon, but they present a number of fundamental challenges from the standpoint of the histopathologist.
There are many unsettled questions concerning classification,
nomenclature, histogenesis, and prognostic significance of
the tumors to be discussed.

Table 1 lists the principal neoplasms that are primary
in the kidneys of children. This list is not complete, and
lists as separate entities a number of tumors that are
closely related to Wilms' tumors.

PRIMARY RENAL TUMORS OF CHILDHOOD

Wilms' Tumor (Nephroblastoma)
Nephroblastomatosis
Congenital Mesoblastic Nephroma
Multilocular Cyst (Cystic Nephroblastoma)
Clear Cell Sarcoma of Kidney (Bone-Metastasizing
  Renal Tumor of Childhood)
Malignant Rhabdoid Tumor
Neurogenic Tumors (Neuroblastoma, Neuroepithelioma,
  Neurofibroma)
Angiomyolipoma
Adenocarcinoma
Sarcomas (Osteosarcoma, Liposarcoma, Rhabdomyosarcoma,
  etc.)
Carcinoid Tumor
Teratoma, Germ Cell Tumors
Transitional Cell Carcinoma

Lymphoma

Table 1. Principal tumor types primary in the child's kidney. Some of the most common synonyms or subtypes are given in parentheses.

Space does not permit discussion of all the entities listed. In this paper we will emphasize the first six lesions on the list, which are much more distinctively pediatric in nature than the remainder.

WILMS' TUMORS

Clinical, epidemiological, and therapeutic aspects of this tumor are discussed by other contributors to this Conference.

In addition to classical triphasic Wilms' tumors, which consist of a mixture of blastemal, epithelial, and stromal tissues, there exist a number of tumors in which only one of these tissues is present. These so-called "monomorphous variants" of Wilms' tumor present a difficult conceptual grey zone between Wilms' tumor and a number of other renal neoplasms. For example, monomorphous tubular Wilms' tumors may be difficult to distinguish from relatively undifferentiated renal adenocarcinoma. It is difficult to be certain whether certain renal sarcomas (e.g. rhabdomyosarcoma or osteosarcoma) should be viewed as monomorphous variants of Wilms' tumor, or as separate tumor categories. Since nearly all parenchymal neoplasms of the human kidney originate from metanephric blastema or its differentiated derivatives, it may be argued that most renal neoplasms, such as adenocarcinoma, are to some extent conceptually related to Wilms' tumor. For practical and therapeutic purposes, however, most of these morphologically distinct entities are best viewed as separate entities.

Monomorphous tubular Wilms' tumors have been viewed by several workers as having a better prognosis than more classical mixed patterns of Wilms' tumor (Chatten 1976, Lawler 1975). Since the therapeutic protocols of the National Wilms' Tumor Study (NWTS) have been associated with very high rates of relapse-free survival, it is difficult for us to confirm or deny this statement. Where a very high cure rate is obtained for any tumor type, the relatively benign end of the spectrum becomes submerged in the cured population, and cannot be separated from lesions of inter- mediate degrees of malignancy (Beckwith 1979). Only the relatively malignant end of the spectrum - those tumors resistant to modern therapy - are likely to be identified. Therefore, it is not surprising that our studies of the histopathology of the NWTS case material has identified, as its principal and most important finding, the most malignant end of the Wilms' tumor spectrum.

Significance of Anaplasia in Wilms' Tumor

Extreme cytological atypism or anaplasia, was found in our studies of NWTS-1 and 2 (Beckwith, 1978, 1980) to be a powerful indicator of unfavorable prognosis. Therefore, it is a major obligation of the pathologist studying a Wilms' tumor, to ascertain whether or not anaplastic cells are present. Anaplasia may involve the epithelial, blastemal, and/or stromal elements of a given tumor. This change is found in approximately 6% of Wilms' tumors. Its incidence increases with age, and it is rarely encountered in tumors from patients under two years of age. We identify cells as anaplastic only when severe atypism is present, as illus- trated in Figure 1. Our minimal diagnostic criteria for anaplasia requires that all three of the following criteria be met:

1) Nuclei are enlarged to at least three times the diameter of nuclei of adjacent, non-anaplastic cells of the same type.
2) The enlarged nuclei are markedly hyperchromatic
3) Multipolar mitotic figures are present.

Table 2 presents the significance of anaplasia in NWTS-1 and 2 combined. This table includes all cases from whom tumor tissue of adequate quality was available for review, with the following exclusions: 1) cases presenting with metastases; 2) cases dying without evidence of tumor, and 3) rhabdoid and clear cell sarcomas, which will be discussed below.

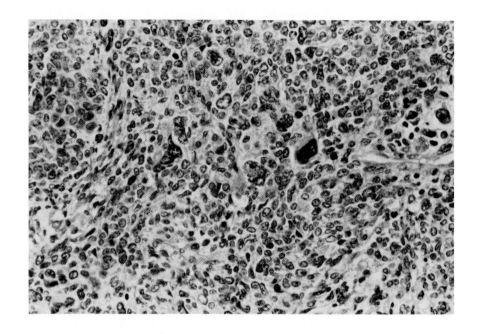

Figure 1: Anaplastic cells in Wilms' tumor. Several enlarged, hyperchromatic nuclei are shown.

	Anaplasia Present	Anaplasia Absent
Total Cases	49	720
Relapses	27 (55%)	101 (14%)
Tumor deaths	23 (47%)	39 (5.4%)

Table 2: Significance of Anaplasia in Wilms' Tumors in NWTS-1 and 2.

Even in those cases where anaplasia was focal, involving only one slide of many taken from a given tumor, the prognosis was markedly worsened. It is therefore apparent that thorough sampling is necessary to ensure that anaplastic cells are not overlooked. We suggest, as minimum guidelines

for sampling, that one generous section be obtained for
every centimeter of tumor diameter. If the tumor is multicentric, each separate tumor should be sampled. Meticulous
care must be taken to ensure excellent histological sections,
in order to avoid artefacts that may be mistaken for anaplasia,
or which may obscure its presence. Thick, poorly fixed,
overstained sections, or tissues subjected to crush artefact,
cannot be reliably evaluated for anaplasia.

NEPHROBLASTOMATOSIS

The term nephroblastomatosis was coined (Hou 1961) to
describe a unique case of massive, diffuse nephromegaly
produced by a generalized proliferation of immature nephrogenic tissue. Subsequently this term has been expanded to
include a variety of more localized abnormalities thought to
represent abnormal persistence and growth of nephrogenic
tissue. Bove and McAdams (1976) introduced the term "nephroblastomatosis complex" to describe this spectrum of lesions,
which ranges from microscopic foci of nephrogenic tissue
(nephrogenic rests, or persistent nodular blastema), to a
variety of grossly obvious masses composed either of discrete
masses of hyperplastic immature tissue to a diffuse "cap"
or "rind", surrounding the entire kidney.

Despite excellent recent reviews of this complex subject
(Bove 1976, Machin 1980), there is general uncertainty as to
the clinical management of cases with nephroblastomatosis.
Much of this confusion arises from the fact that there is no
sharp dividing line between hyperplastic precursor lesions of
Wilms' tumor, and the tumor itself. One is therefore faced
with the same morphological dilemma encountered in other
tumor systems where there is a gradual, or multi-step progression from precursor lesions to tumors, as in carcinomas of
the cervix, endometrium, breast, adrenal, and gastrointestinal
tract. In some ways the problem is reminiscent of the
dilemmas posed by uncertainty as to the relationships of
renal adenomas to adenocarcinomas.

When an unequivocal Wilms' tumor is found to have associated lesions of the nephroblastomatosis complex in the
resected kidney, what are the therapeutic implications? Dr.
Jeffrey Bonadio, working with me in the NWTS Pathology Center,
has recently reviewed this subject, using material from
NWTS-2. 27.1% of cases for which renal tissue was available

to us had some form of nephroblastomatosis, usually consisting
of persistent nephrogenic rests (persistent nodular blastema).
Cases which were associated with nephroblastomatosis had
similar rates of recurrence as for unilateral tumors without
nephroblastomatosis, when stratified according to grade and
stage of tumor. Only 5 cases on NWTS-2 have to date
developed metachronous bilateral Wilms' tumors, suggesting
that this risk is very low, even when the lesions of nephroblastomatosis are present, provided that therapy comparable
to that of NWTS-2 is administered.

   Though final answers are not yet available, we offer the
following general considerations as guidelines for therapy in
cases with nephroblastomatosis:
1)   Nephroblastomatosis is not a malignant tumor per se,
     but a lesion with malignant potential. Therefore, a
     decision to treat this lesion (in the absence of a
     demonstrated Wilms' tumor) should be clearly understood
     to be for purposes of eradicating a precursor lesion, not
     for treating an established cancer. Such therapy should
     not be more deleterious to the patient than the lesion
     itself.
     a)   Recent advances in diagnostic imaging make a policy
          of close followup without therapy reasonably safe
          for some patients. If a tumor develops while the
          patient is receiving frequent examinations by good
          imaging techniques, it should be detected at an early
          stage when an excellent response to conventional
          therapy would be likely.
     b)   When lesions of nephroblastomatosis seem to be
          growing rapidly, chemotherapy similar to that used
          for Stage I Wilms' tumors may be indicated in order
          to preserve uninvolved renal parenchyma. It is
          possible, but as yet unproven, that such therapy might
          lessen the chance of developing a Wilms' tumor.
2)   Nephroblastomatosis diagnosed in one kidney justifies
     the presumption of bilateral involvement. However, as
     discussed above, the subsequent development of contra-
     lateral Wilms' tumor is not commonly encountered using
     modern therapy.

CONGENITAL MESOBLASTIC NEPHROMA (CMN)

This imporant and distinctive entity was first clearly
delineated by Bolande, who later provided a comprehensive
review of the subject (Bolande 1973). CMN is virtually
limited in occurrence to the early infantile period, and
most cases are diagnosed before six months of age.

Histopathologically, CMN is composed of a monomorphous
proliferation of spindle cells that usually interdigitate
with the surrounding kidney and extend outward into the
perirenal and periureter fat, often in the form of long,
delicate fingers of tumor that are easily left behind unless
a wide margin is obtained. Ultrastructurally, CMN is composed
of fibromyoblasts. Thus, the resemblance in both cell type
and growth pattern to infantile fibromatosis is very great,
and it is quite possible that this entity should properly
be included as one of the fibromatoses. In our experience,
skeletal muscle fibers are not seen in CMN, and lesions
containing skeletal muscle are classified as Wilms' tumor.
Entrapped glomeruli and tubules often undergo a distinctive
retrogressive and hyperplastic change, becoming hyperchromatic and sometimes showing papillary overgrowth. This
change has suggested to some workers that CMN is a combined
stromal and epithelial tumor, perhaps, as Bolande suggests,
representing a cytodifferentiated variant of Wilms' tumor.

This tumor is clinically benign with few exceptions.
However, several clinical points cannot be overemphasized:
(1) A complete nephrectomy with exceptionally wide excision
     of perinephric soft tissues is required to remove not
     only the main tumor, but those "tongues" of prolifera-
     ting cells that may radiate for at least 1.0 cm. beyond
     the grossly apparent surface of the tissue, especially
     on the hilar aspect of the kidney. If residual tumor
     remains, recurrences can develop (Beckwith 1974).
     Careful pathological study of margins is essential.

(2) High cellularity and high mitotic rate are not neces-
     sarily adverse prognostic indicators, at least in young
     infants. Relatively little information exists as to
     the significance of moderate to high cellularity in
     the patient over 6 months of age, but at least one
     case of moderately high cellularity, diagnosed at 7
     months of age, developed a pulmonary metastasis
     (Gonzalez-Crussi 1980).

Based upon these principles, we advocate a policy of conservative therapy for all cases where there has been an apparently complete removal of tumor, without spillage, and with no evidence of tumor at or near the margins. When doubt exists as to the completeness of resection, the options are either (a) to provide adjunct therapy or (b) to withhold therapy but watch extremely closely for recurrences, with consideration of a "second look" operation in a few months. In the infant over about six months of age at diagnosis, a high degree of cellularity may be of concern, and adjunct therapy may be indicated. The one reported case that did develop a pulmonary metastasis was successfully retrieved by a combination of Actinomycin D, radiotherapy, and eventual resection of the recurrent lung nodule (Gonzalez-Crussi, 1980).

A final note of caution: CMN is capable of being confused morphologically with two extremely malignant renal tumors of infants - clear cell sarcoma and malignant rhabdoid tumor, as discussed below.

MULTILOCULAR CYST OF KIDNEY (CYSTIC, PARTIALLY DIFFERENTIATED NEPHROBLASTOMA)

Recent advances in diagnostic imaging techniques have led to a heightened clinical interest in the subject of predominantly cystic tumors of the child's kidney. (This discussion considers only localized masses or tumors of the kidney that are cystic, and does not include the various cystic disorders, localized or diffuse, of the renal parenchyma). From the standpoint of the morphologist, a continuous morphological spectrum exists between Wilms' tumors containing one or more cystic spaces at the one extreme, and multilocular cysts consisting of multiple cystic cavities separated by thin, completely differentiated mesenchymal septa at the other extreme. Most predominantly cystic renal masses in the pediatric age range fall into the latter end of this spectrum - the so-called "multilocular cyst of kidney". Not uncommonly, however, small foci of incompletely differentiated epithelial or stromal cells, and even blastema, may be found. For these, the appropriate term "cystic, partially differentiated nephroblastoma" has been suggested (Joshi 1980). All authors have emphasized the benign clinical behavior of such lesions, and some have suggested that when this diagnosis is indicated by modern imaging methods, a partial nephrectomy may be sufficient (Banner 1981). While this approach should usually prove safe, we have pointed out elsewhere (Beckwith 1981) that there are several potential problems:

(a) Occasionally a Wilms' tumor in which cysts are a fairly prominent feature has recurred locally or metastasized.

(b) Clear cell sarcomas, a highly malignant tumor to be discussed below, may be quite cystic.

(c) Over 60% of mesoblastic nephromas in our experience have grossly apparent cysts, and occasionally these are abundant. As discussed above, mesoblastic nephroma is an entity deserving complete nephrectomy with aggressive efforts at obtaining a wide margin.

Based upon these considerations, we would suggest that conservative surgical approaches for predominantly cystic masses in the kidney of infants and children be restricted to those cases in which imaging techniques reveal an over-whelming preponderance of cystic spaces, separated by very delicate septa, without evidence of solid regions in part of the lesion. When solid regions are present, there is the possibility of a potentially metastasizing or recurring lesion, which should be approached with appropriate caution. In many ways, this morphological continuum with malignancy at one end of the spectrum and benignancy at the other, is comparable to the neuroblastoma-ganglioneuroma spectrum of tumors.

CLEAR CELL SARCOMA OF KIDNEY (BONE-METASTASIZING RENAL TUMOR OF CHILDHOOD)

This distinctive renal tumor was encountered indepen-dently and more or less simultaneously by us (Beckwith 1978) in the course of reviewing the pathological specimens of the NWTS and by English pathologist (Marsden 1978, 1980) during review of materials from the MRC Wilms' tumor study. Earlier, Kidd (1970) had recognized the same lesion but did not report the finding in detail until later (Morgan 1978). All three groups have employed different names for this lesion, no one of which is satisfactory. When the cell of origin of this neoplasm becomes established, it will become possible to provide a name for this tumor that will be more meaningful.

Clear cell sarcoma of kidney (CCSK) comprises about 4%

of childhood renal tumors entered on the NWTS. It is composed
of polygonal to stellate cells with poorly outlined pale
cytoplasm that often possesses large vacuoles. Nuclei are
round to oval with finely granular chromatin and inconspicu-
ous nucleoli. The mitotic rate usually appears low. The
growth pattern is distinctly trabecular, with columns of
cells separated by a rather evenly spaced system of capillaries with their delicate supporting stroma. Tubules with
basophilic, cuboid to columnar lining cells are often found
in the tumor, but never, in our experience, are they present
in extrarenal extensions or in metastatic deposits of CCSK.
Thus, there is at the present time no reason to view CCSK
as a variant of WT, and it should be viewed as a separate and
distinctive tumor. To date we are aware of no analogous
neoplasm arising outside the kidney. Ultrastructural studies
on 12 cases, being completed by my associate, Dr. Joel Haas,
reveal a paucity of cytoplasmic organelles, and few clues
to the nature of its intrinsic cells. Candidate cells of
origin include vascular pericytes, renomedullary interstitial
cells, and perhaps blastemal cap cells.

In some specimens of CCSK fibrovascular septa become
widened and densely hyalinized. In our earlier report
(Beckwith 1978) we referred to an "osteosarcomatoid" variant
of renal tumor in children. This category can now be discarded, as all specimens we included have subsequently been
identified as either CCSK or malignant rhabdoid tumors, to
be described below, in which hyalinization had become a
prominent histologic feature. Occasionally, some regions of
a CCSK may exhibit palisading of nuclei in a manner resembling neurilemmoma (Beckwith 1978). Cysts, either arising
from dilatation of entrapped tubules, or from coalescent areas
of mucopolysaccharide accumulation in the tissue interstitium,
may occasionally be quite prominent grossly. In a few specimens
the cell columns and cords, rather than having the usual
delicate, pale, vacuolated cytoplasm, may become quite
compact and darker stained, superfically resembling tubular
differentiation. This "epithelioid" appearance can lead to
confusion with Wilms' tumor, unless the typical pattern of
CCSK is identified in other fields. Fortunately, those potentially misleading histological features are quite uncommon.

CCSK may occur in infants, and in our experience
approximately 50% of cases are diagnosed before two years of
age. Several times we have seen cases originally misdiagnosed as CMN - a potentially disastrous error. A distinctive

feature, present in all large series of cases, is a striking male preponderance, ranging from 3:1 in the NWTS to 7.6:1 in the recent series of Marsden (1980).

Among 31 cases of CCSK in NWTS-1 and 2, there have been 20 relapses and 15 deaths, illustrating the malignancy of this lesion. Cases diagnosed before two years of age fared no better than those in older children. A distinctive clinical feature is the frequency of bone metastases in CCSK. These occurred in 13 of 31 NWTS cases (42%).

CCSK is therefore a distinctive renal tumor of childhood having a high degree of malignancy and a predilection for bone metastases. It is important to distinguish CCSK from Wilms' tumor and from CMN. NWTS-3 is currently testing whether aggressive multimodal therapy can improve the outlook for this tumor.

MALIGNANT RHABDOID TUMOR OF KIDNEY

Another distinctive tumor, identified for the first time in our review of the first NWTS (Beckwith 1978), was initially considered to represent a Wilms' tumor variant, which we termed "rhabdomyosarcomatoid" because of the strong resemblance of the tumor cells to rhabdomyoblasts. Subsequently it has become clear that this distinctive neoplasm is not a Wilms' tumor variant, and that it may occur as a primary tumor in extrarenal sites, including thymus, subcutis, and central nervous system.

Malignant rhabdoid tumor of kidney (MRTK) is composed of cells with abundant acidophilic cytoplasm resembling that of skeletal muscle cells. However, there are no cross striations, and electron microscopy has so far shown no evidence of skeletal muscle cells (Haas 1981). The cell cytoplasm often contains an eosinophilic, globular, hyaline-like inclusion, which ultrastructurally consists of a whorled mass of fine filaments (Haas 1981). Nuclei characteristically possess a prominent single "owl-eye" nucleolus. The growth pattern may be either diffuse or trabecular. The latter may impart a somewhat epithelioid appearance, and may lead to confusion with Wilms' tumor.

MRTK is even more rare than CCSK, comprising about 2% of NWTS cases to date. It has a definite predilection for

the infant and younger child. Of 21 cases on NWTS-1 and 2,
the age range at diagnosis was 3 - 56 months, with a mean of
18 months and median of 13 months. In private consultation I
have seen a case diagnosed at 5 days of age. Therefore,
confusion with CMN can occur due to overlapping age distribution curves, and several times we have seen MRTK mistak-
enly identified as CMN. This is an especially unfortunate
event, since MRTK is one of the most malignant of all childhood tumors. Of 21 NWTS cases, 19 relapsed and 18 have died.
Young age does not improve this grim outlook. NWTS-3 is
attempting to evaluate the efficacy of intensified therapy
for this extremely aggressive neoplasm.

In our consultation experience, we have observed a
total of 16 cases in which MRTK was associated with a tumor
of the posterior fossa that resembled a medulloblastoma.
This latter tumor apparently represents a separate primary
tumor, and may precede the development of the renal tumor.
While cerebral metastases of MRTK may occur, one should
consider the possibility of a second primary if evidence of
a midline posterior fossa tumor develops in a patient with
MRTK. The possibility that MRTK is of neuroepithelial
origin is currently being considered (Haas 1981).

SUMMARY

1)   While Wilms' tumor comprises the vast majority of renal
      tumors in children, a number of other neoplastic
      entities must be considered. Several of these have been
      only recently defined, and have distinctive clinico-
      pathological features.
2)   Wilms' tumors can be subdivided histologically into a
      small group with extreme cellular pleomorphism (ana-
      plasia), which have a relatively poor prognosis, and
      a much larger group lacking anaplasia, for whom the
      prognosis, using modern therapy, is generally excellent.
3)   Precursor lesions of Wilms' tumor, known collectively
      as nephroblastomatosis, constitute a morphological
      spectrum with a variably increased risk of developing
      Wilms' tumor. When a Wilms' tumor develops in a kidney
      with nephroblastomatosis, the prognosis for that tumor
      does not apparently differ from that of a Wilms' tumor
      without evidence of nephroblastomatosis.
4)   A relatively benign infantile renal tumor, the congen-
      ital mesoblastic nephroma, should be treated by a

    complete nephrectomy with an aggressive effort to obtain a wide margin of uninvolved perinephric soft tissue, because of its infiltrative pattern.

5)   Cystic Wilms' tumors are closely related to multilocular renal cysts. These comprise a morphological spectrum and some Wilms' tumors with cysts have metastasizing potential.

6)   Clear cell sarcoma of kidney, or bone-metastasizing renal tumor of childhood, is a recently recognized entity, apparently not related to WT, that has a very malignant potential, and a high rate of bone metastasis.

7)   Malignant rhabdoid tumor of kidney, another destructive and recently described entity, is exceptionally malignant. Some cases develop an apparently separate primary medulloblastoma-like tumor of the posterior fossa. Young age of patients does not reduce the degree of malignancy of this tumor.

8)   Care must be taken not to mistake malignant rhabdoid tumor of kidney, or clear cell sarcoma of kidney, with congenital mesoblastic nephroma.

REFERENCES

Banner MP, Pollack HM, Chatten J, Witzleben C (1981). Multilocular renal cysts: radiologic-pathologic correlation. Am J Roengenol 136:239.

Beckwith JB (1974). Mesenchymal renal neoplasms revisited. J Pediat Surg 9:803.

Beckwith JB, Palmer NF (1978). Histopathology and prognosis of Wilms' tumor. Results from the first National Wilms' Tumor Study. Cancer 41:1937.

Beckwith JB (1979). Grading of pediatric tumors. In Care of the Child with Cancer. American Cancer Society, p 39.

Beckwith JB (1980). The pathology of renal tumors in children: Recent results of the National Wilms' Tumor Study. In Kobayashi N (ed): Recent Advances in Management of Children with Cancer. Children's Cancer Association of Japan, Medical Information Services, Inc, Tokyo, p 75.

Beckwith JB, Kiviat NB (1981). Multilocular renal cysts and cystic renal tumors (Editorial) Am J Roentgenol 136:435.

Bolande RP (1973). Congenital mesoblastic nephroma of infancy. Perspect Pediat Pathol 1:227.

Bove KE, McAdams AS (1976). The nephroblastomatosis complex and its relationship to Wilms' tumor. Perspect Pediat Pathol

3:185.

Chatten J (1976). Epithelial differentiation in Wilms' tumor: A clinico pathological appraisal. Perspect Pediat Pathol 3:225.

Gonzalez-Crussi F, Sotelo-Avila C, Kidd JM (1980). Malignant mesenchymal nephroma of infancy. Report of a case with pulmonary metastases. Am J Surg Pathol 4:185.

Haas JE, Palmer NF, Weinberg AG, Beckwith JB (1981) Ultrastructure of malignant rhabdoid tumor of kidney. A distinctive renal tumor of children. Hum Pathol 12:646.

Hou L-T, Holman RL (1961). Bilateral nephroblastomatosis in a premature infant. J Pathol Bacteriol 82:249.

Joshi VV (1979). Cystic partially differentiated nephroblastoma: An entity in the spectrum of infantile renal neoplasia. Perspect Pediat Pathol 5:217.

Kidd JK (1970). Exclusion of certain renal neoplasms from the category of Wilms' tumor. (Abstract) Amer J Pathol 59: 16a.

Lawler W, Marsden HB, Palmer MK (1975). Wilms' tumor: Histologic variation and prognosis. Cancer 36:1122.

Machin GA (1980. Persistent renal blastema (Nephroblastomatosis) as a frequent precursor of Wilms' tumor: A pathologic and clinical review. Am J Pediat Hematol Oncol 2: 165, 253, 353.

Marsden HB, Lawler W (1978). Bone metastasizing renal tumor of childhood. Br J Cancer 38:437.

Marsden HB, Lawler W (1980). Bone metastasizing renal tumor of childhood. Histopathological and clinical review of 38 cases. Virchow's Arch A Pathol Anat and Histol 387:341.

Morgan E, Kidd JM (1978). Undifferentiated sarcoma of the kidney. A tumor of childhood with histopathologic and clinical characteristics distinct from Wilms' tumor. Cancer 42:1916.

Renal Tumors: Proceedings of the First International Symposium on Kidney Tumors, pages 15–41
© **1982 Alan R. Liss, Inc., 150 Fifth Avenue, New York, NY 10011**

AN EXPERIMENTAL WILMS' TUMOR

Gerald P. Murphy, M.D., D.Sc.

Roswell Park Memorial Institute
666 Elm Street
Buffalo, NY 14263

In recent years there has been a dramatic improvement in the survival rate of children with Wilms' tumor which has been attributed primarily to the combined utilization of surgery, radiotherapy, and chemotherapeutic agents (Smith et al. 1973, Sutow et al. 1970, and Uson et al. 1971). With increased interest in the efficacy of combined therapeutic modalities, the need for model systems akin to the human situation for testing various regimens at different stages of the disease has its obvious advantages in preclinical trials (Tomashefsky et al. 1971). As a prelude to chemotherapeutic trials we have characterized a rat Wilms' tumor model in terms of incidence and growth rate, optimal site of tumor transplant, degree of metastases and lethality, and also to evaluate biochemical parameters that might be used as an index of drug efficacy.

GENERAL

Our first attempts over 10 years ago to transplant the tumor were made with Wistar/Lewis rats. The incidence of tumor acceptance in this strain of rats was approximately 6 to 10 percent. Tumor tissue from these animals when transplanted to Furth/Wistar rats resulted in a 100 percent tumor acceptance. This difference between animal strains was considered to be due to specific strain genetic differences and is not attributed to any other known factor. The incidence of 100 percent tumor acceptance in Furth/Wistar rats has been consistent regardless of the route of tumor transplant (Table 1). In gross appearance the tumor developed

TABLE 1

SURVIVAL TIME ACCORDING TO SITE OF TUMOR TRANSPLANT
IN WISTAR/FURTH WILMS' TUMOR RATS

Transplant Site And No. of Animals	Survival Time (X ± SE)	Tumor Wt. (X ± SE)
	Days	Grams
Intrarenal (19)	27.5 ± 0.8	27.1 ± 4.6
Intraperitoneal (13)	30.4 ± 1.4	28.1 ± 3.8
Subcutaneous (subaxilla) (15)	37.7 ± 1.9	129.7 ± 14.8
Intramuscular (interfiber) (15)	41.1 ± 1.8	57.6 ± 7.2
Intramuscular (trocar) (10)	44.4 ± 1.9	43.9 ± 4.4

as an encapsulated soft, smooth mass. With increased growth
the central region became necrotic. As shown in Figure 1,
it has a close histologic resemblance to the Wilms' tumor
as seen in man, both in its primary site appearance and in
the patttern of metastatic spread. Mitotic figures were
observed and were associated with other aspects of the
functional state of tumor growth. In most locations the
neoplasm retained its undifferentiated character. Maturation
into either tubular or glomerular structures was virtually
absent. The neoplasm showed evidence of vascular invasion
chiefly in the form of clumps of tumor cells plugging
capillaries (Fig. 1). The tumor in our laboratory is now
after 10 years in its 170th tumor transplant generation.

SURVIVAL TIME

When the tumor was transplanted to different sites and
the animals were maintained until death intervened, it was
observed that the most lethal transplant route was intrarenal (Table 1). All of the animals autopsied had
evidence of metastases to the lungs, and in some animals
there were additional metastases to the intestines. In
animals receiving the tumor intraperitoneally it was found
that invariably the tumor invaded the mesentery, although only
one-third of the animals had lung metastases. Animals
receiving the tumor transplant subcutaneously have had
evidence of lung metastases. Evidence of lung metastases
is generally found in over half of the animals with tumor
transplanted intramuscularly. These circumstances in our
opinion, appeared to be independent of whether the tumor
was implanted surgically between the muscle fibers or by
puncture with trocar. In most animals receiving the
tumor transplant intramuscularly, a secondary primary
tumor was frequently found that was approximately equal
in size and indistinguishable from the original implant.
This consistent multinodule finding is evidently
characteristic of this site of implantation and would be
difficult to explain on the basis of cellular tumor
contamination at the time of inoculation.

TUMOR GROWTH

The typical rapid rate of subcutaneous (subaxilla) tumor

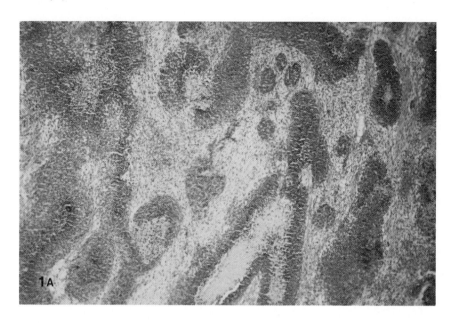

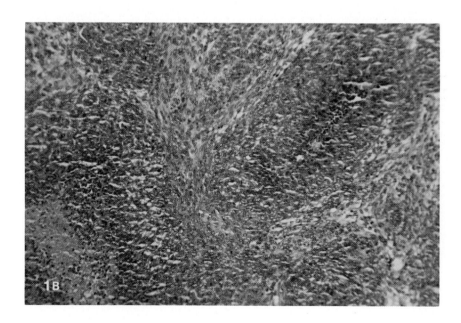

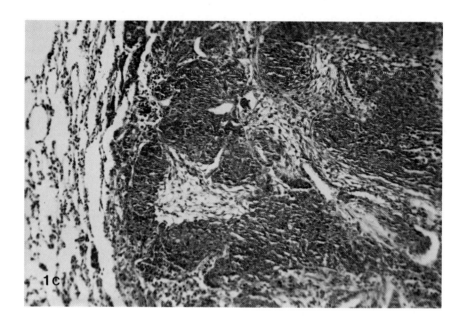

Fig. 1. A. General view of tumor from subcutaneous
transplant. Haphazard arrangement of undifferentiated tumor
cells in a background of immature mesenchymal tissue.
Hematoxylin and eosin, X77. B. Closeup of same tumor.
Notice "blending" of immature tumor elements and areas of
central necrosis. Hematoxylin and eosin X200. C. General
view of metastatic lesion to the lung showing some resemblance
to primary growth. Hematoxylin and eosin, X200.

growth weight is shown in Figure 2.

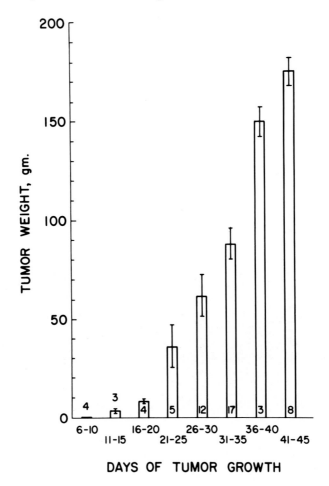

Fig. 2. Growth of subcutaneous tumor transplant in 5-day periods. The number of animals for each time period is indicated above or within the bars of the graph. Values are expressed as $\bar{X}$ + SEM.

The coefficient of correlation between weight and tumor volume in a typical experiment was 0.49 (p<0.05). Because of this finding, tumor weight was used in other experiments as an index of growth. The tumor was readily palpable by the time it reached a mass of 3 g (11 to 15 days post-implant). During this period of growth, tumor total protein and arginase levels remained unchanged. However, for example, in tumor samples assayed 21, 28, 34, and 41 days after tumor transplant the enzyme activity of 5α-reductase progressively increased from 2.50 to 5.69 mμM of testosterone reduced per g of tissue. The regression coefficient was 0.05 ($p<0.05$). Over a longer time period (typically 14 to 42 days of tumor transplant), the DNA level of tumor tissue increased from 5.0 to 6.7 mg. per g of tissue. As tumor growth progressed, there was an increase in the incidence of lung metastases, the animals were observed to be grossly weak, and hematocrit levels declined. Serum calcium and phosphorus levels generally remained unchanged during tumor growth and are comparable to levels obtained in age-matched controls. However, after the tumor had grown for 28 days the alkaline phosphatase level in experimental animals could become 2 to 4 times that found in controls. Isoenzyme studies by L-phenylalanine and urea inhibition revealed a normal mixed pattern in all control animals and in the younger tumor-bearing rats. With increased tumor growth the liver isoenzyme increased quantitatively.

This rat Wilms' model was described by Tomashefsky and his colleagues and could be confirmed as being morphologically and histologically identical to the human tumor (Tomashefsky et al. 1971). It was also similar to the human condition in terms of its preferential metastatic spread to the lungs, demonstrating once more the potential of this tumor to extend into other organs by a double mechanism of lymphatic and vascular invasion. The incidence of tumor acceptance did not vary according to the site of tumor transplant. Implantation to the subaxilla region had as its advantage visibility of tumor growth and surgical ease of transplant. Although obviously involving more work, an implant to the kidney had the advantage of similarity to the human condition and also made available the contralateral kidney for comparative study. For either route of tumor transplant the mean survival time and rate of development was advantageous for introducing therapeutic regimens.

Although the total LDH activity increased with progressive growth of the tumor, this had not been reflected in the LDH liver isoenzymes. Macroscopic examination of the livers

from the animals had failed to reveal metastatic involvement
or noticeable changes in liver size. However, metabolic
changes in the liver are possibly reflected by the increasing
alterations in alkaline phosphatase liver isoenzymes.

METASTATIC POTENTIAL

Additional growth characteristics, such as metastatic
spread and survival times were further evaluated in
transplantable Wistar/Furth rat Wilms' tumor models (Murphy
et al. 1975). Tumor suspension of various tumor cell
dosages were injected in an attempt to find the optimum
level of tumor take. Lung metastases were frequent
following tumor injection by all routes. However, tumor
spread to the lungs was the least frequent following
subcutaneous (SC) injection of the tumor. Survival time for
the intramuscular (IM) group was statistically longer at all
tumor dose levels. For the 1×10^5 tumor dosage, survival
time ranged from a mean of 27 days for the intrarenal (IR)
group to a mean 42 days for the IM group. For the 1×10^4
dosage, survival time ranged from a mean of 37 days for the
intraperitoneal (IP) group to a mean of 51 days for the IM
group. It was concluded that this animal tumor closely
resembles the human Wilms' tumor, and that the point at
which the transplanted tumor fails to be successfully
transplanted is below the dosage level of 1×10^3 tumor cells.

Smith et al. (1973) have done extensive work on a rat
model of Wilms' tumor. The transplanted (axillary) tumor
implants established a vascular supply within a few days,
and the majority of the metastases were blood borne
(Saroff et al. 1975). Within a few weeks the growing
subcutaneously transplanted tumor could be measured, as at
this site it evidently did not directly invade the
musculature or skin until the terminal stages (Saroff et al.
1975). The majority of the early experiments reported involved
transplanting the tumor by means of trocar (Saroff et al.
1975). A small chunk, approximately one to two millimeters
on each edge, was introduced into the recipient rat. With
this procedure, the dosage of tumor cells being used in
each tumor generation was, therefore, not likely to be the
same. Viable tumor cell suspensions were used instead of
chunks to minimize the variability between tumor generations.
Transplantability, survival, tumor cell kinetics, and mode
of disease induction were evaluated on a quantitative basis

and correlations were made with histological determinations and macroscopic observations throughout the duration of the experiments. These studies have provided important information on the growth characteristics of this tumor.

CELL STUDIES

Saroff reported that the incidence of tumor take with a trocar technique in Wistar/Furth rats was 100% regardless of the route of tumor transplantation (Saroff et al. 1975). Thus, the results of this study added the factor of cell number to tumor transplant data. Since the suspension method in such experiments enables the researcher to make a more precise cell count, it is apparently the better controlled method of the two. At first, it was thought that the lower limit of the cell tumor take was at a dosage slightly higher than 1×10^3 tumor cells/cc, but three of the four routes, even at that level, still showed evidence of tumor growth 42 days after transplant (Table 2). It would appear, however, that a 1×10^5 tumor dose will produce a more reproducible and prompt reaction. It has been reported that an occasional animal did not have a palpable tumor until several months after the transplant date (Tomashefsky et al. 1974 and Smith et al. 1973). They speculate that most of the tumor cells had died and that there was a long period before rapid growth began (Smith et al. 1973). The results from the cell suspension type of quantitative experiments have not yet detected such variations. Babcock and Southam injected a Wilms' tumor suspension in young rats via different routes and found that the IP route killed at a slightly faster rate than the SC route (Babcock and Southam 1961). This is in direct agreement with our results.

Smith et al. in 1973 pointed out that the Wilms' tumor line they had was faster growing than it was a few years before, thus killing the host before widespread metastases were evident (Smith et al. 1973). They found that the rats with lung metastases were the ones who survived longer than the average survival time (Smith et al. 1973). This correlation did not seem to be detectable in our study.

Yeakel (1948) also has reported that in general, tumor bearing rats have enlarged livers. We could

TABLE 2

METASTATIC SPREAD TO THE LUNGS OF THE
TRANSPLANTED WILMS' TUMOR

| | Number of Injected Tumor Cells | | |
	1×10^5	1×10^4	1×10^3
SC	10% (10)	0% (9)	0% (10)
IM	50% (10)	66% (9)	66% (10)
IP	100% (10)	100% (9)	60% (10)
IR	50% (10)*	99% (9)**	28% (10)

*100% of animals had ascites.   SC = subcutaneously
**88% of animals had ascites.   IM = intramuscularly
( ) = number of animals.   IP = intraperitoneally
  IR = intrarenally

not substantiate his observation (Murphy et al. 1975). We could, however, confirm that this tumor model can be studied with merit in a variety of ways which are readily quantifiable in terms of the growth of the tumor, its transplantability, and host reactions (Murphy et al. 1975).

METABOLIC EFFECTS

In vitro carbon dioxide was shown to have a regulatory effect on cell growth and in different concentrations may either arrest or stimulate the growth of a malignant cell (Kieler and Bicz 1962). This was also dependent on glycolytic activity of tumor cells, which provides less dependency on carbon dioxide concentrations, thus avoiding the regulatory effect of high carbon dioxide growth of the malignant cells (Kieler and Bicz 1962).

In our studies on the effects of exposure of experimental murine Wilms' tumor to increased atmospheric concentrations of carbon dioxide (West et al. 1978), we found that local tumor growth was not affected by concentrations of 76% and 55% of carbon dioxide applied for 10 and 30 minutes. There was no difference in survival of animals and weight of the tumor between the control and the experimental groups. Ten percent of the animals treated with concentrations of 55% and 76% carbon dioxide developed metastases in contrast to 30% of metastatic growth detected in the control group. This observation, although without statistically significant difference, indicates a need for further study of the carbon dioxide effect in different tumor models and different animal species.

Erythropoietin (ESF) levels were also assayed in rats bearing the Wistar-Furth Wilms' transplantable tumor (Murphy et al. 1976). Sites of tumor inoculation varied from subcutaneous, intramuscular, intrarenal (subcapsular), to intraperitoneal. Two-thirds of the animals exhibited ESP elevations without polycythemia, or severe anemia (HCT<30.0 vol %). The elevations in ESF were not detectably related to the time of sacrifice (age of the animal), size of the primary tumor, or number of gross metastatic foci. The diminished

ESF response noted in animals given intramuscular tumor implantations is believed to reflect differences in tumor blood and lymphatic supply at the various sites of inoculation (Murphy et al. 1976). The pattern of ESF responses in Wistar-Furth Wilms' tumor model was thus quite similar to that which we have observed in man, and appears to represent an animal model for tumor-related ectopic hormone release. The nature of the hormone is believed to differ from that seen in normal physiological states (Murphy et al. 1976).

IMMUNOLOGICAL FACTORS

In 1971 Renoux (Renoux and Renoux 1971) described the effect of antihelmintic Levamisole on potentiation of the bacterial vaccine in mice. Since then the immunological properties of this compound were extensively studied (Symoens 1977). It has been suggested that Levamisole restores the depressed cell mediated immunity (Sampson and Lui 1976) and some apparently successful clinical trials have been reported (Debois 1977). On the other hand, an enhancement of tumor growth was noted (Johnson et al. 1975) and recently Peters and associates (Peters et al. 1977) have observed that the dose of Levamisole may be of critical importance in clinical trials, since in different doses it may either suppress or enhance tumor growth. We also studied this in the animal model of Wilms' tumor. No tumoricidal effect of Levamisole could be documented in this tumor model, and no effect was shown on prevention of tumor, when Levamisole was given before tumor implantation (Wajsman et al. 1978).

It should be recalled in previous experiences with Wilms' tumor model, a good correlation between the human and animal tumor was found in regard to treatment with different drugs (Wajsman et al. 1978). The fact that Levamisole has no effect on our animal model and its reported immunosuppressive effect at some doses should be considered in planning future clinical trials.

ADJUVANT STUDIES

In other studies we have evaluated the effect of surgery, postoperative radiotherapy and postoperative combination chemotherapy on animal survival (Kedar et al. 1981). A total

of 73 rats were studied. They were divided into four
groups (fig. 3).

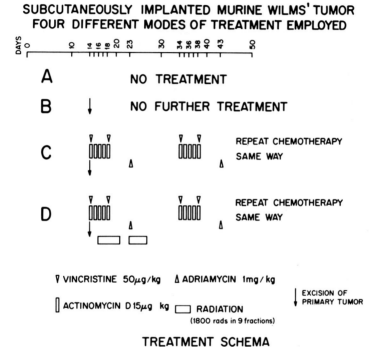

Fig. 3. Subcutaneously implanted murine Wilms' tumor. The
different therapy modalities given to the various groups.

Group A, a control group (18 animals), was given no treatment. Group B (15 animals) had surgical excision of the primary transplanted tumor on day 14. On the same day they received intraperitoneal chemotherapy consisting of actinomycin D 15µ/kg/day for 5 consecutive days, vincristine 15µg/kg/day on the 1st and 5th day of actinomycin D administration, and adriamycin 1 mg/kg 5 days later. This cycle was repeated every 10 days. Group D (20 animals) underwent excision and received chemotherapy in the same fashion as group C. In addition, they received radiotherapy starting on day 16. We used a ^{60}Co source at 50 cm source-to-target distance to deliver 1,800 rads in nine daily fractions of 200 rads each through one anterior port to an area of 1 x 1 cm. The radiation treatment was given 5 days a week. A special radiation cage was devised by us for this purpose (fig. 4). All of the animals in group A, the control, died of tumor with a median survival of 44 days (Table 3, fig. 3). Group B (excision only) had a median survival of 77 days with 40% tumor-free long-term survivors. Group C (excision followed by chemotherapy) had a median survival of 61 days with 35% tumor-free long-term survivors.

Statistical evaluation of the survival pattern for these four groups (Table 4) yielded a very high statistical significance ($p < 0.05$), respectively. Further tests comparing groups B and C indicated no statistical significance. All the animals that died in groups B through D had a recurrence of their primary tumor. Lung metastases were found in 14 out of 18 (77%) of dying rats in group A, 8 out of 9 (88%) dying animals in group B, and in 3 out of 9 (30%) dying animals in group D. In addition, an abdominal wall tumor mass was found in 1 animal of group B, 3 of group C, 2 of group D and in none of group A (fig. 5).

Our experimental study showed that, in the animal model, excision of the primary tumor on the 14th day after implantation leads to long-term survival in 40% of the cases.

Administering postoperative chemotherapy in our tumor model failed to control recurrence of the primary tumor, and thus failed to improve the overall survival. This is in contrast to the results of the National Wilms' Tumor Study 2, where the relapse-free survival of patients with group I Wilms' tumor was above 90% if actinomycin D and vincristine were given in combination for 6 or 15 months postoperatively (D'Angio et al. 1979).

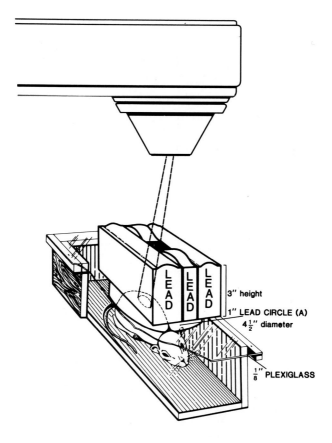

Fig. 4. Subcutaneously implanted murine Wilms' tumor. Cage used to deliver radiation. The lead placement was calculated to provide 90% reduction in exposure to shielded areas. The radiation was given from above through an opening within the shielding.

TABLE 3

SURVIVAL OF THE RATS BY GROUPS

Treatment Groups	Number of Rats	Median Survival Days	Number of Long-Term Survivors[1]
A Control	18	44	0
B Surgery Only	15	77	6 (40%)
C Surgery + Chemotherapy	20	61	7 (35%)
D Surgery + Chemotherapy + Radiotherapy	20	Not Yet Reached[1]	13 (55%)

[1]All surviving animals were sacrificed on day 175

TABLE 4

BRESLOW TEST SURVIVAL COMPARISON FOR
THE FOUR GROUPS OF ANIMALS STUDIED

Group Comparison	Statistical Significance
A vs. B vs. C vs. D	$P<0.001$
A vs. B+C+D Combined	$P<0.001$
B+C vs. D	$P<0.07$ (Borderline)
B vs. C	None
B vs. D	$P<0.08$ (Borderline)
C vs. D	$P<0.05$

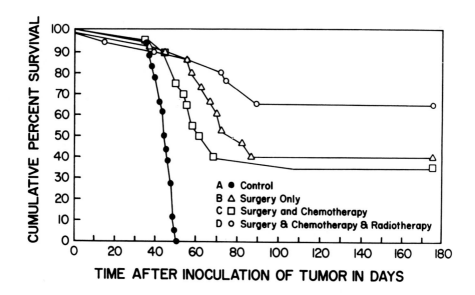

Fig. 5. Subcutaneously implanted murine Wilms' tumor survival. Survival curves according to the various treatment groups. ● =control. Δ=surgery only; □ =surgery + chemotherapy and o=surgery + radiotherapy.

The chemotherapy regimens of the National Wilms' Tumor Study were, however, different from our experimental protocol. The addition of radiation therapy resulted in a better control of the primary tumor in our animal model and increased the number of long-term survivors to 55%. In the National Wilms' Tumor Study the 2-year survival rate for postoperative irradiated children with localized tumor was 97% (D'Angio et al. 1978). In the National Wilms' Tumor Study, however, systemic single agent chemotherapy achieved a similar result (D'Angio et al. 1978).

The presence of abdominal wall involvement in all treated groups while absent in the control group is intriguing. Perhaps our surgical manipulation caused dissemination to the abdominal wall, or perhaps the tumor was altered in some negative fashion by chemotherapy or radiotherapy.

CHEMOTHERAPY SCREENING

Table 5 records the results noted following low-dose adriamycin chemotherapy. A single dose of adriamycin significantly ($p<0.001$) increased survival, reduced the weight of the tumor primary, and decreased the number of metastases noted at autopsy (Table 5). Minimal toxicity in this group was evident as judged by body weight (Table 5). When the low-dose adriamycin was given on a multiple drug basis, an even greater effect ($p<0.001$) was noted on the weight of the primary tumor at death, as well as a decrease in the number of metastases. However, the animals did not live for a significantly longer period of time. Drug toxicity as defined by body weight reduction was evident at this dose, both in tumor-bearing animals, and in nontumor-bearing drug-treated animals, who all succumbed to drug treatment following twenty-four days of therapy (Table 5). Based on other results the reduction in tumor primary weight noted in this study as well as the number of metastases are significant when compared with untreated tumor-bearing animals sacrificed at a similar period.

The higher doses of adriamycin in single or multiple dose had a significant effect on the tumor primary weight, and were associated with decreased metastases (Table 6). However, by all criteria, including microscopic examination of myocardial tissue which demonstrated characteristic necrosis, drug toxicity resulted in immediate general debility and ultimately death. These studies suggested that adriamycin (doxorubicin hydrochloride) could be effective in human therapy.

Chemotherapy is usually associated with some degree of toxicity. This has been clinically evident in human Wilms' tumor cases for some time (Wolff et al. 1974, Wolf et al. 1968 and Kenny et al. 1969). There are, however, also limits in extrapolating the results of an animal tumor model to man. It is still true today that despite the best surgical regimens as well as radiation treatment and chemotherapy, in some patients with Wilms' tumor metastases ultimately occur (Hrushesky and Murphy 1973). At this point a therapeutic dilemma is faced. What next? Despite grave and life-threatening toxicity, certain agents must

TABLE 5

LOW-DOSE ADRIAMYCIN TREATMENT OF EXPERIMENTAL

TRANSPLANTABLE WILMS' TUMOR

Experimental Group	Drug Dosage	Body Weight (Grams) Pretreatment	Body Weight (Grams) Post-Treatment	Tumor Weight (Milligrams)	Survival (Days)	Metastases (Per Cent)
1. Adriamycin	5 mg. per kg. (single dose)	181 ±4	197 ±14	134 ±19	50 ±2	40 ...
2. Adriamycin	5 mg. per kg. (multiple dose)	159 ±3	118 ±7	2.6 ±1.2	31 ±5	10 ...
3. No Treatment No Tumor	...	152 ±11	311 ±9	(Sacrificed at 70 days)		
4. Adriamycin No Tumor	5 mg. per kg. (single dose)	147 ±5	184 ±33	... ...	63* ±3	... ...
5. Adriamycin No Tumor	5 mg. per kg. (multiple dose)	128 ±7	104 ±5	... ...	23 ±1	... ...
6. No Therapy Tumor	... ...	170 ±6	198 ±15	181 ±27	43 ±2	80 ...

*Sacrificed at 63 days.

TABLE 6

HIGH-DOSE ADRIAMYCIN TREATMENT 10 MG. PER KILOGRAM OF

EXPERIMENTAL TRANSPLANTABLE WILMS' TUMOR

Experimental Group	Drug Dosage	Body Weight (Grams) Pretreatment	Post-Treatment	Tumor Weight (Milligrams)	Survival (Days)	Metastases (Per Cent)
1. Adriamycin	10 mg. per kg. (single dose)	213 ±7	153 ±8	27.6 ±17.7	18 ±4	0 ...
2. Adriamycin	10 mg. per kg. (multiple dose)	200 ±4	134 ±3	0.06* ...	12 ±1	0 ...
3. No Treatment No Tumor	... ...	131 ±8	225 ±8	(sacrificed at 21 days)		... ...
4. Adriamycin	10 mg. per kg.	170 ±5	126 ±5	... ...	79 ±8	... ...
5. Adriamycin	10 mg. per kg.	168 ±3	124 ±6	... ...	13 ±1	... ...
6. No Therapy Tumor	... ...	199 ±6	214 ±12	139.4 ±8.5	46 ±2	90 ...

*Small tumors were noted in all animals and were minimally visible grossly.

then be considered. At the time of this animal study, some time ago, we were unaware of any published cooperative study results suggesting that doxorubicin hydrochloride had a beneficial effect. Based on the animal model results in the present study and in others, on a low-dose schedule for a brief period, it appeared that doxorubicin hydrochloride would have a remarkable and heretofore unreported broad spectrum effect. Under suitable conditions the toxicity of a multiple course might be less in man. Doxorubicin hydrochloride at that time we felt should be considered as a candidate agent in these guarded conditions. In our opinion subsequent human trials have somewhat confirmed this point (Murphy and Williams 1975).

BILATERAL TUMORS

This animal model was also further studied in an attempt to review the effect of bilateral Wilms' Tumor. There was no significant improvement in survival, primary tumor growth or incidence of metastases to the lungs demonstrated in the study. Regrowth at the site of nephrectomy was significantly less in the group having nephrectomy performed at day 3 rather than day 7 (Tables 7 and 8). It is possible for this animal tumor to serve as a model of Wilms' tumor for future evaluation of varied surgical interventions in conjunction with chemotherapy. These studies demonstrated that regrowth of tumors at the site of unilateral nephrectomy could be prevented by the use of chemotherapy when nephrectomy was performed on day 3 after tumor implantation. A consideration of the renal counterbalance function in the presence of experimental bilateral tumors is possible in these experiments. Nephrectomy of itself, as expected, results in increased growth of the contralateral tumor bearing kidney. This type of study merits further investigation. Moreover, it suggests that radiation of the nephrectomized tumor bed may be an important consideration. On the other hand it also suggests that radiotherapy of patients with tumor in the remaining kidney merits reconsideration in that it might be deleterious.

SUMMARY AND CONCLUSION

This review reports the various experiments that we have completed to date to characterize a Wilms' tumor model

TABLE 7

EVALUATION OF TRIPLE DRUG THERAPY WITH AND WITHOUT
RIGHT NEPHRECTOMY DAY 3 ON BILATERAL MURINE WILMS' TUMOR

Group	Right Kidney Wt (Gm)	Left Kidney Wt (Gm)	Days of Survival	%Metastases
Sham - Control	$\bar{X}$1.2	$\bar{X}$1.2	40	
Normal Saline	±0.1	±0.1	(Sacrifice)	
Tumor - Control	$\bar{X}$44.2	$\bar{X}$1.2	$\bar{X}$31	50%
Right Kidney Implant	± 2.0	±0.1	± 2	
	N=14	N=14	N=14	
Bilateral Tumor	$\bar{X}$21	$\bar{X}$25	$\bar{X}$27	63%
Implant	± 2	± 2	± 1	
	N=11	N=11	N=11	
Bilateral Tumor Implant	*$\bar{X}$11.2	$\bar{X}$30.0	$\bar{X}$28	46%
Right Nephrectomy day 3	± 1.6	± 2.6	± 2	
	N=7	N=12	N=12	
Bilateral Tumor Implant	$\bar{X}$19.1	$\bar{X}$20.5	$\bar{X}$31	78%
Vincristine 50µg/kg day 7	± 3.0	± 2.0	± 1	
Actinomycin D 75µg/kg day 12	N=14	N=14	N=14	
Adriamycin 1 mg/kg day 17				
Bilateral Tumor Implant	*$\bar{X}$4.3	$\bar{X}$27.7	$\bar{X}$32	57%
Right Nephrectomy day 3	±	± 2.8	± 2	
Vincristine 50µg/kg day 7	N=1	N=12	N=14	
Actinomycin D 75µg/kg day 12				
Adriamycin 1mg/kg day 17				

*Regrowth at site of right kidney post total right nephrectomy.
Values are expressed as $\bar{X}$± SEM.
N=Number of animals evaluated.

TABLE 8

EVALUATION OF TRIPLE DRUG THERAPY WITH AND WITHOUT

RIGHT NEPHRECTOMY DAY 7 ON BILATERAL MURINE WILMS' TUMOR

Group	Right Kidney Wt (Gm)	Left Kidney Wt (Gm)	Days of Survival	%Metastases
Sham - Control Normal Saline	$\bar{X}$1.2 ±0.1 N=15	$\bar{X}$1.2 ±0.1 N=15	40 (Sacrifice)	-
Tumor - Control	$\bar{X}$53.8 ± 2.0 N=12	$\bar{X}$1.2 ±0.1 N=12	$\bar{X}$28 ± 1 N=12	83%
Bilateral Tumor Implant	$\bar{X}$22.4 ± 2.8 N=13	$\bar{X}$27 ± 4 N=13	$\bar{X}$29 ± 1 N=13	30%
Bilateral Tumor Implant Right nephrectomy day 7	*$\bar{X}$9.4 ±5.0 N=2	$\bar{X}$33.7 ± 5.7 N=10	$\bar{X}$26 + 2 N=10	70%
Bilateral Tumor Implant Vincristine 50µg day 7 Actinomycin D 75µg/kg day 12	$\bar{X}$23.2 ± 3.8 N=14	$\bar{X}$21.3 ± 2.8 N=14	$\bar{X}$28 ± 1 N=14	57%
Bilateral Tumor Implant R Nephrectomy day 7 Vincristine 50µg/kg day 7 Actinomycin D 75µg/kg day 17 Adriamycin 1mg/kg day 17	*$\bar{X}$18.0 ± 6.0 N=6	$\bar{X}$27.8 ± 4.1 N=10	$\bar{X}$28 ± 2 N=10	100%

*Regrowth at site of right kidney post total right nephrectomy.

Values are expressed as $\bar{X}$± SEM.

N=Number of animals evaluated.

relevant to the human clinical situation. As one can see, the model itself has reproducible features. Its growth characteristics have been defined. Hormonal capacities such as ectopic erythropoietic release have been described. Other metabolic effects of the tumor have been studied and can be further pursued to perhaps define the various roles of mechanisms of metastases. Immune enhancement in this model to date has not been successful. Postoperative chemotherapy and radiotherapy similar to the clinical situation have been studied and show both successes and failures similar to reported national clinical trials. Specific agents such as doxorubicin hydrochloride have dose related effectiveness in this model. In addition to the study of the unilateral tumor model by serial transplant, a bilateral tumor situation can be successfully induced and the roles of surgery and chemotherapy studied. We have completed these studies over a ten year period at Roswell Park Memorial Institute. Our transfer generations are currently beyond 170. The tumor is available to those interested in further analyses and investigations.

Babcock VI, Southam CM (1961). Transplantable renal tumor of the rat. Cancer Res. 21:130.

D'Angio GJ, Beckwith JB, Breslow N, Sinks L, Sutow W, Wolff J (1979). Results of the second national Wilms' tumor study (NWTS-2) Proc. ASCO/AACR 20:309.

D'Angio GJ, Tefft M, Breslow N, Meyer JA (1978). Radiation therapy of Wilms' tumor. Results according to dose, field, postoperative timing and histology. Int. J. Radiat. Oncol. Biol. Phys. 4:769.

Debois JM (1977). Preliminary experience with levamisole in cancer patients, and particularly in breast cancer. Prog. Cancer Res. Ther. 2:175.

Hrushesky WJ, Murphy GP (1973). Investigation of a new renal tumor model. J. Surg. Res. 15:327.

Johnson RK, Houchens DP, Gaston MR, Goldin A (1975). Effects of levamisole and tetramisole in experimental tumor systems Cancer Chemother. Rep. 59:697.

Kedar A, McGarry M, Moore R, Williams P, Murphy GP (1981). Effect of postoperative chemotherapy and radiotherapy on the survival of subcutaneously implanted Furth Wilms' tumor. Oncology 38:65.

Kenny GM, Webster JH, Sinks LM, Gaeta JF, Staubitz WJ, Murphy GP (1969). Results from treatment of Wilms' tumor at Roswell Park 1927-1968. J. Surg. Oncol. 1:49.

Kieler J, Bicz W (1962). Biological interactions in normal

and neoplastic growth, a contribution to host-tumor problems. A symposium. Little, Brown, and Churchill. Waltham, MA. p 89-100.

Murphy GP, Williams PD, Klein R (1975). The growth characteristics of the metastatic Wistar/Furth Wilms' tumor model. Res. Comm. in Chem. Pathol. and Pharm. 12:397.

Murphy GP, Williams PD, Mirand EA (1976). Erythropoietin levels in Wistar-Furth Wilms' tumor rats. J. Surg. Oncol. 8:131.

Murphy GP, Williams PD (1975). Beneficial effects of adriamycin on Wistar-Furth Wilms' tumor. Urology 5:741.

Peters TG, Sampson D, Lewis JD, Fuhrman TM (1977). Critical dose in levamisole-mediated regression of mammary carcinoma. Surg. Forum 28:153.

Renoux G, Renoux M (1971). Effet immunostimulant d'un imidothiazole dans l'immunisation des souris contre l'infection par Brucella abortus. C.r. Acad. Sci. 272:349.

Sampson D, Lui A (1976). The effect of levamisole on cell-mediated immunity and suppressor cell function. Cancer Res. 36:952.

Saroff J, Chu TM, Gaeta JF, Williams P, Murphy GP (1975). Characterization of a Wilms' tumor model. Invest. Urol. 12:320.

Smith AM, Priestley J, Tomashefsky P, Tannenbaum M, Lattimer J (1973). Current therapy of Wilms' tumor. Investigational background. N.Y. State J. Med. 73:1652.

Sutow WW, Gehan EA, Heyn RM, Kung FH, Miller RW, Murphy ML, Traggis DG (1970). Comparison of survival curves, 1956 versus 1962, in children with Wilms' tumor and neuroblastoma. Pediatrics, 45:800.

Symoens J (1977). An antianergic chemotherapeutic agent. Prog. Cancer Res. Ther. 2:1.

Tomashefsky P, Furth J, Lattimer JK, Tannenbaum M, Priestley J (1971). The Furth-Columbia rat Wilms' tumor. Trans. Am. Assoc. Genitourin. Surg. 63:28.

Uson AC, Wolff JA, Tretter P (1971). Current treatment of Wilms' tumor. Trans. Am. Assoc. Genitourin. Surg. 63:28.

Wajsman Z, Williams PD, Murphy GP (1978). The value of levamisole in a Wilms' tumor animal model. Oncology 35:212.

West CR, Wajsman Z, Williams PD, Murphy GP (1978). A study of the effect of environmental CO_2 on experimental Wilms' tumor. J. Med. 9:91.

Wolff JA, D'Angio GJ, Hartmann J, Krivit W, Newton WA, Jr. (1974). Long-term evaluation of single versus multiple courses in actinomycin D of Wilms' tumor. N. Engl. J. Med.

290:84.

Wolff JA, Krivit W, Newton WA, Jr., D'Angio GJ (1968).
Single versus multiple dose actinomycin therapy of
Wilms' tumor, ibid. 279:290.

Yeakel EH (1948). Increased weight of the liver in Wistar
albino rats with induced and transplanted tumor. Cancer
Res. 8:392.

Renal Tumors: Proceedings of the First International Symposium on Kidney Tumors, pages 43–57

WILMS' TUMOR: GENETIC ASPECTS AND ETIOLOGY

A Report of the National Wilms' Tumor Study (NWTS) Committee for the NWTS Group*

Certain constellations of findings have been identified that are associated with Wilms' tumor.

Congenital anomalies

Overgrowths. The first clear association between enlargements of parts of the body and Wilms' tumor was hemihypertrophy, reported by Miller et al in 1964.(1) This observation since has been confirmed in multiple studies, including that reported by Pendergrass, who reviewed the National Wilms' Tumor Study (NWTS) experience. He found hemihypertrophy in 2.9 percent of the 547 NWTS patients reviewed by him.(2)

*G.J. D'Angio, MD and A.E. Evans, MD, Children's Hospital Cancer Research Center, Philadelphia, PA; E. Baum, MD, Children's Memorial Hospital, Chicago, IL; J.B. Beckwith, MD, Children's Orthopedic Hospital, Seattle, WA; Norman Breslow, PhD, Fred Hutchinson Cancer Research Center, Seattle, WA; Alfred deLorimier, MD, University of California, San Francisco, CA; Donald Fernbach, MD, Baylor College of Medicine, Houston, TX; Ellen Hrabovsky, MD and Barbara Jones, MD, West Virginia University, Morgantown, WV; P. Kelalis, MD, Mayo Clinic, Rochester, MN; H.B. Othersen, Jr., MD, Medical University Hospital, Charleston, SC; Melvin Tefft, MD, Rhode Island Hospital, Providence RI; Patrick Thomas, MD, Washington University, St. Louis, MO.

Other conditions marked by tissue and organ over-growth have been reported in association with a higher frequency of Wilms' tumor. These include the Beckwith-Wiedemann syndrome (macro-glossia, gigantism, umbilical hernia, and kidney and pancreatic hyperplasia),(3) and the Klippel-Trenaunay syndrome (multiple nevi, hemangiomas, mental retardation, seizures).(2)

Genito-urinary. An increased frequency of genito-urinary (G-U) anomalies ranging from duplex collecting systems to gross malformations of the external genitalia has been reported in association with Wilms' tumor. Pen-dergrass, for example, found GU abnormalities in 4.4% of his cases.(2) Whether this truly represents an increase is uncertain because an accurate estimate of minor G-U anomalies in the general population is difficult to as-certain. Nonetheless, there is general agreement that G-U malformations are more frequent in Wilms' tumor patients.(4)

A subset of these patients is characterized by pseudohermaphrodism and nephropathies of various types (e.g., nephrosis, glomerulonephritis.)(2)

Aniridia. This malformation of the iris of the eye occurs in the familial and in the sporadic form. It is the non-familial type that is associated with Wilms' tumor, a finding that was included in the initial report by Miller et al which also recorded the observation con-cerning hemihypertrophy.(1) It was present in about 1% of the NWTS cases reviewed.(2)

Familial

The frequency of Wilms' tumor in siblings is not high. In a recent review by Carli et al of cancer in siblings, there was one Wilms' tumor sibship with con-cordant tumors (the only time) among 27 families col-lected by them.(5) The Pendergrass review found 6 chil-dren who were one of twins, with no Wilms' tumors in the co-twins. Three families reported nephroblastoma in other family members. Thus, the familial frequency was less than 1%. Two were in siblings and the third in an extraordinary family with 2 and probably 3 family members with Wilms' tumor.

Associations with other neoplastic and paraneoplastic conditions

Neurofibromatosis. An association between Wilms' tumor and neurofibromatosis has been suggested by Stay and Vawter.(6) They found 3 patients with neurofibromatosis among 342 children with Wilms' tumor, a 29-fold higher incidence than would be predicted by chance events. Stay and Vawter point out "... the close parallels in associative lesions ... suggest a genetic basis for both entities which may have elements in common."

Nephroblastomatosis. The appearance of foci of primitive nephroblastic elements, usually subcortical in location, and of nodular renal blastema has been found to have a high association with the subsequent appearance of Wilms' tumor itself. The potential for bilateral involvement must therefore be kept in mind when such findings are recorded in a nephrectomy specimen.(7,8)

Mesoblastic nephroma. The lesions, known by several other names (e.g., renal hamartoma) has been identified as a separate entity.(9) Occurring in younger children, it has a distinctive histologic appearance with an almost invariably benign course. There are, however, mesoblastic nephromas with histologic features that place it on the borderlands of Wilms' tumor, and there are recorded instances of local relapse of the mesoblastic nephroma as well. It therefore would appear that this tumor may be at one end of a spectrum of Wilms' tumor histologic types, or that there may be forms of nephroblastoma that have histocytologic features that make it indistinguishable from mesoblastic nephroma, the latter still to be considered a benign neoplastic process.

Sub-types of Wilms' tumor according to cyto-histologic characteristics are being identified.(10) Tumors located centrally in the kidney have features that are reminiscent of tumors derived from the neural crest. Indeed, certain indubitable Wilms' tumors contain ganglion cells.(11) It therefore would seem that much remains to be done in the future to categorize and sub-classify the nephroblastoma complex. Major advances, of course, have already been made along these lines. The clear cell sarcoma, also known by other names, and the "rhabdoid" tumors, once thought to be Wilms' tumor variants, are now clearly identified as being

separate entities.(10) It may be that there are major
sub-types of the nephroblastoma, one derived from renal
anlage, and one from neural crest elements. The latter
would help explain the additional observation, now abun-
dantly verified, that neuroblastomas can occur intrarenally
and be indistinguishable roentgenographically from Wilms'
tumor itself.(12)

Etiology

The nitrosamines have been identified as being etiologic factors in the production of multiple tumors in
opossums, among them lesions typical of Wilms' tumors.(13)
Other etiologic clues, derived from epidemiologic studies,
point to lead; but there is as yet no clearly identified
causative factor.(14) Studies of pre-natal maternal and
paternal influences are underway, and are needed.

At the molecular level, a fairly specific aberration
of chromosome 11 has been identified by several investigators in familial as well as non-familial cases of the
aniridia-Wilms' tumor syndrome, pointing to a possible
genetic basis.(15)

Pathology

Beckwith and Palmer have subdivided the Wilms' tumor
into two broad categories based on histopathologic characteristics.(10) The first, which makes up more tham 85%
of cases, they termed Favorable Histology (FH). The others
are grouped as Unfavorable Histology or UH. Patients with
FH tumors are not necessarily risk-free, but their chances
for survival are much better. Two year survival rates
in NWTS-2, for example, were 90% for FH and 54% for UH.
(p<0.0001).(16)

UH tumors are further subdivided into the anaplastic
lesions, which appear to be more malignant variants of
Wilms' tumor and the rhabdoid and clear cell sarcomas. The
latter two are currently believed to be separate entities,(17) and some of their clinical characteristics have
been discussed above.

NATURAL HISTORY AND METASTATIC PATTERNS

The tumor usually grows as a single mass without predilection for either kidney, nor for either pole. The size of the tumor is not a major prognostic factor. Very small lesions, such that the kidney with its associated tumor did not exceed 250 grams, appeared to be associated with a better prognosis in the first National Wilms' Tumor Study (NWTS-1). Age under 24 months also had favorable connotations in Group 1 NWTS-1 patients.(18)

Multi-focal disease is found in 7% of the patients, and is not different in prognosis, age distribution, nor outlook from children with a single tumor mass.(19) Bilateral tumors, however, occur in younger patients, and the clinical outlook is generally more favorable for these patients, who make up about 5% of the total.(19,20)

Local spread occurs by direct invasion of the tumor through the renal capsule to infiltrate the parieties, usually in the retroperitoneal regions. Penetration through the peritoneal surface and peritoneal seeding occurs rarely. The tumor may propagate as an intralumenal thrombus extending into the renal vein, sometimes into the inferior vena cava, and on occasion into the right atrium. Such a thrombus, unattached to the walls of a major vessel or the heart, does not confer an unfavorable prognosis.(18) Obviously, care is needed at the time of operation not to dislodge the thrombus. When that occurs, minute embolization into the lungs can occur or, in certain instances, the pulmonary artery can be choked by a massive embolus with its obvious associated problems. More ominous is tumor penetration through the wall of the renal vein or inferior vena cava, the tumor demonstrating thereby its more aggressive characteristics. There are anecdotal reports to suggest that such patients fare less well than those who have a free-floating thrombus.

Lymph node metastases. Lymph node metastases, when present, are associated with a lower survival rate. Two-year relapse-free survival rates for NWTS-2 patients with and without nodal metastases was 54% and 82% respectively (p<0.001).(16) It may be that lymph node involvement restricted to the renal hilum may not be so unfavorable, and studies are underway to elucidate this question.

Peritoneal seeding occurs rarely before diagnosis, and usually is thought to represent a prediagnosis tumor rupture into the peritoneal cavity. Spillage of tumor at the time of surgery, when massive, heightens the risk of peritoneal seeding; in girls, the pouch of Douglas has a higher predilection for such recurrences.

Distant metastases are present in 11% of cases at diagnosis.(16) They most commonly are first found in the lungs, with or without other sites involved in 95% of patients with metastases at the time of diagnosis and are the first site of distant dissemination in more than 80% of children after primary surgery.(16,21) The patterns of metastases to other sites differ according to histologic type (See below).

STAGING

Various staging systems have been proposed over the years. The factors described above, and others found to have prognostic implications, have been incorporated in the staging system used in the third NWTS.(16,18) It promises to provide better discrimination among patients than the NWTS grouping method previously employed.

CLINICAL SIGNS AND SYMPTOMS

Most children with Wilms' tumor appear to be healthy when first seen. The tumors usually are found incidentally during a well-baby examination, or are noted by a family member during bathing or dressing. Associated signs and symptoms are infrequent and often non-specific. The most common are pain, hematuria and fever. Hypertension is present in perhaps half the patients. Sukarochana et al found elevations of the systolic pressure with or without diastolic elevations in 29 of the 46 patients (63%) they studied.(22) Other clinical findings are relatively uncommon. It is rare, for example, to have a patient with Wilms' tumor diagnosed because of dyspnea caused by extensive pulmonary metastases.

Trauma to the flank may lead to rupture of a Wilms' tumor, and the attendant pain and signs of blood loss must be differentiated from rupture of the spleen, liver, or, indeed, a normal kidney.

Ramsay et al have described a specific complex of signs and symptoms that can be found in Wilms' tumor patients.(23) These stem from an intracapsular hemorrhage which can occur spontaneously or after trauma. There is a sudden appearance of a tumor mass, and the patient may be febrile, hypertensive, and anemic. Such a hemorrhage some time prior to diagnosis probably accounts for the arcuate, peripheral calcifications seen in some Wilms' tumor specimens. The appearance is to be differentiated from that found in the neuroblastoma, where the radio-opacities tend to be minute and scattered throughout the tumor to give the so-called "pepper and salt" appearance.

DIFFERENTIAL DIAGNOSIS

The differential diagnosis of children with a flank mass includes both benign and malignant conditions.

Benign. Cystic lesions of the kidney can produce clinical and roentgenographic findings similar to those of the Wilms's tumor. Differentiation usually is easy by sonography, revealing a solid mass on the one hand, and a cystic process on the other. Due caution must be exercised, however, in that some Wilms' tumors occur in association with cystic lesions.(24) The mesoblastic nephroma can produce roentgen changes identical to the Wilms' tumor, and differentiation by means of angiography, sonography and presumably by computerized tomography is not possible.(25) Other conditions that produced confusing clinical and imaging patterns in the first NWTS include renal carbuncle, hemorrhage into the suprarenal gland, the congenital renal vein thrombosis, and dysplastic kidney.(12)

Malignant. The intrarenal neuroblastoma is the most frequent source of error in diagnosis, having been encountered in 9 among 30 "wrong diagnoses". Various sarcomas accounted for an additional 4 errors, and there were 3 renal cell carcinomas as well.(12)

The errors in pre-operative diagnosis are of relatively minor importance because surgery is usually performed promptly and the correct diagnosis is thus established. The situation is different when pre-operative therapy is contemplated. Then, irradiation or chemotherapy may be given inappropriately for a benign condition, or the chemotherapeutic agent administered is not best for the malignant lesion actually present (e.g., actinomycin D for a neuroblastoma).

DIAGNOSIS

Pre-operative. The work-up of children with flank masses makes for a text-book example of cost-benefit considerations. Excretory urography (intravenous pyelogram or IVP) and chest films may suffice. Pulmonary deposits found in association with an intrarenal mass virtually make the diagnosis; any other malignant lesion would be rare indeed. The diagnosis may be less clear if the lungs are normal. There is no doubt that present-day diagnostic procedures, including sonography, computerized tomography, and angiography could identify with greater precision the presence or absence of a neoplastic process within an enlarged kidney. The point is whether these extra studies are worth the extra time, money, and x-ray exposure. A surgeon confronted with a flank mass must explore the child, whether the mass pre-operatively is thought to be of benign or of malignant nature. The main value of such studies lies in establishing that the mass is, in fact, intrarenal, and that there is a second kidney. Studies of the affected side in addition to an IVP are therefore seldom indicated.

Inferior vena cavography. It is the practice in some centers to visualize the inferior vena cava as a preliminary to obtaining the IVP. The opaque material is injected through a foot or ankle vein while the venous return from the opposite leg is occluded. Films are taken as the bolus passes through the main vessels. Films for a routine IVP follow. This method has not found wide favor. It not uncommonly produces incomplete or false information. The Valsalva maneuver associated with a crying child produces artifactual under-opacification of the inferior vena cava, and "streaming" effects also produce confusing patterns.(26) It is therefore preferable to undertake a formal inferior vena cavogram using percutaneous catheter techniques in patients where the procedure is thought especially indicated; e.g., the child with a non-visualized kidney on routine IVP, or with prominent collateral venous pattern on the anterior abdominal wall when main venous channel obstruction can be suspected.

Sonography. Recent technical advances have made this imaging method more attractive than before. Its major role would seem, at this juncture, to be in the visualization of the renal vein and inferior vena cava. Information regarding the patency of these structures can be obtained accurately, simply and without radiation exposure. The renal mass, of course, is also visualized and its nature (cystic or solid) determined with some precision, but the study is felt to be complementary to the IVP and has not supplanted excretory urography. The sensitivity and accuracy of the method for identification of other abnormalities (e.g., positive lymp nodes) remains to be established.

Computerized axial tomography (CT). Striking displays of the regional anatomy are obtained by CT, but it has not been established that the study is of routine value. It can be used to provide supplementary information, for example, when the IVP suggests the presence of bilateral disease or when liver involvement is suspected.

Renal arteriography. Opacification of the arterial tree is not indicated as a routine measure. It can be used to delineate the size, number and distribution of lesions identified on the opposite side at the time of initial surgery so that the response to treatment can be gauged, and "second look" operations planned. It is probable that sonography and computerized tomography will supercede renal arteriography in most cases.

Radioactive isotope scans. Radionuclide images of the kidneys or the liver are seldom indicated in Wilms' tumor patients. The necessary information is obtained with greater precision by the other imaging techniques mentioned above. In any case, liver involvement at diagnosis is rarely found.(27)

Supplementary studies may be useful in certain clinical situations; for example, if the diagnosis lies between a post-traumatic hematoma or renal carbuncle and Wilms' tumor. Even here, however, additional diagnostic procedures cannot always be conclusive. There could be a hematoma around a Wilms' tumor, for example. Studies of the opposite side may be more rewarding, but no imaging method can be expected to identify the small, sessile lesions barely protruding from the cortex that sometimes are found at the time of surgery. It therefore is imperative that the entire surface of the contralateral kidney be examined at the time of surgery to rule out the presence of bilateral tumors. This is especially worthwhile when the affected kidney shows gross signs of nephroblastomatosis, or when there are overt clinical malformations such as the Beckwith-Weidemann syndrome which has a higher correlation with bilaterality. Diagnostic studies of the contralateral kidney are more useful in the post-operative period, therefore, when bilateral disease has been identified than they are pre-operatively. They can supply useful guidelines to follow the response of the tumor to chemotherapy, radiation therapy, or the combination. Angiography, and sonography have been helpful for this purpose. The eventual role of computerized tomography remains to be elucidated, but may well serve as an effective substitute for angiography in the future.

Follow-up studies. The most rewarding investigations are careful physical examinations and chest radiographs. Frequent post-operative IVP's have not always been successful in identifying contralateral kidney disease before it became palpable.(28) Palmer and co-workers provided additional relevant data.(29) Their report concerned 13 children with non-familial aniridia who were followed closely because they were known to be at risk for developing Wilms' tumor. The tumor was detected roentgenographically in only 1 of 9 who had had frequent IVP's. The others developed clinical signs (mass in 6 and hematuria in 2) rather suddenly, and in some cases shortly after a negative IVP. The authors concluded that careful physical examination was the most valuable means of following patients at risk. Thus, excretory urography not more often than once a year for the first 3 post-operative years is employed in NWTS-3. Follow-up excretory urography in the future may well be supplanted by sonography which is a simpler and perhaps more accurate method. Chest films are another matter. The lungs are the most frequent sites of metastases, and frontal and lateral views of the chest are requested prior to each course of chemotherapy in NWTS-3, every 6 months thereafter to the third year, and yearly thereafter. Oblique views and CT scans at each of these times would surely increase the yield, but it is doubtful that earlier detection (within these intervals) would substantially affect outcome. The extra cost and exposure would therefore not seem to be

warranted. Urinalyses to coincide with the chest films are
easily obtained and may provide useful information. Microscopic hematuria may be the first sign of contralateral
involvement or, when coupled with proteinuria, of combined
therapy nephropathy.

Special considerations. The renal clear cell sarcoma
is associated with bone metastases.(30) Skeletal lesions
are rare in any of the other childhood tumors primary in
the kidney. There are anecdotal reports (including one of
our own) that roentgenographic skeletal surveys are more
useful than bone scans in identifying early clear cell
sarcoma skeletal metastases. By contrast, brain metastases
and independent posterior fossa small cell brain tumors,
are found in association with the "rhabdoid" tumor of the
kidney.(31) Computerized tomography or brain radionuclear
scans therefore are worthwhile in any child who has such a
lesion diagnosed; studies of the brain otherwise are unlikely to be rewarding. Liver metastases are found in
about 1% of patients at diagnosis.(27) They are perhaps
twice as common in children with the unfavorable forms of
Wilms' tumors. Appropriate diagnostic (imaging) examinations of that organ are thus more likely to be rewarding in
the follow-up of such patients, and not recommended for
those with FH tumors.

Sub-classification of the primary tumors of the kidney
has thus provided useful information regarding which diagnostic studies should be carried out, eliminating from
routine work-up the radiation exposure and costs entailed
in expensive routine imaging surveys, while targeting according to the histology of the tumor those studies most
likely to be useful adjuncts to the standard procedures.

Renal sinus. The significance of protrusion of the
tumor into the renal sinus remains to be elucidated.
Beckwith and co-workers have identified this region of the
kidney as being extra-capsular, and therefore having potentially unfavorable clinical significance. However, in a
recent review by Bonadio and Beckwith of National Wilms'
Tumor Study cases, it was found that renal sinus involvement in patients who had Stage I tumors did not confer a
worse prognosis.(32) Studies of this finding in association
with Stage II and III specimens is underway.

FUTURE GOALS

Some of the problems remaining for the pathologist to solve are the further subclassification of tumors into sets with specific clinical connotations, as they have done so brilliantly up to now, (7-11, 33-35) and in identifying which child with multiple tumor nodules in one kidney or nephroblastomatotic changes in either or both kidneys is likely to develop an overt Wilms' tumor on the opposite side. The need for such is pointed up by the patient, reported by Rosenfield et al(36) who had regressing changes of nephroblastomatosis, yet developed a frank Wilms' tumor.

Other challenges for the future, lie in devising more effective treatments for patients with metastatic disease and with the unfavorable histologic types. On the other end of the scale, they lie in identifying patients who are at low risk through painstaking studies of the myriad cytohistologic patterns that are seen in Wilms' tumors, and correlating these with more refined staging criteria. Such identification is required so that treatments can be reduced to the bare minimum for these children.

Careful, comparative studies are needed in order to determine the usefulness of the newer sonographic and computerized tomographic imaging methods so that indications for their use can be established. Not only is better diagnostic accuracy being sought, but also the means of reducing radiation exposure and expense. Meanwhile, the search for a sensitive diagnostic chemical or biologic test goes on; it has been unsuccessful to date.

The real challenges, however, lie in identifying the genetic and environmental factors that contribute to the development of Wilms' tumor. Important leads are being developed. Studies of these factors are needed, because true success will come in Wilms' tumor management, not when survival rates climb towards 100%, but when incidence rates approach zero.

ACKNOWLEDGEMENTS

The authors acknowledge the contribution made by the many members of the NWTS Group without whom the study would have been impossible. They also thank past members of the

NWTS Committee and Dr. R. Shalek and the staff of the Radiological Physics Center, and the staff of the NWTS Data and Statistical Center.

Supported in part by USPHS Grant No. CA-11722.

1. Miller RW, Fraumeni JF, Jr and Manning MD (1964) Association of Wilms' tumor with aniridia, hemihypertrophy, and other congenital malformations. N Engl J Med 270:922-927.
2. Pendergrass TW (1976). Congenital anomalies in children with Wilms' tumor. Cancer 37:403-409.
3. Beckwith JB (1969). Macroglossia, omphalocele, adrenal cytomegaly, gigantism, and hyperplastic visceromegaly. Birth Defects: Original Article Series 5; No. 2, 188-196.
4. Jagasia KH and Thurman WG (1965). Congenital anomalies of the kidney in association with Wilms' tumor. Pediatr 35:338-340.
5. Carli M, Cordero di Montezemolo L, DeRossi G, et al: An Italian survey of cancer in siblings. (Unpublished observations).
6. Stay EJ and Vawter G (1977). The relationship between nephroblastoma and neurofibromatosis (Von Recklinghausen's disease). Cancer 39:2550-2555.
7. Bove KE, Koffler H and McAdams AJ (1969). Nodular renal blastema. Definition and possible significance. Cancer 24:323-332.
8. Bove KE and McAdams AJ (1976). The nephroblastomatosis complex and its relationship to Wilms' tumor: a clinico-pathologic tretise. Perspect Pediatr Pathol 3:185-223.
9. Bolande RP, Brough AJ, Izant RJ (1967). Congenital mesoblastic nephroma of infancy. A report of eight cases and the relationship to Wilms' tumor. Pediatrics, 40:272-278.
10. Beckwith JB and Palmer NF (1978). Histopathology and prognosis of Wilms' tumor. Cancer 41:1937-1948.
11. Llombart-Bosch A, Peydro-Olaya A and Cerda-Nicolas M (1980). Presence of ganglion cells in Wilms' tumours: A review of the possible neuroepithelial origin of nephroblastoma. Histopathology 4:321-330.
12. Ehrlich RM, Bloomberg SD, Gyepes MT, Levitt SB, Kogan S, Hanna M, and Goodwin WE (1979). Wilms' tumor misdiagnosed pre-operatively. A review of 19 National Wilms' Tumor Study I Cases. J Urol 122:790-792.

13. Jurgelski W, Hudson PM, Falk HL, and Kolin P (1976). Embryoma neoplasms in the opossum: A new model for solid tumors of infancy and childhood. Science 193: 328-332.

14. Zack M, Cannon S, Loyd D, Health CW, Falletta JM, Jones B, Housworth J, Crowley S (1980). Cancer in children of parents exposed to hydrocarbon-related industries and occupations. Am J Epidemiology 111:329-336.

15. Yunis JJ and Ramsay NKC (1980). Familial occurence of the aniridia-Wilms' tumor syndrome with deletion 11. J Pediatr 96:1027-1030.

16. D'Angio GJ, Evans A, Breslow N, Beckwith B, Bishop H, Farewell V, Goodwin W, Leape L, Palmer N, Sinks L, Sutow W, Tefft M, and Wolff J (1981). The treatment of Wilms' tumor: Results of the Second National Wilms' Tumor Study. Cancer 47:2302-2311.

17. Beckwith JB (1979). The pathology of renal tumors in children. Recent results of the National Wilms' Tumor Study. In: "Recent Advances in Management of Children with Cancer." Tokyo, p 73-87.

18. Breslow NE, Palmer NF, Hill LR, Buring J, and D'Angio GJ (1978). Wilms' tumor: Prognostic factors for patients without metastases at diagnosis. Cancer 41: 1577-1589.

19. Breslow NE, Beckwith JB, Palmer NF, Jacobson S and Sim DA (In press). Epidemiological features of Wilms' tumor. Results of the National Wilms' Tumor Study. J Nat'l Cancer Inst.

20. Bishop HC, Tefft M, Evans AE, D'Angio GJ (1977). Survival in bilateral Wilms' tumor - review of 30 National Wilms' Tumor Study cases. J Pediatr Surg 12:631-638.

21. Sutow WW, Breslow NE, Palmer NF, D'Angio GJ, Takashima J (In press). Prognosis in children with Wilms' tumor metastases prior to or following primary treatment. Results from the First National Wilms' Tumor Study (NWTS-1). Cancer Clin Trials.

22. Sukarochana K, Tolentino W, and Kiesewetter WB (1972). Wilms' tumor and hypertension. J Ped Surg 7:573-578.

23 Ramsay N, Dehner L, Coccia P, D'Angio GJ, Nesbit M (1977). Acute hemorrhage into Wilms' tumor. Ped 91: 763-765.

24. Beckwith JB, Kiviat NB (1981). Multilocular renal cysts and cystic renal tumors. Am J Roentgenol 136: 435-436. (Editorial)

25. Hartman DS, Lesar MSL, Madewell JE, Lichtenstein JE, Davis CJ, Jr (1981). Mesoblastic nephroma: Radiologic-pathologic Correlation of 20 cases. Am J Roentgenol 136:69-74.

26. Rosenberg H, Mahboubi S, Ring E, Chatten J, D'Angio G (1979). Proc XI Meeting of the International Society of Pediatric Oncology, Lisboa, p 7.51. (Abstract).

27. Tefft M (1980). Liver metastases as initial site of failure in Wilms' tumor: A report from the National Wilms' Tumor Study (NWTS). Proc of ASCO, 21:385.

28. Cohen MD, Siddiqui A, Weetman R, Baehner R, Weber T, Grosfeld JL (In press). A rational approach to the radiologic evaluation of children with Wilms' tumor. Cancer.

29. Palmer NF, Evans A and Meyer JA. Wilms' tumor in sporadic aniridia. A report from the NWTS. Proc of XI meeting of the International Society of Pediatric Oncology, p. 7.9. (Abstract).

30. Sutow WW, Breslow N, Palmer NF, D'Angio GJ, Takashima, JR (1979). Prognosis after relapse in children with Wilms' tumor. Results from the First National Wilms' Tumor Study Group. Proc of AACR 20:68. (Abstract).

31. Palmer NF, Beckwith JB (1981). Multiple primary tumor syndrome in children with rhabdoid tumor of the kidney. Proc of ASCO 22:406.

32. Bonadio JF, Beckwith JB. The prognostic significance of renal sinus involvement in Wilms' tumor. (In preparation).

33. Chatten J (1976). Epithelial differentiation in Wilms' tumor: A clinico-pathological appraisal. Perspect Pediatric Pathol 3:225-254.

34. Kidd JK (1970). Exclusion of certain renal neoplasms from the category of Wilms' tumor. Am J Pathol 59:16a.

35. Marsden HB and Lawler W (1980). Bone metastasizing renal tumour of childhood. Histopathological and clinical review of 38 cases. Virchows Arch A Path Anat and Histol 387:341-351.

36. Rosenfield NS, Shimkin P, Berdon W, Barwick K, Glassman M and Siegel NJ (1980). Wilms' tumor arising from spontaneously regressing nephroblastomatosis. Am J Roentgenol 135:381-384.

Renal Tumors: Proceedings of the First International Symposium on
Kidney Tumors, pages 59–66
© 1982 Alan R. Liss, Inc., 150 Fifth Avenue, New York, NY 10011

EVALUATION OF NEPHROBLASTOMAS

Sylvia Neuenschwander, M.D., Jean Philippe
Montagne, M.D., Clément Fauré, M.D.
Hôpital Trousseau
26, av. Dr. A. Netter   75571 Paris Cedez 12

Radiologic and echographic examinations have a prominant
place for the diagnosis of an abdominal mass in children.
They are able to determine whether the lesion is intra or
extra renal and whether it is solid or cystic. When the
diagnosis of a solid intrarenal tumor is made, they are
used to determine the extent of the lesion. Under therapy,
they are useful to follow the effects, to detect complications, metastases or recurrences.

CONVENTIONAL RADIOLOGY

The plain films of the abdomen, frontal and lateral
views usually show a flank mass of water density, which
shadows the psoas muscle margin and displaces the bowel
gas. The mass is rarely calcified (10 to 20%). When
present, the calcifications are spotlike or ringlike.
They are different from the stippled or flaky densities
of neuroblastomas (Grossman 1977; Kaufman et al. 1978).
Despite new techniques of imaging, intraveinous pyelography continues to be the basic examination for the
diagnosis of nephroblastoma. It has to be performed with
good technique (Bardon et al. 1967; Cope et al. 1972;
Horodniceanu et al. 1981). For us, in order to find
a displacement or a thrombosis we start the examination
by the opacification of the inferior vena cava (IVC).
Some authors advocate an injection in the IVP itself
to avoid a false diagnosis of thrombosis. We think
that such a procedure may be hazardous. Our technique is
to inject the contrast medium through a vein of the
foot with a small needle and to take a lateral and a

frontal view of the IVC (Fig. 1).

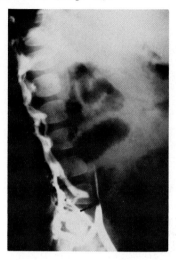

Fig. 1. Inferior vena cava thrombosis. Lateral view: ↗
total obstruction of the inferior vena cava. Collateral
veinous drainage is noted.

Among our last 30 nephroblastomas, 20 had an opacification of the IVC. We were able to demonstrate 3 cases
of IVC thrombosis which were confirmed at surgery. We
had no false positive nor false negative. Then being
at the total body opacification phase we take a front film
of the whole abdomen (Kurlander, Smith 1967). In our
experience, the lesion increased its density non-homo-
genously (12/20 cases).

To study the excretory phase of the IVP, we advocate
frontal oblique and lateral views. Typically an intrarenal tumor causes splaying and displacement of pyelocalyceal cavities (Fig. 2). Dilation of one or several
calyces or varying degrees of hydronephrosis is quite common (Grossman, 1977). The ureter is displaced medially
and/or anteriorly depending on the extent of the lesion.
Tomographies usually do not add useful information. The
involved kidney may not be secreting (16%), 2/30 cases in
our series. The opposite kidney needs to be carefully
evaluated for bilateral involvement.

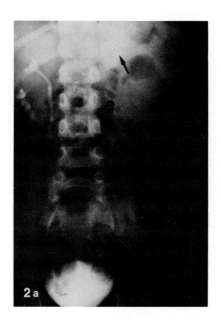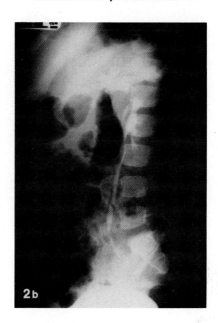

Fig. 2 a and b: Left nephroblastoma.
a) anterior view.
b) lateral projection: mass of the lower pole of the left
kidney displacing and splaying the collecting system (↗).

ECHOTOMOGRAPHY

For us, echotomography is a systematic adjunct to the
excretory urography. The following results of echography
are based on our experience (30 cases) and a review of the
literature (Horodniceanu et al. 1981). The mass is
always echogenic but echogenicity may be homogenous
(9/30 cases) or non-homogenous with several large (10/30)
or with few (11/30) anechogenic areas. Such lesions
correspond to necrosis (Fig. 3).

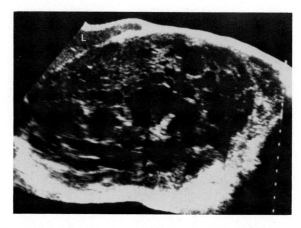

Fig. 3. Left nephroblastoma. Longitudinal sonogram of
the left kidney in supine position. Large left renal mass
with multiple anechogenic areas: pseudo cystic nephroblastoma prior to chemotheraph (L: left lobe of the liver).

Echography gives the location, size and limits of the
lesion (Fig. 4). It also gives the relationship with the
renal pelvis and calyces, with the liver, the diaphragm,
with the midline the great vessels in paticular (inferior
vena cava and aorta). Out of our 30 cases, IVC was normal
in 15, dislocated by a retrocaval extension in 7,
thrombosed in 4 (Fig. 5), and not seen in 4 due to a poor
technique.

Enlarged lymph nodes around the renal vessels, aorta
and IVC do not give a well defined lesion but a hyperecho-
genic area with widening of the distance between the
vessels or of the distance between the vertebrae and the
great vessels (Fig. 6). In 15 cases, the area of the
great vessels looked normal in six, five were normal at
surgery, and one had a pathologically enlarged node but
it was located below the renal vessels. In three cases
this area was not seen, in two cases it was due to bowel
gas shadowing and in one case the scan was poor due to a
non cooperative baby. Enlarged nodes were diagnosed in
six cases and were confirmed at surgery. But at pathology
three were metastatic and three showed only inflammatory
changes.

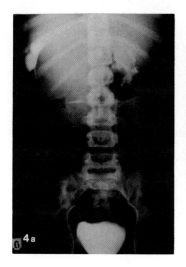
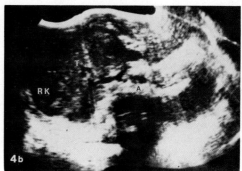

Fig. 4 a and b: Right nephroblastoma
a) excretory urography, anteroposterior view shows a
mass of the medial aspect of the right kidney displacing
and partially obstructing the collecting system. The
right ureter is displaced laterally.
b) echotomography, transverse scan in supine position:
the right kidney (R.K.) is displaced laterally by an
echogenic mass (T) which does not cross the midline (A:
aorta).

Following an intravenous pyelography echotomography
confirms the diagnosis of solid intrarenal tumor and
defines the extension. Echotomography is used to
follow the evolution under chemotherapy. In seven cases
ultrasound showed an increase of necrosis. In one case
IVP returned to normal after chemotherapy. A tumor
remnant was discovered by ultrasound (Fig. 7).

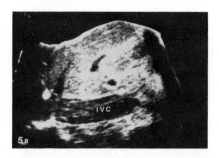 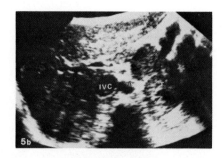

Fig. 5 a and b. left nephroblastoma with IVC thrombosis.
a) echotomography. Longitudinal scan in decube position.
The inferior vena cava (IVC) is enlarged and filled with
echoes.
b) transverse scan in decube position. The inferior vena
cava (IVC) is not displaced, its lumen is enlarged and
filled with echoes (A: aorta, T: tumor, ↗ :dilated
collecting system).

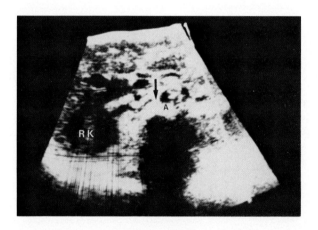

Fig. 6. Right nephroblastoma with enlarged lymph nodes.
R.K.: right kidney, A: aorta, ↗ : clumps of echoes
between inferior vena cava and aorta.

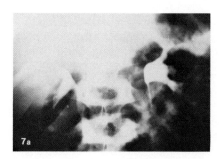 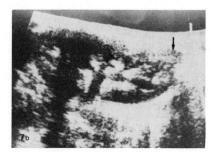

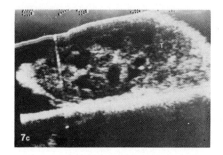

Fig. 7.   Left nephroblastoma
a)   normal looking IVP after chemotherapy.
b)   echotomography, left kidney longitudinal scan in prone
position: small clump of echoes at the lower pole (↗).
c)   echotomography of the specimen: small tumor remnant
at the lower pole (T).

ARTERIOGRAPHY

Arteriography has limited indications and was previously
used in cases of non secreting kidney, but it has been
replaced by ultrasonography.   Ultrasound is also diagnostic
in cases of a pseudotumor (Cremin, Kaschula 1972; Grossman
1977).

Indications of arteriography can be reduced to bilateral involvement or solitary kidney. In our series we performed angiographies in order to exclude a neuroblastoma in two cases, because of bilateral involvement in three cases and we did an hepatic arteriography in one case of liver metastasis. Radiographic evaluation is completed by frontal and lateral films of the chest. We do not recommend routine lung tomography.

Berdon WE, Baker DH, Santulli TV (1967). Factors producing spurious obstruction of the inferior vena cava in infants and children with abdominal tumors. Radiology 88:111.

Cope JR, Roylance J, Gordon IRS (1972). The radiological features of Wilms' tumor. Clin Radiol 23:331.

Cremin BJ, Kaschula RDC (1972). Arteriography in Wilms' tumour - the results of 13 cases and comparison to renal dysplasia. Brit J Radiol 45:415.

Grossman H (1977). Wilms' tumor in Parker BR, Castellino RA, Pediatric oncologic radiology. Saint Louis. The CV Mosby Company. p 237.

Horodniceanu C, Neveu P, Sagui M, Gruner M, Neuenschwander S, Montagne JPh (1981). Echotomographie des néphroblastomes et des sympathoblastomes de la fosse lombaire chez l'enfant. Arch Fr Pediatr 38:345.

Kaufman RA, Holt JF, Heidelberger KP (1978). Calcification in primary and metastatic Wilms' tumor. AJR 130: 783.

Kurlander GL, Smith EE (1967). Total body opacification in the diagnosis of Wilms' tumor and neuroblastoma. AJR 89:1075.

Renal Tumors: Proceedings of the First International Symposium on Kidney Tumors, pages 67–70
© 1982 Alan R. Liss, Inc., 150 Fifth Avenue, New York, NY 10011

COMPUTERIZED TOMOGRAPHY AND NEPHROBLASTOMAS

Dominique Couanet, Anne Geoffray, Francoise Le
Bras, Jean Daniel Piekarski, Daniel Vanel,
Jacques Masselot
Institut Gustave Roussy, rue Camille Desmoulins
94805 Villejuif Cedex

This study is based on 39 cases of nephroblastomas on which 65 computerized tomography scans CT were performed. We have concluded that CT does not generate more diagnostic information than IVP and echotomography. We base this on 10 cases of unilateral nephroblastoma. CT is indicated only in cases of poor echography (gas artefacts, restless baby) and in cases of a huge tumor disturbing the anatomical landmarks of echography.

We have evaluated twelve bilateral nephroblastomas and in our experience, on initial evaluation, CT never gave more information concerning the number and location of tumors than IVP and echotomography. In one case angiography disclosed a cortical nodule missed by other examinations. On follow-up, after chemotherapy and surgery, excretory urography may not show the margins of the kidneys very well. Ultrasonography may be unsatisfactory due to bowel gas. It is not possible to repeat angiographies. Computerized tomography is thus indicated. The size limit is 1 cm in diameter.

Post surgical evaluation of 19 cases suggested to us that CT may be the best procedure for post surgical evaluation. We use oral diluted contrast medium to identify the bowel (Fig. 1). Recurrences in the renal fossa or intraperitoneal are recognized if their size is superior to 2-3 cm (Fig. 2).

Two pitfalls that we observed are post surgical fibrosis and hematoma of the renal fossa (Fig. 3). The evaluation of the liver can be adequately done either by echotomography or by computerized tomography.

In conclusion, CT does not give additional information for the initial evaluation. But after surgery it is the method of choice for the follow-up.

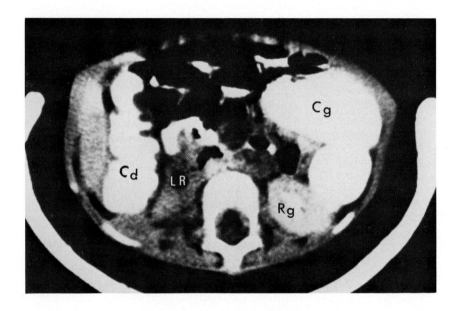

Fig. 1: Computerized tomography after right nephrectomy. (Cd: right colon, Cg: left colon, Rg: right kidney, LR: right renal fossa occupied by bowel loops).

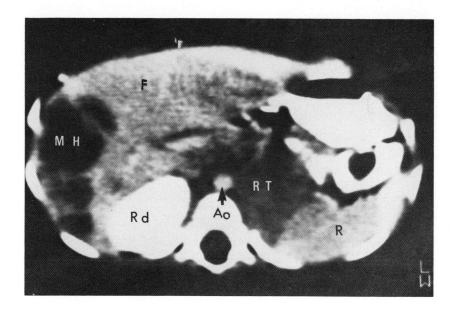

Fig. 2: Tumor recurrency (RT) after left nephrectomy.
(Rd: right kidney, R: spleen, Ao: aorta, F: liver,
MH: metastases

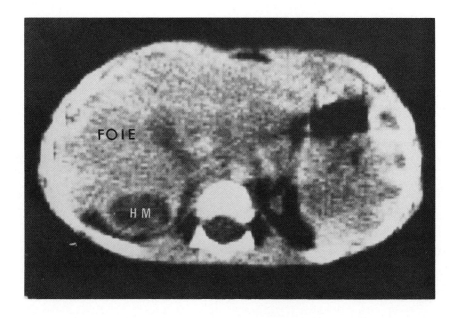

Fig. 3: Post operative hematomy (HM) in the upper part
of the right renal fossa (foie: liver).

Renal Tumors: Proceedings of the First International Symposium on Kidney Tumors, pages 71–81
© **1982 Alan R. Liss, Inc., 150 Fifth Avenue, New York, NY 10011**

EVALUATION OF UNUSUAL NEPHROBLASTOMAS AND DIFFERENTIAL
DIAGNOSIS

Jean Philippe Montagne, Sylvia Neuenschwander,
Clément Fauře
Hôpital Trousseau

26, av. du Dr A. Netter
75571 Paris Cedex 12

Some tumors grow outside of the kidney. On excretory
urography they look like an extrarenal lesion, the kidney
is dislocated, the pyelocalyceal system shows no distorsion.
We have encountered such a case (Fig. 1). Echotomography,
computerized tomography and angiography may be helpful for
the diagnosis.

Extrarenal nephroblastomas are extremely rare (Fried et
al, 1980; McCauley et al, 1979). They develop outside of the
pathway of the fetal kidney. When it is separated from the
normal kidney it is impossible to make the differential
diagnosis with neuroblastoma on excretory urography and
echotomography .

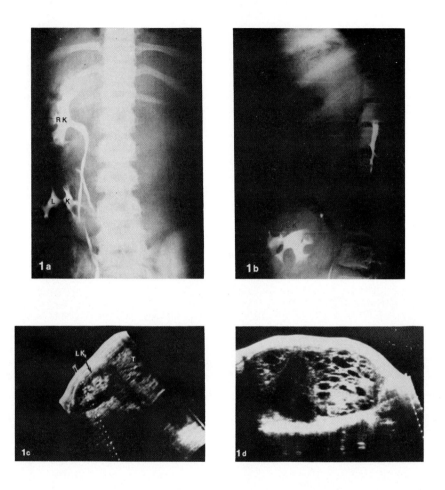

Fig. 1a, b, c and d. Exorenal left nephroblastoma (a and b) intravenous pyelography anteroposterior and lateral views. The left kidney (LK) is displaced in the right iliac fossa (RK: right kidney).

c) echotomography, transverse scan on the right iliac fossa in decube position; the internal margin of the left kidney (LK) is close to the right margin of the tumor (T).

d) echotomography, longitudinal scan on the midline; the tumor is heterogenous with large anechogenic areas.

Bilateral nephroblastomas occur in 5 to 10% of cases (Garret, Donohue, 1978; Grossman, 1977). Bilateral tumors are more likely to be of multifocal origin than metastatic disease. They are reported to be more frequent in case of Wilms' tumor associated with congenital malformations. Intravenous pyelography (IVP) rarely shows typical appearance of involvement of both kidneys (Fig. 2). Usually one has to look carefully for an irregularity of a calyx or for a calcification. Ultrasound is a help for the diagnosis and allows to differentiate from an enlargement of a septum of Bertin. Selective angiography (frontal view and profile) need to be performed. All those examinations may be negative and the involvement of the opposite kidney is only discovered at surgery.

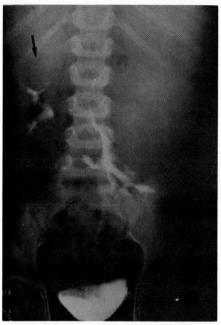

Fig. 2. Bilateral nephroblastoma. Intravenous pyelography. The left kidney is displaced inferiorly and medially by a mass of the upper pole. The calyces of the upper pole of the right kidney are slightly displaced by a mass (↗).

So called small and localized subcapsular nodules or sheets of primitive metanephric epithelium are incidental findings in one out of every 200 or 400 autopsies of infants

under age 4 months (Bar-Ziv et al, 1975; Gruner et al, 1981;
Rosenfield et al, 1980). It is called nodular renal blastoma.
If the nodules are large, confluent and if they replace the
normal renal cortex it is called nephroblastomatosis. Nephroblastomatosis is frequently associated with congenital
abnormalities (hemihypertrophy, trisomy 18, gigantism and
macroglossia). Clinical examination shows two enlarged
kidneys. Excretory urography shows bilateral renal enlargement and distorsion of the calyces (looking like polycystic
kidney disease adult type). Untrasound may be confusing
showing nodular lesions which appear totally or partly cystic.
If angiography is performed, it shows a decrease of perfusion
of the renal cortex which is thickened. Interlobar arteries
and arcuate vessels are stretched and distorted. There are
several publications on the progression from nephroblastomatosis to Wilms' tumor (Fig. 3). Under chemotherapy,
nephroblastomatosis without Wilms' tumor totally disappears.

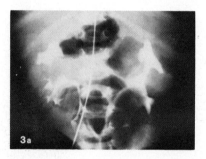

Fig. 3 a, b, c and d. Bilateral nephroblastomatosis and
left nephroblastoma.
a) intravenous pyelography. The upper part of the right
calyceal system is slightly dilated, mass effect in the
medial part of the left kidney.

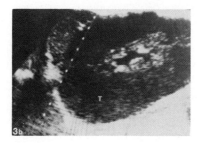

b) echotomography, longitudinal scan on the left kidney in supine position. Echogenic mass (T) in the posterosuperior aspect of the left kidney.
c) echotomography, longitudinal scan on the right lumbar fossa in prone position. The renal cortex is irregularly thickened (↓).

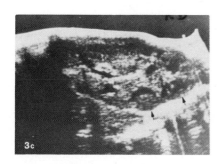

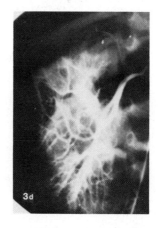

d) arteriography right kidney anteroposterior view. The arteries of the upper pole are stretched.

Extrarenal tumors,especially neuroblastomas (Grossman,
1977),are usually easy to differentiate. Plain film findings
show that calcifications are present in 2/3 of cases. They
appear to be finely stippled or less frequently like coalescent larger clumps of amorphour calcium. The spinal
pedicles and the thoracoabdominal paravertebral region
should be checked carefully. For excretory urograms, we
use the same technique as for nephroblastomas. Intravenous
pyelography (IVP) is usually displaced forwards and laterally.
During the total body opacification phase, the lesion may
blush. Typically a neuroblastoma will displace the kidney
downwards and laterally but it may be displaced upwards if
the tumor arises from below the kidney. Neuroblastomas
frequently cross the midline. They do not distort the
calces. The diagnosis may be more difficult especially in
case of a tumor invading the kidney. Echography, computerized tomography, angiography may be non contributive (Fig.
4). Laboratory tests are of great value; an excess of
catecholamine metabolites in the urine is found in about
95% of patients.

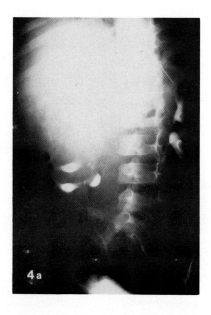

Fig. 4 a and b. Neuroblastoma invading the right kidney.
a) intravenous pyelography, oblique view: tumor mass in
the upper pole of the right kidney.

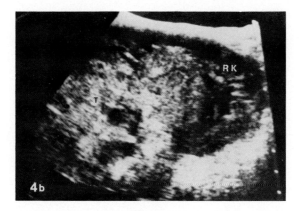

b) echotomography, longitudinal scan in prone position.
The tumor (T) impinges upon the excretory cavities of the
right kidney (RK).

An hematoma, subcapsular or in the perineal space may
be confusing. But there is a history of trauma. Echotomography is contributive showing a typically fluid filled
lesion (Fig. 5). An urinoma is detected by ultrasound as
well.

In cases of an enlarged non secreting kidney, it is
easy with ultrasound to make the diagnosis of hydronephrosis,
uretero-hydronephrosis, multicystic dysplasia or renal vein
thrombosis. In case of an intrarenal lesion, ultrasound
may show a typically fluid single cavity which is more
likely to be a renal cyst. If the cavity is separated with
a solid component one must think of a cystadenoma but the
differential diagnosis with a cystic nephroblastoma is not
possible (Crouzet et al, 1980). In case of a pseudotumor
(Gooding, 1971), echography is able to show the enlarged
septum of Bertin (Fig. 6). Congenital mesoblastic nephroma
ultrasound, computerized tomography and arteriography are
of no help to distinguish from nephroblastoma. The diagnosis
has to be suggested in young babies (87% are discovered
before 1 year of age) to avoid radiation or chemotherapy.

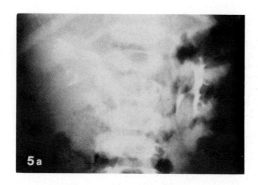

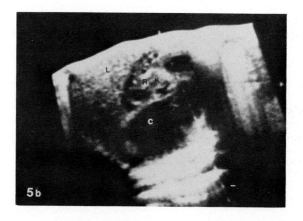

Fig. 5 a and b.   Subcapsular hematoma of the right kidney.
a) intravenous pyelography: the collecting system of the
right kidney is displaced medially.
b) echotomography, longitudinal scan in prone position: the
right kidney (RK) appears normal pushed anteriorly by a
cystic mass.(c). (L: Liver).

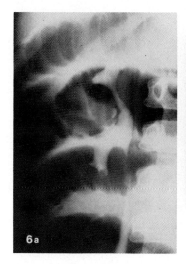
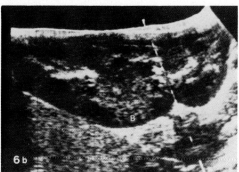

Fig. 6 a and b. Enlargement of a septum of Bertin (the baby boy has a left nephrectomy for nephroblastoma two years earlier.
a) intravenous pyelography: intra-renal mass effect.
b) echotomography, longitudinal scan in prone position: clump of echoes (B) whose echogenicity is similar to the normal cortex.

Half of the angiomyolipoma are seen in tuberous sclerosis. At IVP and ultrasound the lesion is heterogenous, it contains fluid and fat. Usually the involvement is bilateral. It is often difficult to affirm the benign nature of the lesion by X-ray or ultrasound.

The age when adenocarcinoma (Fig. 7) is discovered is older (mean 8 years; nephroblastoma, 3.5 years). Hematuria is more frequent (56% versus 25% in case of nephroblastoma). Usually the mass is not palpable. When calcified, the deposits are usually on the periphery of the lesion. At arteriography they present arterio-venous fistulae.

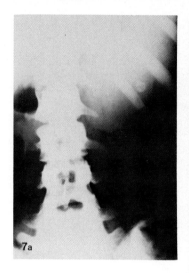
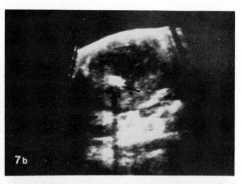
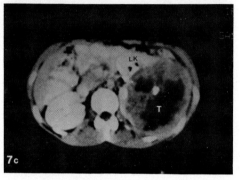

Fig. 7 a, b and c. Adenocarcinoma of the left kidney.
a) plain film of the abdomen. The inferolateral margin of
the left kidney is enlarged, there is a dense calcification
in the same area.
b) echotomography, transverse scan in supine position. The
tumor is inhomogenously echogenic, a clump of echoes with
posterior shadowing (↗) represents the calcification.
c) computerized tomography after intravenous contrast
medium. The tumor (T) develops in the posterior part of the
left kidney (LK) the calcification is well seen.

References

Bar-Ziv J, Hirsch M, Perlman M (1975). Bilateral nephro-
  blastomatosis. Pediatr Radiol 3:85.
Crouzet A, Pasquier D, Dyon JF, Bost M, Baudin Ph (1980).
  Kyste multiloculaire ou nephroblastome plurikystique.
  Pediatrie 35:359.

Fried AM, Hatfield DR, Ellis GT, Fritzgerald KW (1980).
  Extrarenal Wilms' tumor: sonographic appearance.
  J Clin Ultrasound 8:360.
Garret RA, Donohue JP (1978). Bilateral Wilms' tumors.
  J Urol 120:586.
Gilly J, Bouvier R, Berard J (1980). Néphromes mésoblastiques.
  A propos de 6 cas Chir Pediatr 21:275.
Gooding CA (1971). Childhood renal pseudotumor. A case
  report. Radiology 98:79.
Grossman H (1977). Wilms' tumor in Parker BR, Castellino RA,
  Pediatric Oncologic Radiology. Saint Louis: The CV
  Mosby Company, p 237.
Gruner M, Guilhaume A, Montagne JPh, Fauré C (1981).
  Néphroblastome et syndrome de Beckwith-Wiedemann,
  Ann Radiol 24:39.
McCauley RGK, Safaii H, Crowley CA, Pinn VW (1979).
  Extrarenal Wilms' tumor Am J Dis Child 133:1174.
Poole CA, Viamonte MJr (1970). Unusual renal masses in
  the pediatric age group. AJR 109:368.
Rosenfield NS, Shimkin P, Berdon NW, Barwick K, Glassman, M,
  Siegel N (1980). Wilms' tumor arising from spontaneously
  regressing nephroblastomatosis. AJR 135:381.

Renal Tumors: Proceedings of the First International Symposium on Kidney Tumors, pages 83–84
© **1982 Alan R. Liss, Inc., 150 Fifth Avenue, New York, NY 10011**

PREOPERATIVE DIAGNOSIS OF WILMS' TUMOR

Denys Pellerin

Professor of Pediatric Surgery, Chief of Department of Pediatric Surgery, Hôpital des Enfants
Malades, Paris

It is probably presumptuous to say that there is no
incorrect diagnosis of nephroblastoma. The precise and
specific results of front and lateral I.V.P. films give
the exact diagnosis of Wilms' tumor in more than 90% of
cases.

In the past, unvisualized kidneys were diagnosed
by arteriography. Today, ultrasonography, perhaps more
than C.T., leads to the exact diagnosis of a solid renal
tumor.

At last, negative biological marker assays (fetuin
of yolk sac tumor, cathecholamines of neural crest tumor)
further augment a precise diagnosis.

For these reasons, a negative diagnosis of Wilms'
tumor indicates need for a biopsy, such that rectification
of incorrect diagnosis during surgery is exceptional.

In our data of 352 nephroblastomas (1951-1981), we
observed 4 incorrect diagnoses which were rectified during
surgery. They are old records. One Wilms' tumor was
not diagnosed in a one-month-old boy. A non-visualization
of the kidney was considered to be a congenital hydronephrosis. Another kidney, without excretion, in a four-
month-old baby was diagnosed as Wilms' tumor. In fact,
it was a pyonephrosis, in spite of there being no clinical
or biological symptoms of urinary tract infection. Exact
diagnosis was made preoperatively by puncture in front of
a very inflammatory adhesion of the tumor to the right

colon and duodenum.

Of course, today, these two incorrect diagnoses would be impossible by routine ultrasonographic examination. Two other incorrect diagnoses were noted in front of an intraparenchymatous solid process. One was a median aortico-renal neuroblastoma; the second was a pararenal mesen-chymatous tumor. It also seems that today ultrasono-graphy and C.T. exams would help to avoid such mistakes. Of course, not included in surgically incorrect diagnosis are the histological varieties of tumor such as meso-blastic nephroma (Boland tumor), clear cell epithelioma or nephroblastomatosis, the diagnoses of which can only be done by the pathologist. However, an experienced pediatric surgeon can frequently make these diagnoses on macroscopic examination.

Thus, in our experience, errors of diagnosis are rare. However, we note in the SIOP I and II reports a surprising list of incorrect diagnoses. Among 719 cases, there were 76 non Wilms' tumors of which 19 were neuroblastomas, 9 were cysts and multilocular cysts and 4 were hydronephrosis. Fortunately, in the 1980 SIOP V report, among 381 cases, there were only 25 non Wilms' tumors, of which 1 was a hydronephrosis, 1 was a multilocular cyst and 4 were neuroblastomas. The other 17 non Wilms' tumors were solid malignancies of various histological types.

The decreasing incidence of incorrect diagnosis probably reflects the reporting of more experienced physicians, surgeons, radiologists and especially the current use of the new investigative procedures. It is a good position which emphasizes that abdominal tumors of children be treated by experienced teams, in special pediatric centers, and not individually by non-specific means.

To conclude, we agree with the last SIOP recommendation: "If the diagnosis of nephroblastoma is uncertain during the operation, avoid taking any biopsy or puncturing the tumor, as there is a grave risk of disseminating tumor cells into the peritoneal cavity." Thus, exact diagnosis of Wilms' tumor must be done preoperatively.

Renal Tumors: Proceedings of the First International Symposium on
Kidney Tumors, pages 85–89
© 1982 Alan R. Liss, Inc., 150 Fifth Avenue, New York, NY 10011

SURGERY OF WILMS' TUMOR

Denys Pellerin

Department of Pediatric Surgery
Hôpital des Enfants Malades, Paris

Nephro-ureterectomy is a satisfactory surgical treatment of Wilms' tumor. Surgery is one of the sequential
steps in care used according to a precise protocol of
treatment. Whenever surgery is performed either primarily
or after chemotherapy or radiation, the surgical methodology
must be scrupulous in order to resect the tumor and all
tissues around it, to prevent malignant cells from dif-
fusing. This also provides material for the pathologist
to precisely characterize the histological type and stage
of the tumor.

Our experience comes from data of 352 nephroblastomas
surgically approached. Most of these cases were performed by myself and some by my surgical team from 1951
to 1981. Most of the patients were treated oncologically
by the Pediatric Department of the Gustave Roussy Institute.
The more recent ones are included in the S.I.O.P. study.
We believe that the experience permits us to express some
personal comments.

A. ANESTHESIOLOGY AND PREOPERATIVE CARE

We should like to emphasize that survery of Wilms'
tumor is risky. The risk does not necessarily correlate with the clinical volume of the tumor. A big
tumor can be easy to resect. A tumor reduced by prior
chemotherapy can still be deeply extended with dangerous
vascular adhesions. Thus, the anesthesiologist must
know the surgeon's approach and needs to preserve an exact
hemodynamic balance. However, the surgeon must also

remember that surgery of Wilms' tumor cannot be a single, simple technique. We believe that excellent cooperation of the surgical and anesthesiologist team is the basis for successful excision of our stage III nephroblastomas. Among these cases no case was noted unresectable. Only one operative death was observed and also the postoperative deaths from septicemia and malignant varicella were noted.

B. CHOICE OF THE ABDOMINAL INCISION

Because of the anterior development of this tumor, and the necessity to approach the primary vascularture, one must not approach such tumor the conventional lumbar way. Two approaches can be used. These are the transversal anterior laparotomy and the antero-lateral laparotomy.

The transversal anterior sub-umbilical laparotomy is an excellent procedure. Its current use in pediatric surgery results from the anatomical development of the abdominal cavity during growth of the baby and the child. The main portion of the abdominal cavity is above the umbilical level. The inconvenience is the exposure of intestinal loops with a higher risk of postoperative occlusive bands, and especially in case of peroperative rupture of the tumor, the intra-abdominal cells diffuse and may require high risk total abdominal radiation post-operatively.

The antero-lateral approach along the rectus muscle and then the oblique muscle is an excellent and anatomically reasonable procedure. One can extend the incision if necessary on the thorax. This gives a wide exposure from the thorax to the pelvis. The spermatic vessels and the low part of the ureter are well controlled. The intestinal loops are well protected by the mesocolon and are unexposed. Any potential rupture of the primary tumor is localized at the retro-colic site. A lateral limit to radiation can be used if subsequently necessary. The occlusive risk is very low (less than 0.30% in our data). We have routinely used this procedure for 25 years. The transversal abdominal approach is reserved for babies less than one year of age in consideration of their special abdominal morphology.

Renal Tumors: Proceedings of the First International Symposium on Kidney Tumors, pages 91–95
© **1982 Alan R. Liss, Inc., 150 Fifth Avenue, New York, NY 10011**

TMM DESCRIPTION AND STAGING OF WILMS' TUMORS
PROGNOSTIC FACTORS

Jean Lemerle M.D.

Chief, Pediatric Department
Institut Gustave-Roussy, 94800 Villejuif, France

T.N.M. AND STAGING

Surgical-pathological staging has been widely used
in Wilms' tumor as a result of large multi-institutional
studies, namely the National Wilms' Tumor Study (NWTS)
in the United States, and the Wilms' Tumor trials and
studies conducted by the International Society of Pediatric
Oncology (SIOP) in Europe. Thousands of cases have been
registered in both organizations, which made it necessary
to use a simple, clear and accurate system to define the
cases falling into the different treatment groups; the
SIOP has adopted the NWTS staging system (D'Angio 1972).
In 1980, the International Union Against Cancer (U.I.C.C.),
the SIOP, and the American Joint Committee (A.C.J.) agreed
upon a TNM and staging system for the most frequent
pediatric tumors (Lemerle 1981).

As far as Wilms' tumor is concerned, the clinical TNM
description, which is a clinical-radiological description
made before treatment, has been found to be useful because of the increasing number of cases where surgery was
preceded by radiotherapy and/or chemotherapy. It is completed by a surgical-pathological assessment called pTNM.
Clinical stages are defined, based on the clinical TNM.
Pathological stages are based on pTNM, and do not differ
from the traditional staging system mentioned above.
When appropriate, the y symbol is added when the description applies to a patient who has received chemotherapy
or radiotherapy before assessment; e.g. y p T1, describes
a tumor which is found to be well encapsulated and competely

resected in a patient who has received chemotherapy prior to surgery.

CLINICAL TNM DESCRIPTION

T   Applies to the primary tumor, N to regional lymph nodes (between diaphragm and bifurcation of the aorta) and M to distant metastases. X is used when information is not available.

T_0:   No evidence of primary tumor.

T_1:   Unilateral tumor, 80 cm^2 or less in area, measured on I.V.P. (including kidney).

T_2:   Unilateral tumor more than 80 cm^2 (area calculated by multiplying vertical and horizontal dimensions of the radiological shadow of the tumor and kidney).

T_3:   Evidence of tumor rupture (unilateral).

T_4:   Bilateral tumor.

N_0:   No evidence of regional L.N. involvement

N_1:   Evidence (assessment seldom relevant in Wilms' tumor).

M_0:   No evidence of distant metastases.

M_1:   Evidence

CLINICAL STAGING

CS I   : T_1 M_0: small unilateral

CS II : T_2 M_0: large, unilateral

CS III: T_3 or N_1, M_0: rupture or nodes

CS IV : M_1, any T, N: unilateral metastatic

CS V   : T_4, any N, M: bilateral

SURGICAL-PATHOLOGICAL TNM DESCRIPTION

p T_0:   No tumor found at histopathological examination

p T_1:   Encapsulated tumor, completely resected

p T_2:   Invasion beyond kidney capsule, complete excision

p T_3:   Incomplete excision, including rupture
     a.   microscopic residue
     b.   macroscopic, or spillage
     c.   unresectable tumor at surgery

p T_4:   Bilateral tumor

p N_0:   Negative nodes

p N_1:   Positive nodes
     a.   considered completely resected
     b.   incompletely resected

p M_0:   No evidence of distant metastases

p M_1:   Evidence - includes those detected clinically.

SURGICAL-PATHOLOGICAL STAGING

p S I   :   p T_1, p N_0, encapsulated, complete excision

p S II   :   p T_2 or p N_{1a}; not encapsulated or positive nodes.
                              complete excision

p S III: incomplete resection, including rupture
     a. p T_{3a},   :   microscopic residue
     b. p T_{3b} or p N_{1b}:   macroscopic residue
     c. p T_{3c} :   unresectable tumor

p S IV :   p M_1, any pT, pN :   metastatic, unilateral

p S V   :   p T_4, any pN, pM :   bilateral

PROGNOSTIC FACTORS

Prognostic factors have been extensively studied in
Wilms' tumor in order to predict outcome and to try to
adapt the treatment to each case (Lemerle et al. 1976).
The following factors have been found to influence independently survival and recurrence free survival.

1) Young age was found to be a good prognostic factor
    in the first studies conducted before active
    chemotherapy was used. It is now less important.

2) Stage is still important. Clinically, the size
    of the tumor measured on I.V.P. is a good indicator.
    The same applies to surgical-pathological stages.
    In the most recent studies, however, stages I and
    II do not significantly differ from each other.
    Lymph node involvement at pathological examination,
    which is a part of stage, is of great prognostic
    value. Recurrence free survival, in SIOP studies
    1 and 2 is 27% and 67%, respectively, according
    to presence or absence of regional node involve-
    ment (Jereb et al. 1980). The histological pat-
    tern of the tumour is also of great importance.
    A group of 10% of all cases are now classified
    as anaplastic or sarcomatous and have a death rate
    considerably higher than the other cases (Beckwith,
    Palmer 1978). Practically, for the purpose of
    the prognosis-oriented SIOP 6 trials, we have
    defined 3 groups of patients according to prognosis:

      Good cases (66%), stage I (pathological) and
                        stage II with negative nodes.

      Bad cases (33%), stage II with positive nodes
                        and stage III.

      Cases with unfavourable histology are considered
                        separately.

Beckwith JB, Palmer N (1978). Histopathology and prognosis
  of Wilms' Tumor. Results of the National Wilms' Tumor
  Study. Cancer 41:1937.
D'Angio GJ (1972). Management of children with Wilms'
  Tumor. Cancer 30:1528.

Jereb B, Tournade MF, Lemerle J, Voûte PA, Delemarre JF, Ahstrom L, Flamant R, Gérard-Marchant R, Sandstedt B (1980). Lymph node invasion and prognosis in mephroblastoma. Cancer 45:1632.

Lemerel J (1981). The TNM classification of Nephroblastoma, Neuroblastoma and Soft Tissue Sarcomas of Childhood. Marseille: SIOP Proceedings p. 13.

Lemerle J, Tournade MF, Gérard-Marchant, R, Flamant R, Sarrazin D, Flamant F, Lemerle M, Jundt S, Zucker J-M, Schweisguth O (1976). Wilms' Tumor, natural history and prognostic factors. Cancer 37:2557.

Renal Tumors: Proceedings of the First International Symposium on Kidney Tumors, pages 97–110
© **1982 Alan R. Liss, Inc., 150 Fifth Avenue, New York, NY 10011**

RADIATION THERAPY OF WILMS' TUMOR
METHODS AND IMMEDIATE COMPLICATIONS

Pierre BEY

Department of Radiotherapy
CENTRE ALEXIS VAUTRIN
54511   VANDOEUVRE LES NANCY (France)

Local radiotherapy has been used in the treatment of nephroblastoma since 1916 (Friedlander 1916). The first published results of post-operative radiotherapy (Gross 1950) showed an increase in survival rate (about 45 %) compared to survival after surgery alone (about 35 %). Radiotherapy has been used subsequently to treat lung metastases. The addition of chemotherapy (actinomycin D and vincristine) increased overall survival rate to about 80 %.

The knowledge of late effects of radiotherapy (fig. 1), (Schweisguth 1979, Jaffe 1980), the effectiveness of chemotherapy and the identification of prognosis factors (Jereb 1980) result in a better definition of radiation indications. Even though the importance of radiotherapy is decreasing (Voute 1979, D'Angio 1980), one can estimate that in 1981 about 50 % of children with nephroblastoma will be irradiated on the tumor bed and/or on the lungs.

Nephroblastoma is a radiosensitive tumor. This was demonstrated by the regression (often considerable) that was observed after small doses of radiation (10 to 20 Gy) given pre-operatively (Margolis 1973, Lemerle 1976), and by the disappearance of lung metastases after 15 to 20 Gy on both lungs.

The dose necessary to sterilize presumptive microscopic disease is not well established but can be estimated from the study of intra-abdominal relapses in different series. Usually, a dose between 20 and 30 Gy given over 2 to 4 weeks (Hussey 1971, Perez 1973, Sutow 1977, Cassady 1978, D'Angio

1980, Jeal 1980, Tefft 1980) in association with actinomycin D and vincristine is sufficient. For eradication of residual macroscopic tumor, at least 30 Gy could be necessary.
On lungs, doses of about 15 Gy with actinomycin D can sterilize microscopic disease (Schweisguth 1979).

A very accurate technic, adapted volumes and doses are
important to minimize acute and late effects of radiotherapy.

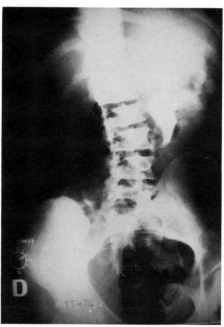

Fig. 1 - Late "historical" sequelae 20 years after right
tumor bed/200 Kv irradiation.
- scoliosis with hemi-hypotrophy of lumbar vertebrae.
- hypotrophy of right ilium.
- sacroiliac chondrosarcoma developed on irradiated bone.

1 - RADIOTHERAPY METHODS

Although exclusive radiotherapy can sometimes give local
cure, it is never recommended. Pre-operative radiotherapy
is no more indicated as chemotherapy is able to play the
same role (results of SIOP trials n°5). In most cases, irra-

diation is focused after surgery on the renal bed on the side of the tumor (stage II and some stage III). No irradiation is needed for stage I. Whole abdominal irradiation, which has been used routinely in all stages by some authors (Pearson 1964, Jeal 1980), is now reserved for stage III in case of peritoneal spillage. Radiotherapy has to be started within 15 days after surgery. In case of diffuse lung metastases, irradiation on both lungs may be indicated. It is rarely necessary to irradiate other metastatic sites (liver, bone). Usually no special set up proceeding is needed during treatment if the child feels confident. For young babies, special immobilization with sedation may be necessary. Great care has to be taken to monitor the reproducibility of the daily irradiation with frequent check-films.

A - Renal Bed Irradiation

The volume including the tumor bed and the retroperitoneal para-aortic lymphnodes is treated by two parallel opposed anterior and posterior fields crossing the midline to cover the entire width of the vertebral bodies (both epiphyseal plates) so as to minimize future scoliotic changes (Margolis 1973, Perez 1973, D'Angio 1978, D'Angio 1980). The external limit extends to the lateral body wall with a tangential abdominal wall shield. Upper and inferior limits of the fields are adapted to the extent of the tumor to encompass the whole area of kidney and of the tumor with a safety margin. These limits are determined by pre-operative clinical and radiological examinations, operative reports and, when available, by per-operative radiograph with a metallic thread to outline the tumor contour.

Special care must be exercised to avoid direct ovarian irradiation, to exclude a part of the liver on right sided tumors and to respect iliac crest (fig. 2).

This volume must be irradiated exclusively by two parallel opposed anterior and posterior fields treated daily, 5 fractions per week. The daily dose given at midplane varies between 1,5 and 2 Gy depending on the volume of liver included and on the size of the fields (1,5 Gy on right sided tumors). The best dose distribution is obtained by 4 to 10 MV photon beam (fig. 3)

Total dose to be given has not been clearly defined

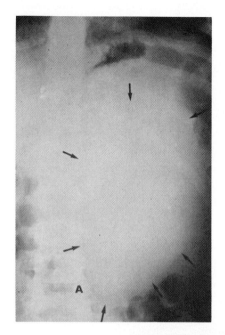
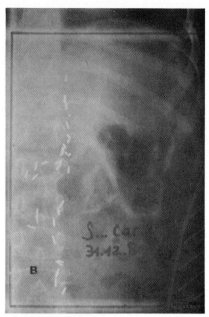

Fig. 2 : A – Left nephroblastoma : pre-operative IVP
        B – Simulator film
        C – Portal film

Fig. 3 : Computerized isodose distributions in grays (Gy) on a transverse section for 2 parallel opposed fields and 30 Gy prescribed at midplane (Fields separation : 14,5 cm) Fields size : 10, 5 x 13 cm)

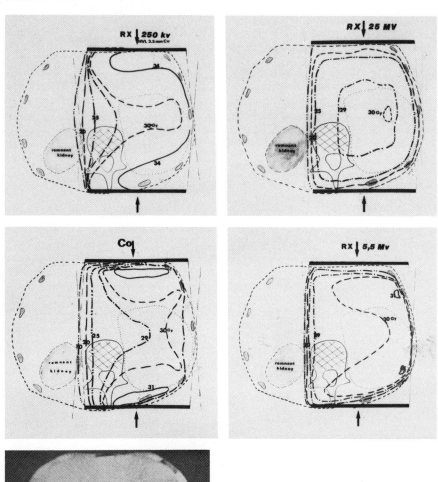

The best distribution is obtained with 5,5 MV Xrays

because of increasing survival rate following chemotherapy (actinomycin D, vincristine which are always associated and sometimes adriamycin). SIOP in its trial n° 6 is presently comparing no radiotherapy versus 20 Gy for stage II with negative lymphnodes ; it recommends 30 Gy for stage II with positive nodes and stage III (with a possible boost of 5 Gy on residual tumor).

The NWTS (D'Angio 1976) in its third study is comparing no radiotherapy versus 20 Gy in stage II and will compare 10 versus 20 Gy in stage III. In stage IV and in unfavorable histologic types, dose is graduated according to age (18 to 35 Gy). For children under one year, doses over 20 Gy are unadvisable.

B - Whole Abdomen Irradiation

The volume includes the whole peritoneal cavity from the dome of the diaphragm to the pelvic floor (lower edge of the pubic symphysis) and laterally to the lateral body wall. Two opposed anterior and posterior fields are utilized. Femoral epiphyses are excluded (fig. 4). The remaining kidney is shielded by a posterior (and sometimes an anterior)

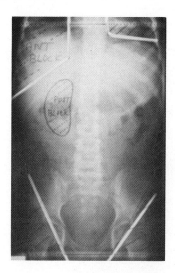

Fig. 4 : Whole abdomen simulator film with anterior and posterior femoral shielding, anterior partial hepatic shielding, posterior right kidney shielding.

individualized block so as not to receive more than 12 Gy (or 15 Gy taking in account scattered radiation). The entire liver is included in the volume and must be partially shielded so as not to receive more than 20 Gy. The two fields are treated daily with a midplane dose of 1,2 to 1,5 Gy, 5 fractions a week by cobalt or high energy photons. Total dose can be 30 Gy (SIOP) or 20 to 25 Gy with a boost on the renal bed to 30 Gy.

Irradiation of the whole abdomen must not be performed on children less than one year old.

C - Bilateral Tumor

In case of bilateral tumor, usually nephrectomy occurs on one side and partial nephrectomy on the other (or partial bilateral nephrectomy). When radiotherapy is indicated, dose on the remaining kidney (or the remaining parts of the kidneys), must not exceed 12 to 15 Gy in 3 to 4 weeks (Malcolm 1980).

D - Lung Irradiation

The volume which comprises both lungs including costophrenic sulci (located on a lateral film) is treated by two parallel opposed anterior and posterior fields (fig. 5).This volume includes the upper portion of the liver. If abdominal

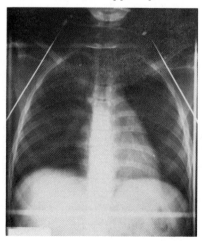

Fig. 5 - Simulator film of lung irradiation.

irradiation has been given before, special care must be exercised for the calculation of the junction between the two volumes to avoid overdosage. Renal bed volume must not be treated in the same time as lung volume. The midplane dose delivered by cobalt or 4 to 10 MV photons is usually 1,5 Gy per day up to a total dose that ranges from 15 to 20 Gy (with air correction). Boost doses up to 30 Gy could be delivered to very restricted areas for residual disease.

Air correction is determined for each case and requires very accurate dosimetry.

E - Other Metastases

Liver metastases should be irradiated by two parallel opposed fields to a maximum total dose of 30 Gy in 4 weeks if irradiation has not been performed previously. Bone metastases require 30 Gy in 2 to 3 weeks on the lesion with a sufficient margin.

F - Irradiation of Nephroblastoma Occuring in Adults

Few data are available for this rare condition. Nevertheless, similar methods and doses of irradiation to the ones used for children have been recommended (Babaian 1980). The place of radiotherapy is greater in adults than in children because late sequelae are less severe and chemotherapy seems to be less effective than in children.

2 - IMMEDIATE COMPLICATIONS OF TREATMENT

They occur mainly during the first three months following the start of radiation therapy. They are related to the volume of normal tissues included in the fields (the main organs involved in early side-effects are the liver, the small bowel, the skin, the hemopoietic system, the lungs, the opposite kidney), the total dose given to the organ, the age of the child and the association of chemotherapy given concurrently with radiation, especially actinomycin D. (D'Angio 1976).

A - Hepatic Complications

(Tefft 1970, Bernard 1974, Tefft 1977, Schultz 1979) Three degrees of hepatic toxicity can be individualized. The symptoms may occur during irradiation or in the first month following irradiation.

- Transient biological changes of liver function tests : transaminases (SGOT), alkaline phosphatases and hypofixation on liver scan.

- Hepatomegaly which is preceded by biological modifications, at first of the non irradiated part of the liver and then of the entire liver. Hypoprotidemia and low cholesterol may be associated. Sudden, sometimes severe thrombocytopenia, due to local intravascular coagulopathy can be associated.

- In very rare circumstances (high dose on the entire liver) hydrosodic retention with ascitis may occur with biological modifications and hepatomegaly with or without thrombocytopenia with possible secondary portal hypertension with jaundice.

The risk factors are :

- the irradiated volume of liver : the higher risk is observed with right sided tumors or with whole abdominal irradiation. It can occur during lung irradiation.

- the total dose $\geq$ 30 Gy received by more than 80 % of hepatic parenchyma.

- partial hepatectomy (less than one month before irradiation).

- the association of actinomycin D.

The treatment of these complications is symptomatic. Corticosteroids may be indicated in case of thrombocytopenia. In the third degree, sodium restriction and diuretics must be used. The regression takes place in a few weeks with partial atrophy of the liver. The mortality is about 1 %.

Some measures can be taken to suppress severe (lethal) hepatic complications and to reduce the other ones.

- to shield a part of the liver in right sided tumors whenever it is possible,
- to deliver no more than 20 Gy with actinomycin D on the
  entire normal liver (maximum 7,5 Gy per week, in 5 fractions),
- to respect a delay of one month after partial hepatectomy
  to start radiotherapy and actinomycin D.

G - Gastrointestinal Complications

Severe abdominal pain, diarrhea with or without vomiting, may appear during the second week of radiotherapy.
These symptoms can be transient or severe with dehydratation
(Cassady 1973, Donaldson 1975) and denutrition. The association with pancytopenia leads to a high risk of septicemia
from gut origin.

The risk factors are :

- the irradiated volume of small bowel. Severe diarrhea occurs especially when the whole abdomen is irradiated,
- the young age of the child,
- the total dose and the dose per fraction (more than 1,5
  Gy on the whole abdomen).

The treatment is :

- intravenous fluids, antispasmodics and antiseptics,
- discontinuation of irradiation,
- elemental diet free of gluten, lactose and milk proteins.

The prevention is :

- avoiding irradiation on the whole abdomen in young children under one year of age,
- using ≤ 1,5 Gy per fraction, 5 fractions per week to no
  more than 30 Gy on the whole abdomen,
- adding a fractionated low residue diet, free of gluten,
  lactose and milk products, sometimes with nasogastric tube
  using a pump with continuous drip at a constant rate
  (Donaldson 1975).

C - Skin Complications

With cobalt or high energy Xrays, severe skin reactions

rarely occur in the field surface even when actinomycin D is associated. No correlation can be found with other toxicities particularly with hepatic toxicity.

The intensity of these reactions rarely needs a transient interruption of the treatment. Local application of an eosin solution is a sufficient treatment. Prevention is to avoid the application of irritating products (like alcoholic solutions) on the irradiated skin.

Such a skin reaction can reappear during the subsequent courses of actinomycin D (recall phenomenon).

D - Kidney Toxicity

Acute toxicity is never observed when doses less than 15 Gy in 4 weeks are delivered to the remnant kidney, even with chemotherapy.

Nephritis, which could appear few months after the end of radiotherapy is not considered as an immediate complication.

E - Hematologic Toxicity

It is related especially to chemotherapy. When whole abdomen is irradiated, the volume of hemopoietic tissue is important and pancytopenia may occur during irradiation, leading to the possible risk of severe infection, such as chicken pox, and irradiation may sometimes be postponed.

F - Pulmonary Toxicity

Some patients experience acute pneumonitis within few weeks following the end of thoracic irradiation. Clinical symptoms are cough, dyspnea and fever. Surinfection is not rare, sometimes leading to death. Pulmonary fibrosis at various degree may appear later.

The risk factors are :

- total dose : high risk if more than 20 Gy (with air correction) are given with actinomycin D,

- previous abdominal irradiation,
- additional dose on residual metastases.

Treatment is symptomatic (steroids, antibiotics and perhaps hyperbaric oxygen).

Prevention consists of :

- respecting a maximum dose of 20 Gy (with air correction), avoiding or limiting boosts,
- avoiding re-irradiation of lungs,
- taking into account previous abdominal irradiation and scattered dose to the inferior part of the lungs.

3 - CONCLUSION

Radiation therapy remains a useful and necessary treatment, to control local disease or lung metastases in about half of the children with nephroblastoma. The technic and the practical achievement must be carefully monitored to avoid severe acute reactions which could be life-threatening and to minimize late sequelae.

Babaian RJ, Skinner DG, Waisman J (1980). Wilm's tumor in the adult patient : diagnosis, management and review of the world medical literature. Cancer, 45:1713.

Bernard O (1974). Etude des lésions hépatiques provoquées par l'irradiation des néphroblastomes de l'enfant (Thèse Paris), n° 203, dactyl.

Cassady JR, Tefft M, Filler R et al. (1973) Considerations on the radiation therapy of Wilms'tumor. Cancer, 32:598.

Cassady JR, Jaffe N, PAED D, FILLER RM (1977). The increasing importance of radiation therapy in the improved prognosis of children with Wilms'tumor. Cancer, 39:825.

Cassady JR, Belli JA (1978). Radiation in the management of children with Wilms'tumor. Int. J. Radiation Oncology Biol. Phys. 4:907.

D'Angio GJ, Evans AE, Breslow N (1976). The treatment of Wilms'tumor. Results of the national Wilms'tumor study. Cancer 38:633

D'Angio GJ, Tefft M, Breslow N, Meyer JA (1978). Radiation therapy of Wilms'tumor. Results according to dose, field, post-operative timing and histology. Int. J. Radiation

Oncology Biol. Phys. 4:769

D'Angio GJ, Beckwith JB, Breslow N et al (1980). Wilms'tumor: an update. Cancer, 45:1791.

D'Angio GJ (1980). Radiation therapy in Wilms'tumor revisited. Int. J. Radiation Oncology Biol. Phys. 6:737.

Donaldson SS, Junot S, Ricour C, Sarrazin D, Lemerle J and Schweisguth O (1975). Radiation enteritis in children. A retrospective review, clinicopathologic correlation and dietary management. Cancer, 35:1167.

Friedlander A (1916). Sarcoma of the kidney treated by the roentgen ray. Amer. J. Dis. Child, 12:328.

Gross RE, Neuhauser EBD (1950). Treatment of mixed tumors of the kidney in childhood. Pediatrics, 6:843.

Hussey DH, Castro JR, Sullivan MP, Sutow WW (1971).Radiation therapy in management of Wilms'tumor. Radiology, 101:663.

Jaffe N, Mc Neese M, Mayfield JK et al.(1980). Childhood urologic cancer therapy related sequelae and their impact on management. Cancer, 45:1815.

Jeal PN, Jenkin RDT (1980). Abdominal irradiation in the treatment of Wilms'tumor. Int. J. Radiation Oncology Biol. Phys. 6:655.

Jereb B, Tournade MF, Lemerle J, Voute PA, Delemarre JF et al. (1980). Lymph node invasion and prognosis in nephroblastoma. Cancer, 45:1632.

Lemerle J, Voute PA, Tournade MF et al. (1976). Preoperative versus postoperative radiotherapy, single versus multiple courses of actinomycin D in the treatment of Wilms'tumor. Cancer, 38:647.

Malcolm AW, Jaffe N, Folkmann MJ, Cassady JR (1980). Bilateral Wilms'tumor. Int. J. Radiation Oncology Biol. Phys. 6:167.

Margolis LW, Smith WB, Wara WM et al (1973). Wilms'tumor – an interdisciplinary treatment program with and without dactinomycin. Cancer, 32:618.

Pearson D, Duncan WB, Rointon RCS (1964). Wilms'tumor. A review of 96 consecutive cases. Brit. J. Radiol., 37:154.

Perez CA, Kaiman HA, Keit J et al. (1973). Treatment of Wilms'tumor and factors affecting prognosis. Cancer, 32:609.

Schultz H, Jacobben B, Jensen KB, Sell A. (1979). Nephroblastoma – Results and complications of treatment. Acta Radiol. Oncol., 18:449.

Schweisguth O (1979). Tumeurs solides de l'enfant, Flammarion ed., 317 p.

Sutow W, Vietti T, Fernbach D (1977). Clinical Pediatric Oncology, 2nd Ed. Mosby, St Louis.

Tefft M, Mitus A, Vawter GF, Miller RM (1970). Irradiation of the liver in children : review of experience in the acute and chronic phases and in the intact normal and partially resected. Amer. J. Roentgen, 108:365.

Tefft M (1977). Radiation - related toxicities in national Wilms'tumor study n° 1. Int. J. Radiation Oncology Biol. Phys., 2:455.

Tefft M, D'Angio GJ, Beckwith B et al. (1980). Patterns of intra-abdominal relapse (IAR) in patients with Wilms'tumor who received radiation : analysis by histo-pathology - a report of National Wilms'tumor studies 1 and 2 (NWTS 1 and 2). Int. J. Radiation Oncology Biol. Phys., 6:663.

Voute PA, Lemerle J, Tournade MF et al. (1979). Advances and new prospects in the treatment of nephroblastoma in "Recent advances in management of children with cancer". Tokyo, p. 231.

Renal Tumors: Proceedings of the First International Symposium on Kidney Tumors, pages 111–118
© **1982 Alan R. Liss, Inc., 150 Fifth Avenue, New York, NY 10011**

CHEMOTHERAPY IN WILMS' TUMOR - INDICATIONS AND EARLY SIDE EFFECTS

Annie Boilletot, M.D.

Service des Maladies du Sang
Hopital de Hautepierre
Strasbourg, France

The use of chemotherapy is certainly one of the most important advancements in the management of nephroblastoma. Before 1956, the two-year survival rate was 40% for patients treated by both surgery and radiotherapy (Figure 1). Actinomycin D was the first chemotherapeutic agent used for Wilms' tumor and improved the two-year survival rate for non-metastatic disease to more than 80% in the 1960's.

Indications for chemotherapy then became progressively wider and it appears today as a full part of multidisciplinary treatment of nephroblastoma, being effective in preoperative reduction of the tumor volume as well as in prevention of relapse or metastases. However toxicity of anticancer drugs may be important and this factor must be considered in chemotherapy protocols. Strong adverse effects must not jeopardize survival and chemotherapy has to be managed by trained medical teams.

Actinomycin D was discovered in 1940. It is a polypeptide antibiotic produced by several streptomyces species. The mechanism of its cytotoxic effect was first studied in 1952. It was shown to form a tight complex with DNA and to have an absolute specificity for guanine residues in DNA. Actinomycin D intercalates between the base pairs of the DNA and binds to two deoxyguanosine residues. It thus interferes with transcription and blocks synthesis of DNA.

In 1959, actinomycin D was shown by D'Angio to enhance the effect of radiation and increased interest was focused

on this drug. Its effectiveness as an anticancer drug for
nephroblastoma was first noted by Farber in 1954 and Gross
in 1955 who reported two cases of complete remission and
prolonged survival in children with lung metastases (d'Angio
1962; Farber 1966; d'Angio et al. 1959).

Between 1956 and 1969, several therapeutic trials proved
clearly the superiority of chemotherapy with actinomycin D
in Wilms' tumor management versus treatment by surgery and
radiotherapy alone. Survival rates of patients treated
with actinomycin D was improved to 75%. However no
statistical difference appeared in survival rates of patients
treated by a single course of the drug and patients treated
by multiple courses, though relapses were more frequent
in the former group (Fernbach, Martyn 1966; Burgert,
Glidewell 1967; Wolff et al. 1968, 1974).

Like most anticancer agents, actinomycin D acts
mainly on replicating cells. This accounts for the nature
of its toxic side effects.

Hematological toxicity is usual, especially thrombocytopenia, which is frequent at the end of the course, and,
to a lesser degree, neutropenia. Although generally
moderate, thrombocytopenia may be important and lead to
bleeding episodes which require the use of lower doses for
subsequent courses. Nausea and vomiting are frequent 4 to
6 hours after injection and stop at the end of treatment.
Complete alopecia occurs frequently and is generally
reversible with cessation of therapy.

Stomatitis and perineal ulcerative lesions may appear
a few days after the end of the courses. Bacterial and
fungal superinfections may occur and require specific
local and general therapy. Recovery is generally complete
in 8 to 10 days but these episodes lead to anorexia and
weight loss.

As it potentiates cytotoxic effects of radiation
therapy, actinomycin D may enhance tumor reduction by
radiotherapy fields. It may reactivate latent radiation
effects in normal tissues, even when it is administered a
long time after completion of radiation therapy, for
instance in skin areas previously treated by X-rays.
Though liver toxicity is usually mild or absent, it may
become important when drug is given with liver irradiation

(d'Angio 1962' d'Angio et al. 1959).

Vincristine sulfate is the second most effective agent in Wilms' tumor. Vincristine is an alcaloid extracted from the periwinkle plant in 1958. Its cytotoxicity mainly results from a direct interaction with the cell microtubule system. It has also been shown to intervene in many biochemical pathways leading to inhibition of DNA, RNA and protein synthesis. It blocks the cells in their passage through metaphase and leads to mitotic cell accumulation. The antitumor effect of vincristine in metastatic Wilms' tumor was demonstrated in 1961 and the drug appeared to be very effective in patients who became resistant to actinomycin D and also when it is used for preoperative tumor volume reduction. However, the effectiveness of vincristine alone seems to become exhausted after a few months of treatment (Sutow et al. 1965; Sullivan et al. 1967; Schweisguth et al. 1970).

Nausea and vomiting are not frequent, nor is alopecia. Bone marrow depression is very moderate when vincristine is used alone.

The main toxicity is observed on the neuromuscular system as the drug combines with proteins of microtubules which have an important role in nerve conduction. Neuromuscular toxic side effects include paresthesia in the fingers and toes, jaw pain, atrophy of distal muscles (hands, feet), diminution and even disappearance of the deep tendon reflexes. Polyneuritis of the lower limbs with foot drop and walking troubles requires immediate cessation of the drug. In children, recovery is progressively obtained after cessation of treatment and B vitamintherapy.

Constipation and even small bowel occlusive syndroms are frequent in pediatric patients and may be misdiagnosed as surgical emergencies. In these cases, surgery must be avoided as spontaneous normal transit reappears in a few days. Occlusive episode duration can be shortened by the use of laxatives, enemas, or subcutaneous prostigmin.

In the 1970's, randomized trials were undertaken by The National Wilms' Tumor Study group in the U.S.A. to test the effectiveness of actinomycin D alone, vincristine alone or both drugs in combination therapy.

As shown by NWTS 1, combination therapy with both drugs
was more effective than therapy with each drug given alone,
which was also found by SIOP trials. Thus this treatment
is now commonly used in Wilms' tumor and cumulative toxicity
is acceptable (d'Angio 1976; Sutow 1973).

Actinomycin D is given in i.v. pulse injections at a
dose of 15 micrograms/kg body weight daily on day 1 to 5;
vincristine is also given in i.v. pulse injections at a
dose of 1 - 1.5 mg/m^2 body surface on days 1 and 5. These
courses are repeated every 6 to 8 weeks and optimal
complete duration of treatment is 6 to 15 months according
to staging of the disease.

After injection, the vein must be washed with saline
or glucose solution. Paravenous injections result in
harmful local reactions such as oedema, erythema, and may
be followed by local necrosis.

Other drugs have been tested among which cyclophosphamide has shown some effectiveness when used in a "high
dosage" schedule. Children given this drug in i.v. pulse
doses of 10 mg/kg body weight have undergone some tumor
regression. This alkylating agent alone is not as effective
as actinomycin D or vincristine, and may be interesting in
combination therapy. Its late side effects upon sterility
however are too important to allow a major role in Wilms'
tumor treatment (Finklestein et al. 1969; Livingston,
Carter 1970).

Since 1974-1975 doxorubicin or adriamycin, a new cancer
antibiotic, was found to be effective in Wilms' tumor
resistant to conventional chemotherapy or in far advanced
cases. This drug belongs to the anthracyclin class or
antibiotics as well as daunorubicin. Adriamycin was
isolated in 1967 from streptomyces peucetius. It binds
to DNA by intercalation, resulting in inhibition of DNA
replication and transcription. Anthracyclin antibiotics
are thought to produce alkylating radicals in vivo and
interfere with the mitochondrial oxido-reduction system.

The anticancer action in pediatric malignant tumors
was investigated first in 1970 by Bonnadonna and in 1971
by Tan et al. Good responses and complete remissions in
Wilms' tumors resistant to actinomycin.D and to vincristine were reported. It was then included in metastatic

disease treatment protocols alone or in association with
actinomycin D and vincristine with good results (Tan
et al. 1973; Wollner et al. 1971; Bonadonna et al. 1970;
d'Angio et al. 1981).

However high immediate and delayed toxicity restricts
its indications to high risk stages of the disease as good
results can be obtained with less aggressive drugs.

Alopecia is almost constant. Stomatitis and oral ul-
cers are more frequent than with actinomycin D and superin-
fection is enhanced by major bone marrow depression.

Anemia is usually moderate, but deep neutropenia and
thrombopenia occur between 8 to 14 days after drug injection in more than 50% of patients. The most toxic side
effect of adriamycin is a delayed cardiotoxicity, which
depends on cumulative doses and leads to progressive
cardiomyopathy and congestive heart failure. Echographic
monitoring may avoid this complication by exhibiting
ventricular dysfunction far earlier than electrocardiogram
and allows discontinuation of the drug before irreversible
lesions occur.

Whether adriamycin cardiomyopathy once present may
recover and to what degree is not known. Mediastinal
radiotherapy seems however to greatly reinforce adriamycin
radiotherapy even in sequential therapy.

Adriamycin is usually given by i.v. pulse injections
at a dose of 40 to 60 mg/m^2 body surface every 3 to 4 weeks.
Harmful local toxic reactions may occur if the injection
is not strictly i.v.

Nevertheless, despite numerous side effects, chemotherapy is a valuable treatment of nephroblastoma and has
allowed a very good improvement of Wilms' tumor prognosis.
Most non metastatic nephroblastomas can now be cured as
two-year survival rates of group I - II - III disease was
nearly 75 to 80% in the last NWTS and SIOP trials, and as
relapses atfer two years are very infrequent.

When managed by well trained medical teams, toxicity
is acceptable provided side effects are controlled by a
good monitoring for infectious and of transfusions. Most
of these treatments can be achieved in ambulatory patients.

Today, the main indications for chemotherapy in Wilms' tumor can be summed up as follows:

A. Preoperatively, it can largely reduce the tumor volume up to 30-40%, as shown in SIOP 5 randomized trial, allowing safe surgical resection. Preoperative chemotherapy seems as effective as preoperative radiotherapy in preventing operative ruptures and tumor spillage. Moreover, histological changes seem to be less important than after radiotherapy, allowing a better histological diagnosis. Preoperative chemotherapy can allow surgery on inoperable tumors. This is of special interest in bilateral nephroblastoma where conservative surgery is made possible (Jacobson et al. 1979; SIOP 5).

B. Regarding metastases, long term relapse free survivals are well known in patients treated by chemotherapy combined with radiotherapy and/or surgery.

The benefit of chemotherapy has been also largely proven by NWTS 2 in residual disease or in treatment of micro metastases as 2-year relapse-free-survival in grade III disease is 90% compared to less than 50% in previously treated patients. These results are confirmed by SIOP trials (d'Angio et al. 1981).

C. Chemotherapy is also effective as adjuvant treatment in low risk patients. For instance actinomycin D and vincristine seem to be as effective as radiotherapy in stage I patients, and may permit one to choose not to irradiate stage I and very young patients and therefore to prevent late spine growth retardation (SIOP 5; d'Angio et al. 1980).

Thus chemotherapy is indicated in all forms of Wilms' tumor. The drugs to be used and their modalities have yet to be further defined by international randomized trials according to the extension of the disease. However one can assume that adriamycin is not to be given to low-risk patients.

In fact, chemotherapy in combination with surgery and radiotherapy will certainly allow future optimal control of the disease with minimal side effects.

D'Angio G (1962). Clinical and biological studies of Actinomycin D and roentgen irradiation. Amer J Roentgen 87:106.

Farber S (1966). Chemotherapy in the treatment of leukemia and Wilms' tumor. JAMA 198:826.

D'Angio GJ, Farber S, Maddock CL (1959). Potentiation of X-ray effects by actinomycin D. Radiology 73:175.

Fernbach DJ, Martyn DT (1966). Role of Dactinomycin in the improved survival of children with Wilms' tumor. JAMA 195:1005.

Burgert EO, Glidewell O (1967). Dactinomycin in Wilms' tumor. JAMA 199:464.

Wolff JA, Krivit W, Newton WA, D'Angio GJ and the CCSGA (1968). Single versus multiple dose Dactinomycin therapy of Wilms' tumor. New Eng J Med 279:290.

Wolff JA, D'Angio GJ, Hartmann J, Krivit W, Newton WA and the CCSGA (1974). Long-term evaluation of single versus multiple courses of Actinomycin D therapy of Wilms' tumor. New Eng J Med 290:84.

Sutow WW, Thurman WG, Windmiller J (1963). Vincristine (leurocristine) sulfate in the treatment of children with metastatic Wilms' tumor. Pediatrics 32:880.

Sullivan MP, Sutow WW, Cangir A, Taylor G (1967). Vincristine sulfate in management of Wilms' tumor. JAMA 202:79.

Schweisguth O, Taris N, Lemerle J, Tchernia G (1970). Action de la Vincristine dans les néphroblastomes. Bull Cancer 57:93.

D'Angio GJ, Evans AE, Breslow N (1976). The treatment of Wilms' tumor. Results of the National Wilms' tumor study. Cancer 38:633.

Sutow WW (1973). Chemotherapy in Wilms' tumor. Cancer 32:1150.

Finklestein JZ, Hittle RE, Hammond GD (1969). Evaluation of a high dose cyclophosphamide regimen in childhood tumors. Cancer 23:1239.

Livingston RB, Carter SK (1970). Single agents in cancer chemotherapy - New York, Washington, London, IFI/PLENUM, pp. 25.

Tan C, Etcubanas E, Wollner N, Rosen G, Gilladoga A, Showel J, Murphy ML, Kradoff H (1973). Adriamycin an antitumor antibiotic in the treatment of neoplastic diseases. Cancer 32:9.

Wollner N, Tan C, Ghavini F, Rosen G, Tefft M, Murphy ML (1971). Adriamycin in childhood leukemia and solid tumors. ASCO 1971 300.

Bonadonna G, Monfardini S, De Lena M, Fossatibellani F, Beretta G (1970). Phase I and preliminary phase II Evaluation of Adriamycin. Cancer Res 30:2572.

D'Angio GJ, Evans AE, Breslow N, Beckwith B, Bishop H, Farewell V. Goodwin W, Leape L, Palmer N, Sinks L, Sutow W, Tefft M, Wolff J (1981). The treatment of Wilms' tumor: Results of the second National Wilms' tumor study. Cancer 47:2302.

Jacobson B, Rubenson A, Hanson G, Sorensen SE, Hagberg S (1979). Regression of Wilms' tumor after preoperative chemotherapy. Acta Paed Scand 68:763.

International Society of Paediatric Oncology Trial (SIOP V) Results - to be published.

D'Angio GJ, Beckwith TB, Breslow NE, Bishop HC, Evans AE, Farewell V, Fernbach D, Goodwin WE, Jones B, Leape LL, Palmer NF, Tefft M, Wolff JA (1980). Wilms' tumor: an update. Cancer 45:1791.

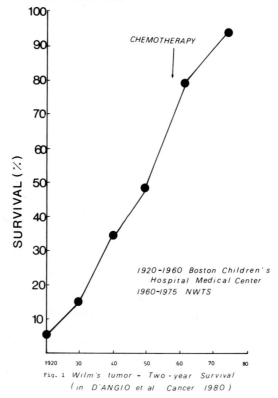

Fig. 1 Wilm's tumor - Two-year Survival
(in D'ANGIO et al Cancer 1980)

Renal Tumors: Proceedings of the First International Symposium on Kidney Tumors, pages 119–121
© **1982 Alan R. Liss, Inc., 150 Fifth Avenue, New York, NY 10011**

COMPLICATIONS AND SEQUELAE OF THE TREATMENT OF WILMS' TUMOR

Jean Lemerle M.D.

Department of Pediatrics

Institut Gustave-Roussy, 94800 Villejuif, France

The treatment of Wilms' Tumor combines in different ways surgery, radiotherapy, and chemotherapy. Each of these procedures, taken separately, may result in acute complications and/or sequelae. Practically, the treatment received by a given patient cannot be divided, and one should rather consider acute complications and long term sequelae of treatment as a whole.

Acute complications

Surgical rupture of the primary tumor during nephrectomy and tumor spillage in the abdomen increases the risk of local recurrences and distant metastases. It therefore often makes it necessary to widen the size of the portals for delivery of irradiation to the whole abdomen. This results frequently in acute intestinal disorders, and usually impairs ovarian function in girls. Tumor ruptures can be prevented by preoperative treatment, radiotherapy and/or chemotherapy, as shown by the 1st and 5th SIOP clinical trials (Lemerle et al, 1976; Lemerle et al, 1981). Abundant bleeding in the tumor may occur before surgery, very seldom raising a surgical emergency problem.

Actinomycin D and Vincristine, when administered according to the Wilms' Tumor protocols, are not very toxic drugs. Blood counts are affected minimally and the infection risk is reasonably small when the protocols are carefully followed. In any case, nausea, vomiting, and alopecia cannot be avoided. The combined use of radiation therapy and chemotherapy, either at the same time or in succession, may be the reason for several rare but eventually serious complications. Radiation enteritis may be observed when a large proportion of the intestine is irradiated and Actinomycin is given concurrently. Vomiting and diarrhea may call for radiotherapy to be interrupted for a few days or sometimes weeks. A low fat, low cellulose, milk free, gluten free diet is used to prevent these disorders. Long term intestinal problems such as chronic diarrhea, or acute or subacute intestinal obstruction may be observed in those patients who had acute intestinal symptoms (Donaldson et al, 1975). Radiation hepatitis is seen in right sided tumors when a large part of the liver is irradiated. Actinomycin D, again, enhances or reveals the radiation damage to the liver. Liver enlargement and thrombocytopenia are the most common symptoms and are associated with a clear reduction of isotope uptake in the irradiated areas of the liver (Lemerle et al, 1975). The frequency and severity of acute radiation enteritis and hepatitis now can be clearly diminished by careful shaping of the portals sparing as much as possible of normal tissue, and by using appropriate dose and time schedules, both for radiotherapy and for chemotherapy, in order to avoid cumulated or enhanced toxicity.

Viral infections, chickenpox and particularly measles, may be severe in patients receiving chemotherapy. We have seen several deaths due to measles pneumonitis. Congestive heart failure is an acute, long term, but now rare, complication of Adriamycin treatment.

Sequelae and delayed complications of treatment

The late effects of radiation therapy on growing children are possibly enhanced in some cases by chemotherapy.

Spinal deformities, especially kyphosis and scoliosis, become obvious at the spurt of growth around puberty. These deformities are related to the irradiation of the primary tumor and can be minimized only by cutting doses Careful follow-up of children having received spinal irradiation is mandatory and orthopaedic treatment (brace) often has to be applied several years after irradiation (Dubousset, 1980). Radiotherapy to both lungs is the only way of curing the majority of the patients with lung metastases. 2000 rads to the whole thorax of young children

impairs growth of the lungs and thoracic wall. Vital capacity of these children, when growing, is reduced by 20 to
40%. We have not been able to demonstrate any evidence
of lung fibrosis, but longer follow-up to adulthood may be
necessary to assess fully the potential deleterious effects
of radiotherapy delivered to growing lungs (Benoit et al,
in press). The renal functions of Wilms' Tumor survivors
have been assessed and have always been found to be within
the normal range. The only exception is for some of those
cases who received extensive abdominal irradiation or were
aggressively treated for bilateral Wilms' Tumor, with very
little kidney tissue left.

Second primary tumors are a threat to those children who
survived a first tumor. In a group of 750 Wilms Tumor
patients, we have seen two cases of AML and one of osteogenic
sarcoma in an irradiated area, and 3 soft tissue sarcomas.

An attempt to minimize long term sequelae is one of the
aims of SIOP Number 6 Wilms' Tumor trial in which the possibility of reducing the treatment of good cases is
being investigated.

Benoit MR, Jean R, Lemerle J. Pulmonary function in
  children irradiated on the chest for metastases of
  Wilms' Tumor. Thorax (in press).
Donaldson SS, Jundt S, Ricour C et al. (1975). Radiation
  enteritis in children. A retrospective review, clinicopathologic correlation, and dietary management. Cancer
  35:1167.
Dubousset J (1980). Déformations rachidiennes post radiothé-
  rapiques après traitement du néphroblastome chez l'enfant.
  Revue Chir Orthopédique 66:441.
Lemerle J, Tournade MF, Sarrazin D (1975). Tumors of the
  kidney. In Bloom HJG, Lemerle J, Neidhart MK, Voute, PA
  (eds): "Cancer in Children: Clinical Management." Berlin,
  Heidelberg, New York: Springer Verlag, p. 262.
Lemerle J, Tournade MF, Voute PA et al. (1976). Preopera-
  tive versus postoperative radiotherapy, single versus
  multiple courses of Actinomycin D in the treatment of
  Wilms' Tumor. Cancer 38: 647.
Lemerel J, Tournade MF, Voute PA (1981). Effectiveness of
  preoperative radiotherapy and/or chemotherapy in Wilms'
  Tumor. A.S.C.O. Proceedings 294: 407.

Renal Tumors: Proceedings of the First International Symposium on Kidney Tumors, pages 123-130
© 1982 Alan R. Liss, Inc., 150 Fifth Avenue, New York, NY 10011

WILMS' TUMOR UPDATED: EVOLUTION OF IDEAS AND TRENDS

A Report of the National Wilms' Tumor Study (NWTS) Committee for the NWTS Group*

The purposes of the National Wilms' Tumor Study at its inception included a desire to understand better

1. the epidemiologic, biologic and clinical features of the tumor,
2. the role of surgery,
3. the role of radiation therapy, and
4. the role of chemotherapy.

The succeeding studies of the NWTS have adhered to these initial goals. Epidemiology information has been accumulated, giving with greater precision the genetic and familial factors inherent in Wilms' tumor patients (Pendergrass 1976; Breslow in press). The biologic and clinical

*G.J. D'Angio, MD and A.E. Evans, MD, Children's Hospital Cancer Research Center, Philadelphia, PA; E. Baum, MD, Children's Memorial Hospital, Chicago, IL; J.B. Beckwith, MD, Children's Orthopedic Hospital, Seattle, WA; Norman Breslow, PhD, Fred Hutchinson Cancer Research Center, Seattle, WA; Alfred deLorimier, MD, University of California, San Francisco, CA; Donald Fernbach, MD, Baylor College of Medicine, Houston, TX; Ellen Hrabovsky, MD and Barbara Jones, MD, West Virginia University, Morgantown, WV; P. Kelalis, MD, Mayo Clinic, Rochester, MN; H.B. Othersen, Jr., MD, Medical University Hospital, Charleston, SC; Melvin Tefft, MD, Rhode Island Hospital, Providence RI; Patrick Thomas, MD, Washington University, St. Louis, MO.

characteristics also have been reported extensively and were summarized recently (D'Angio 1980).

Treatment considerations are reviewed here.

Surgery. The role of surgery needs sharper definition. Some of the dicta of the surgical literature require constant re-examination in the modern era of multimodal therapy. It has often been emphasized that the renal hilus must be approached first; yet, a retrospective review of data from the NWTS by Leape et al failed to substantiate this as an important surgical variable (Leape 1978). Also, the significance of minor capsular rents, created at surgery or antedating the operation, also were found to be of minor prognostic significance. This is not to condone careless or non-meticulous surgery; rather, it is to put in perspective some of the factors that have led surgeons to be either excessively cautious or overly aggressive under certain sets of circumstances. Awareness of the true significance (or insignificance) of these contingencies will sharpen surgical judgment at the operating table. Meanwhile, there is no substitute for a transabdominal approach that provides adequate exposure, permitting a thorough exploration of the abdominal contents and the opposite kidney as well as a sweeping dissection of the affected renal fossa for removal of the involved kidney and any associated lymph nodes. Careful attention to the renal vein and inferior vena cava is needed so as not to dislodge tumor propagating intraluminally.

For the future, the role of surgery in the management of patients with metastatic disease in the lungs requires redefinition. The NWTS has not addressed this question. Because new NWTS trials are built on the one preceeding, bilateral pulmonary irradiation has remained standard therapy for lung metastases. The results of other approaches such as those being used by some members of SIOP and others are awaited with interest. Chemotherapy is employed by them to reduce the number of pulmonary metastases and thus perhaps make them more amenable to surgical excisions. This may well disrupt pulmonary function less than bilateral pulmonary irradiation. The latter clearly is associated with demonstrable pulmonary deficits when appropriate tests are made (Littman 1976). The fact these deficits are subclinical gives little comfort because it can be expected these patients will develop pulmonary problems prematurely, especially if extraneous, noxious influences such as smoking are added.

Radiation therapy (RT). The role of RT has been addressed in sequential studies (Breslow 1980; D'Angio, 1980; D'Angio 1981). First, it has been found that the routine post-operative administration of flank irradiation to Stage I patients receiving adjuvant chemotherapy is not necessary -- certainly, not for those under two years of age. An interesting and ancillary finding in this regard has been the demonstration in NWTS-2 that vincristine added to actinomycin-D appears to "substitute" for post-operative RT (D'Angio 1981). Figure 1 shows the excellent result obtained in these non-irradiated patients whether the two drugs are given for 6 or for 15 months. The statistically worse result obtained in NWTS-1 in children over two years of age who were not irradiated has not been seen since the routine use of double-agent chemotherapy in NWTS-2. The efficacy of such chemotherapy has also colored thinking with respect to the need for routine administration of post-operative radiation therapy in children with more advanced stages of the disease. This is being put to the test for Stage II tumors in NWTS-3. Meanwhile, rad dose-response data are being sought in Stage III patients (D'Angio 1980).

Chemotherapy. The use of double-agent chemo-therapy routinely for 15 months was found to be advanta-geous when compared to results with use of either actino-mycin D (AMD) or vincristine (VCR) alone given over a similar period (D'Angio 1980). This has established these two agents as the minimum therapies needed post-operative-ly. They are well-tolerated, and there is little reason to forego their use in the vast majority of children with nephroblastoma. NWTS-2 established that adriamycin (ADR) is of value when added to AMD and VCR (Figure 2)(D'Angio 1981). In keeping with the spirit of the NWTS, however, attempts are being made to discover whether more intensive use of AMD and VCR will give equally good results. This is because the long-term effects of ADR are unknown. It is feared that the microscopic myocardial changes induced by even low doses of ADR may result in precocious heart dis-ease in Wilms' tumor survivors.

Meanwhile, the results are not good in patients with Stage IV tumor and those classified as "Unfavorable

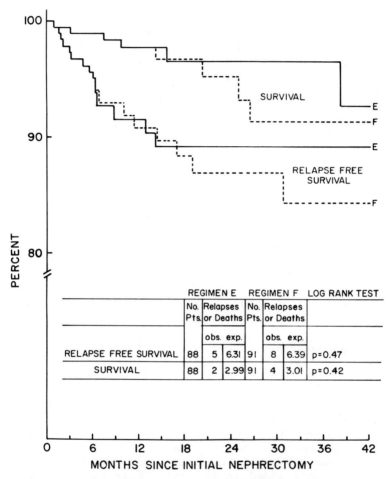

Figure 1. Relapse-free survival and survival curves for National Wilms' Tumor Study-2 Group 1 patients by randomized treatment Regimen. Reg. E = postoperative actinomycin D + vincristine for 6 months without irradiation. Reg. F = same as E, but chemotherapy for 15 months. Early portions of both sets of curves show deaths and relapses for patients experiencing those events prior to the 6 months' randomization. These are not counted in the treatment comparisons.

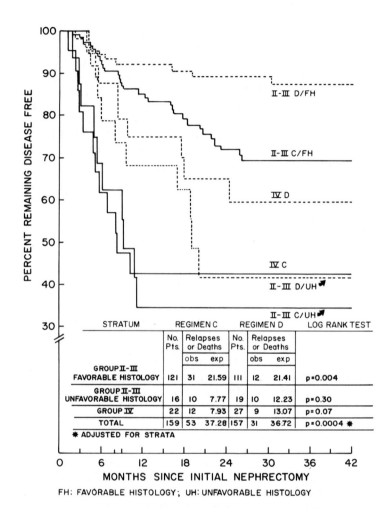

The following data table appears within the figure:

STRATUM	REGIMEN C			REGIMEN D			LOG RANK TEST
	No. Pts.	Relapses or Deaths		No. Pts.	Relapses or Deaths		
		obs	exp		obs	exp	
GROUP II-III FAVORABLE HISTOLOGY	121	31	21.59	111	12	21.41	p=0.004
GROUP II-III UNFAVORABLE HISTOLOGY	16	10	7.77	19	10	12.23	p=0.30
GROUP IV	22	12	7.93	27	9	13.07	p=0.07
TOTAL	159	53	37.28	157	31	36.72	p=0.0004 ✱

✱ ADJUSTED FOR STRATA

FH: FAVORABLE HISTOLOGY; UH: UNFAVORABLE HISTOLOGY

Figure 2. Relapse-free survival curves by randomized treatment regimen and histology for National Wilms' Tumor Study-2 Gp. II-III pts. and for Gp. IV pts., any histology. Reg. C = postoperative irradiation + actinomycin D and vincristine for 15 months. Reg. D = same as Reg. C except that adriamycin was added to the other 2 agents.

Histology" (UH) D'Angio 1981). Better forms of therapy are
needed. There are very few promising agents on the horizon
that, when added to AMD, VCR, and ADR, might yield better
results. Cyclophosphamide has been found useful in the
past. It is undergoing tests in NWTS-3 where it is added
to AMD, VCR and ADR. To date, there is no better outcome
with the four-agent regimen then with the three drugs.
These are aggregated results, however, and are not necessarily indicative of what might be happening within any of
the four specific sub-types grouped under UH. Continuing
study of the role of cyclophosphamide is therefore needed
in order to ascertain whether it might or might not be
useful in the anaplastic or the clear cell sarcoma groups,
for example, even though it might be of little value
against the other cell types.

Special considerations. Beckwith has well pointed
out that when treatment improves, patients at highest risk
stand out more clearly while those at low risk are ob-
scured. (Beckwith 1979) One of the goals of the NWTS has
been to reduce therapy to the barest minimum. There is
therefore a continuous cautious search underway within the
NWTS to identify the children who are at low risk. This
has been done by decreasing the length of treatment in
Stage I patients and in pilot studies where only single
para-operative courses of chemotherapy are being given to
Stage I/FH patients. It may well be that there is a group
of children who require only surgical excision in order to
enjoy a high likelihood of continuous relapse-free survival. Prolonged and pains-taking trials are needed in
order to identify these patients with precision. Such
studies are probably better suited to single large institu-
tions than to cooperative groups. This is because the
several extraneous variables can be kept to a minimum when
the team members can be in constant contact. Gross and
cytohistologic studies of tumors no doubt will make their
contributions to these attempts.

Succeeding NWTS studies have also made clear a truism.
Prognostic criteria change as treatments improve. Thus,
factors found to be of importance in earlier NWTS studies
such as age and tumor size have disappeared as more effective forms of therapy have been added. (D'Angio 1981). This
is a corollary to what has just been said with respect to
obscuring patients who are at low risk. Thus, staging

systems must change as treatments become more efficient if they are to serve as guides to therapy.

Data from cooperative trials can and should be used for purposes other than those strictly related to the therapeutic investigations. The accumulated information can be used to test statistical as well as medical hypothesis, or to exploit the gathered ancillary information in other ways. For example, there was a question some years ago that the potency of actinomycin D might have changed. The NWTS was able to show, through a search of its toxicity files, that the severity of bone marrow depressions had not changed during the suspect years, thus negating the suggested potency change. The NWTS has also reported analyses modelling the new NWTS staging system (Farewell, D'Angio, Breslow 1981), the hypothetical results had historical rather than concurrent controls been used in NWTS-2, (Farewell 1981), and epidemiologic studies of such factors as familial incidence, congenital anomalies and multicentricity (Pendergrass 1976; Breslow in press).

ACKNOWLEDGEMENTS

Figures 1 and 2 are reproduced through the courtesy of the journal CANCER.

The authors acknowledge the contribution made by the many members of the NWTS Group without whom the study would have been impossible. They also thank past members of the NWTS Committee and Dr. R. Shalek and the staff of the Radiological Physics Center, and the staff of the NWTS Data and Statistical Center.

Supported in part by USPHS Grant No. CA-11722.

REFERENCES

Beckwith JB (1979). Grading of pediatric tumors. In: "Care of the Child with Cancer," New York: American Cancer Society, pp 39-44.
Breslow NE, Beckwith JB, Palmer NF, Jacobson S, Sim DA (In press). Epidemiological features of Wilms' tumor. Results of the National Wilms' Tumor Study, J Nat'l Cancer Inst.

Breslow NE, Palmer MB, Hill LR, Buring J, D'Angio GJ (1978). Wilms' tumor: Prognostic factors for patients without metastases at diagnosis. Results of the National Wilms' Tumor Study. Cancer 41:1577-1589.

D'Angio GJ, Beckwith JB, Breslow NE, Bishop HC, Evans AE, Farewell V, Fernbach D, Goodwin WE, Jones B, Leape L, Palmer NF, Tefft M, Wolff JA (1980). Wilms' tumor: An up-date. Cancer 45:1791-1798.

D'Angio GJ, Evans AE, Breslow N, Beckwith B, Bishop H, Farewell V, Goodwin W, Leape L, Palmer N, Sinks L, Lutow W, Tefft M, Wolff J (1981). The treatment of Wilms' tumor: Results of the Second National Wilms' Tumor Study. Cancer 47:2302-2311.

Farewell VT, D'Angio GJ (1981). A simulated study of historical controls using real data. Biometrics 37:169-176.

Farewell VT, D'Angio GJ, Breslow N, Norkool P (1981). Retrospective validation of a new staging system for Wilms' tumor. Cancer Clin Trials 4:167-171.

Leape LL, Breslow NE, Bishop HC (1978). The surgical treatment of Wilms' tumor: Results of the National Wilms' Tumor Study. Ann Surg 187:351-356.

Littman P, Meadows AT, Polgar G, Borns P, Rubin E (1976). Pulmonary function in survivors of Wilms' tumor; Patterns of impairment. Cancer 41:1577-1589.

Pendergrass TW (1976). Congenital anomalies in children with Wilms' tumor. Cancer 37:403-409.

Renal Tumors: Proceedings of the First International Symposium on
Kidney Tumors, pages 131-144
© 1982 Alan R. Liss, Inc., 150 Fifth Avenue, New York, NY 10011

PREOPERATIVE CHEMOTHERAPY IN WILMS' TUMOUR
RESULTS OF CLINICAL TRIALS AND STUDIES ON NEPHROBLASTOMAS
CONDUCTED BY THE INTERNATIONAL SOCIETY OF PAEDIATRIC
ONCOLOGY (SIOP)

For the Trial Committee: J.de Kraker, P.A. Voûte,
J. Lemerle, M.-F. Tournade, H.J.M. Perry

INTRODUCTION

The most frequent malignant tumour of the kidney in
children is the Wilms' tumour or nephroblastoma. This
tumour was described for the first time by Wilms (Wilms,
1899). The tumour derives from embryonal kidney tissue
or blastema. Earlier American studies report an 8% cure
rate with surgery alone. These results were achieved in
a period of poor anaesthesia and poor pre- and postoperative care. With better techniques the cure rate
increased to 30%. Radiotherapy of the tumour region
after surgical extirpation brought the cure rate to 40%
and by adding actinomycin D as a chemotherapuetic agent
50% of the patients were cured. Combination chemotherapy
with actinomycin D and vincristine brought the cure rate
up to 80%. It is difficult to assess what the different
treatments contributed to the progress from 30% to 40%
to 50%, because at the same time the supporting care with
anaesthesia and pre- and postoperative care became
considerably better.

NEPHROBLASTOMA TRIAL AND SIOP STUDY No. 1

In the United States the National Wilms' Tumor Study
started in 1969. They used a staging system which is outlined in Table 1. This same staging system was used in
the SIOP studies. From September 1971 to October 1974,
the SIOP conducted a study comparable to the NWTS. The
questions asked in this study, SIOP No. 1, were:

1. Is it better to operate immediately or is it better to
    start treatment with radiotherapy to diminish the
    tumour volume and to devitalize the tumour cells.
2. Are multiple courses of actinomycin D better than a
    single course to prevent the development of metastases.
    This trial is outlined in Fig. 1. A total of 395
    patients with a Wilms' tumour from 42 clinics in
    Europe were registered. Of these, 192 patients were
    suitable for the controlled clinical trial, and 203
    patients were excluded because they were younger than
    1 year of age, or had been treated before or had a
    stage IV or V tumour.

Table 1

Staging System
National Wilms' Tumour Study

stage I Tumor limited to the kidney and completely
         excised.
         The renal capsule is intact. The tumour has not
         ruptured nor had it been punctured before its
         excision. No tumour is observed in the renal
         bed, and histological examination confirms that
         the capsule is intact.

stage II Tumour extends outside the kidney, but is completely
         excised.
         There is a local extension of the tumour, includ-
         ing in particular:
         - penetration of the tumour into the perirenal
           tissues beyond the false capsule of the tumour;
           "adhesions" that are confirmed histologically
           to be due to tumour.
         - invasion of the paraaortic nodes, confirmed
           histologically; the pathologist must make a
           careful search of all the excised nodes for
           foci of tumour cells.
         - invasion of the renal vessel walls outside the
           kidney or thrombosis caused by tumour in these
           vessels. Thrombosis which is apparently
           nonneoplastic may contain islands of tumour
           cells; they need to be examined very carefully.
         - invasion of the renal pelvis and ureter.

stage III Incomplete excision, without haematogenous
          metastases.
          This stage occurs if one or several of the
          following conditions are present:
          - a tumour biopsy was taken before or during
            surgery, tumour rupture before or during
            surgery.
          - peritoneal metastases, as distinguished from
            the simple tumour adhesions of stage II.
          - invasion of lymph nodes beyond the local
            regional nodes.
          - complete excision impossible (for example,
            infiltration of the vena cava).

stage IV Haematogenous metastases.
          Involving lungs, liver, bones, brain, etc.

stage V   Bilateral renal tumours.

Fig. 1

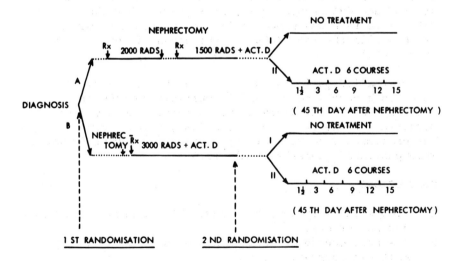

The disease free survival of the total group of 192
patients was 52%. The other 48% of the children developed
a recurrence of metastases. The latter were treated with
vincristine and actinomycin D and lung irradiation
resulting in cure for a considerable number. A survival
percentage of 71% was reached in the total group.

The results of this trial were updated in May 1981.
Survival and recurrence rates are not significantly different in the two groups. But tumour ruptures, minimal
and massive, during surgery occurred in 32% of those
patients who were operated first (group B) and in 4% only
of those who had received radiotherapy prior to surgery
(group A), a difference which is statistically significant
(p = 0.001). Eleven of the 19 ruptures in group B were
massive ruptures with tumour spillage in the abdomen.
The consequences of the tumour ruptures are the following:
11 children, including 7 girls, had to receive whole
abdomen irradiation to prevent tumour regrowth. The
ovaries were located in the radiation fields, which must
have resulted in gonadal destruction, while severe
testicular damage probably occurred in boys. Survival
in the 2 groups with or without ruptures was equivalent
at 58%, and 68% respectively, at 8 years. But the
metastatic rate was higher (73%) in the tumour-rupture
group versus the rate (49%) in the cases without rupture
(p = 0.001).

Of the 158 patients who received chemotherapy, 79
received a single course and 79 multiple courses of
actinomycin D. The disease free survival and the total
survival for the two groups were 50% and 70%, respectively.
The preliminary results of this trial and SIOP study No. 1,
were published (Lemerle et al. 1976).

CONCLUSIONS

1. Preoperative treatment is advisable to prevent ruptures
   during surgery.
2. A single course of actinomycin D is as good as
   multiple courses.
3. Combination chemotherapy with vincristine and actinomycin D administered in metastatic patients gives such
   a high cure rate, that it should be used from the
   beginning.

NEPHROBLASTOMA TRIAL AND SIOP STUDY No. 2

In a second study, SIOP No. 2, the above mentioned conclusions were applied in a non-randomized study comparing 6 months versus 15 months combination chemotherapy. Preoperative radiotherapy was given except in cases where a stage I tumour was expected. From the first study we had the strong impression that radiotherapy was not necessary for stage I tumours. These are the patients with a very small tumour.

From October 1974 to January 1977, 246 patients were entered by 36 clinics. Of these, 138 were treated according to the protocol. Disease free survival was 79% and total survival was 84% (Figs. 2 and 3). No difference could be found in the two groups of 37 and 101 patients, respectively.

The patients from the SIOP No. 1 and No. 2 studies were grouped by stage according to disease free survival and survival. As is demonstrated in Table 2, stage I and II patients show a good prognosis in response to the treatment scheme used. Disease free survival and survival are nearly the same. Patients with a stage III tumour did not benefit significantly concerning survival in comparison to the first SIOP study, although disease free survival was much better.

Table 2

	Number of patients	Disease free survival	Survival
SIOP 1			
Stage I	57	54%	78.5%
Stage II	84	59%	73 %
Stage III	51	37%	59 %
SIOP 2			
Stage I	56	87%	93 %
Stage II	36	91%	94 %
Stage III	41	57%	63 %

Fig.2.

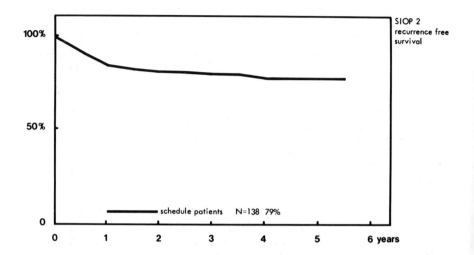

Fig.3.

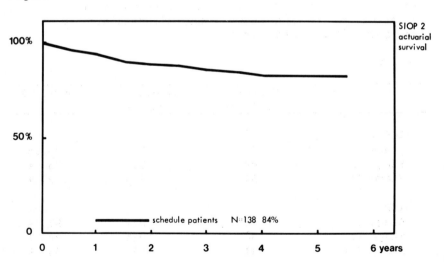

CONCLUSIONS

1. There is a considerable difference in survival data between stage I and II, and stage III.
2. It is not necessary to give chemotherapy for a longer period than 6 months especially in stage I and II patients.

ANALYSIS OF SIOP No. 1 and No. 2

Further analysis of the material has shown that the difference between the stages is due to the presence or absence of metastatic regional lymph nodes. One can make a division between normal risk group (NRG) and high risk group (HRG), NGR consisting of stage I and stage II patients with negative lymph nodes, and HRG consisting of stage II patients with positive regional lymph nodes and stage III (Table 3).

On the question of the lymph nodes in the patients included in the 2 studies, a publication was presented by the committee which confirmed the importance of the lymph nodes (Jereb et al. 1980).

A second study in the SIOP No. 2 patients was a comparison in duration of postoperative combination chemotherapy (6 months versus 15 months). No difference could be found between the two groups in terms of recurrence free survival and actuarial survival (Fig. 4).

The results demonstrated the benefit brought by preoperative radiotherapy. Chemotherapy has been shown to be effective by these studies on micro metastases as it is known to be effective on clinically detectable metastases. The question was then raised as to whether preoperative chemotherapy could be as efficient as preoperative radiotherapy. This formed the basis of the SIOP No. 5 trial and study.

Table 3

	Number of patients	Disease free survival	Survival
SIOP 1			
NRG	215	61%	78%
HRG	99	34%	59%
SIOP 2			
NRG	135	87%	92%
HRG	61	62%	71%

Fig. 4

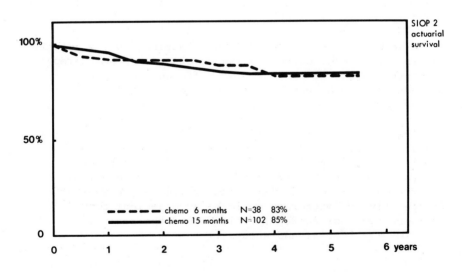

NEPHROBLASTOMA TRIAL AND SIOP STUDY No. 5

The third SIOP nephroblastoma trial and study addressed the question of whether preoperative chemotherapy is as good as preoperative radiotherapy to avoid tumour ruptures during surgery. This was also to be evaluated in relation to survival and disease free survival.

It was decided not to give radiotherapy to patients with a stage I tumour at surgery. In addition, this could generate further useful information on this group of patients. In other words, a careful attempt was made to demonstrate that chemotherapy could completely replace radiotherapy in patients with a nephroblastoma.

To be sure that no selection on patients included in trial was made by the participating centers, all of their patients with a Wilms' tumour had to be registered.

The protocol is shown in Fig. 5. At diagnosis, the eligible patients were randomized into treatment groups C and R.

Group C received preoperative chemotherapy with 4 injections of vincristine (1.5 mg/m^2), and 2 x 3 injections of actinomycin D (15 µg/kg). Group R received preoperative radiotherapy (Gray 20 in 2 weeks), and only 5 injections of actinomycin D (15 µg/kg). Following nephrectomy, radiotherapy was given according to stage. Stage I patients received no postoperative radiotherapy. Group R and Group C stage II and III patients received Gray 15 and Gray 30, respectively. Postoperative chemotherapy was the same as that given to patients in SIOP Study No. 2.

Maintenance chemotherapy was given after the induction therapy and lasted 6 months, and consisted of a combination of vincristine and actinomycin D.

Patients in the trial and study. From January 1977 to July 1980, 406 histologically proven cases of Wilms' tumour from 34 participating centers in Europe have been registered, of which 168 were randomized and were suitable for the trial.

Fig.5.

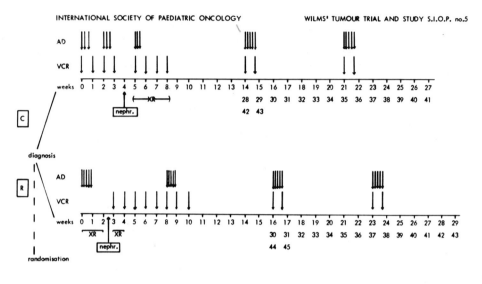

AD = Actinomycin D   15 µg/kg
VCR = Vincristine   1,5 mg/m2

Fig.6.

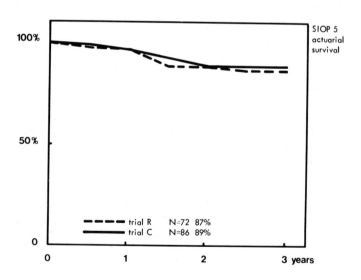

RESULTS

1. Randomization. The 2 randomized groups C and R are
   identical in terms of age at nephrectomy, size of the
   tumour measured on IVP at diagnosis, sex, side affected,
   site of the tumour and number of tumour nodules at
   pathological examination.
2. Treatment. The treatment protocol has been given with
   no great deviations. It could be followed easily and
   resulted in no significant toxicity.
3. Tumour ruptures. Ruptures were seen in 7 cases. Most
   were minimal ruptures without tumour spill. In each
   arm of the protocol was one patient with a major tumour
   rupture.
4. Survival. Survival curves are shown on Figures 6 and 7.
   The 3 years actuarial survival of the 158 trial patients
   with complete information is 88%, with no difference
   between Groups C and R (Fig. 6). The recurrence free
   survival at 3 years is 71%, with no significant difference in the two curves (Fig. 7). In July 1981, 38
   patients had recurrent disease. Evenly distributed in
   both arms of the protocol were 22 patients with lung
   metastases. Intra-abdominal recurrences were as
   follows: in arm C, there were two abdominal recurrences, one associated with liver and the other with
   liver and lung metastases, and there was one case of
   liver metastases associated with lung involvement.
   In arm R, there were two cases of metastases confined
   to the liver. It should be emphasized that out of the
   37 stage I patients in arm C who received no radiotherapy at all, none had abdomenal recurrence.
   Seventeen patients in the trial have died this far,
   13 of progressive disease, and 4 of treatment-
   related toxicity (1 sepsis; 1 undefined encephalitis;
   1 postoperative death; 1 gastrointestinal toxicity
   due to radiotherapy).

Fig. 7

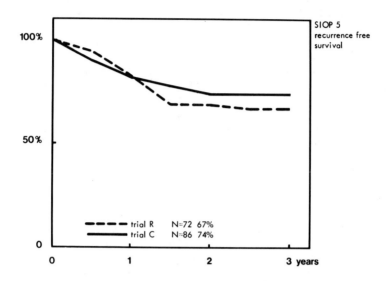

DISCUSSION

We have shown that preoperative chemotherapy is as efficient as preoperative radiotherapy.

Preoperative chemotherapy is demonstrated to have several advantages in the treatment of Wilms' tumour.

a) Preoperative treatment increases the proportion of stage I tumours. In SIOP No. 5, we reach the level of 43% stage I after preoperative chemotherapy. None of these patients has received any radiotherapy to the tumour bed, and none has recurred locally. If these results are confirmed, chemotherapy given prior to surgery would allow us to give no radiotherapy at all to half of the patients. This advantage is considerable, especially in places where adequate paediatric radiotherapy is not yet available.

b) Histological changes induced by preoperative chemo-therapy are significantly less important than the radiotherapy-induced changes. This makes it possible to recognize tumours for special treatment based on unfavourable histology.

CONCLUSION

1. Preoperative chemotherapy is as good as preoperative
    radiotherapy in terms of prevention of tumour rupture,
    but does not have its drawbacks. No toxicity is added
    by this technique since, if one compares it to primary
    surgery, it only changes the date of nephrectomy which
    is postponed 4 weeks in the protocol used. It has been
    shown that with this treatment 50% of the patients can
    be cured without receiving radiotherapy.

2. Overall results during the period of the SIOP No. 1.
    No. 2, and No. 5 trials and studies show. a significant
    increase in cure rates and decrease of metastatic rates
    when comparing Wilms' tumour studies SIOP No. 1 to SIOP
    No. 2, and No. 5.

    SIOP No. 5 shows that the same results may be achieved
    with less radiotherapy given to the patients, and there-
    fore with fewer sequelae of treatment.

    In the current 4th trial and study on Wilms' tumour
    (SIOP No. 6), which was activated July 1981, these
    results have been taken into account. Patients are
    divided in a normal risk group (NRG) and a high risk
    group (HRG).

    NRG is comprised of stage I and stage II patients
    with negative lymph nodes.

    HRG is comprised of stage II patients with positive
    lymph nodes and patients with stage III tumours.

    In stage I NRG a trial is conducted on duration of
    chemotherapy.

    In stage II NRG a trial is done if postoperative radio-
    therapy is necessary, with the aim of finding out if
    the number of patients with a nephroblastoma that
    can be cured without receiving radiotherapy can be
    increased.

    In the HRG, which also includes the unfavourable histo-
    logy group, the trial compares a chemotherapy scheme of
    intensified vincristine medication to a chemotherapy
    scheme with adriamycin.

    As of August 1981, 131 patients have been included in
    the trial and study. Of these, 38 are in the stage I
    trial, 14 in stage II NRG and 11 in HRG. At this
    moment it is too early to draw any conclusions.

Jereb B, Tournade MF, Lemerle J, Voûte PA, Delemarre JF, Ahström L, Flamant R, Gerard-Marchant R, Sandstedt B (1980). Lymph node invasion and prognosis in nephroblastoma. Cancer 45:1632.

Lemerle J, Voûte PA, Tournade MF, DeLemarre JFM, Jereb B, Ahström L, Flamant R, Gerard-Marchant R (1976). Preoperative versus postoperative radiotherapy, single versus multiple courses of Actinomycin D, in the treatment of Wilms' tumour. Preliminary results of a controlled clinical trial conducted by the International Society of Paediatric Oncology (S.I.O.P.). Cancer 38: 647.

Wilms M (1899). Die mischgeschwülste der Niere. Leipzig Verlag von Arthur Georgi.

This work was supported by a grant from the Koningin Wilhelmina Fonds, Dutch organization against cancer (The Netherlands) and a grant (ATP no. 1, 714 431) from the INSERM (France).

Renal Tumors: Proceedings of the First International Symposium on Kidney Tumors, pages 145–154
© **1982 Alan R. Liss, Inc., 150 Fifth Avenue, New York, NY 10011**

WILMS' TUMOR: HISTOLOGIC GRADING AS A PROGNOSTIC FACTOR IN
TUMORS BEYOND 10CM IN DIAMETER

Julio Pow-Sang M.D., Graciela Ramírez M.D. and
Víctor Benavente M.D.
Instituto Nacional Enfermedades Neoplásicas
Av. Alfonso Ugarte 825. Lima 1. Perú

Inspite of efforts developed in the study of Wilms'
tumor, there are many factors not clearly established about
its behavior. Our previous studies showed a definitive
correlation between the size of the tumor and prognosis of
the disease (Pow-Sang et al, 1975; Pow-Sang, Benavente 1980).

It is not yet clear if histologic grading of the tumor
might influence the prognosis of the disease, independent of
the presence or absence of Rhabdomyosarcoma of the kidney
(Breslow et al, 1978). An assertion was made that considering the normal weight of kidneys at autopsy (26 gm at birth;
100 gm at 3 years of age and 178 gm at 10 years of age)
Wilms' tumors under 12.8 cm in diameter do not show more than
26% relapse and no more than 17% mortality two years after
initial diagnosis (Breslow et al, 1978).

Histologic grading of Wilms' tumor is a parameter which
has not been considered extensively in previously published
studies. According to Breslow et al (1978), 12% of the NWTS
population had Rhabdomyosarcoma of the kidney. The poor
outcome in this group of patients is fortunately limited to
a distinct minority of cases. Histologic type is of limited
prognostic value for the remaining 88% of the patient
population (Breslow et al, 1978).

Taking into account these considerations we decided to
study a group of patients bearing Wilms' tumor with a diameter
size greater than 10 cm in order to see what the correlation
might be with the histological grade of the tumor.

The particular set of patients presented in this paper are grouped in accordance to the criteria set forth by Lawler and Kheir as prognostic factors (Lawler et al, 1975; Kheir et al, 1978).

MATERIALS AND METHODS

Sixty selected cases of Wilms' tumor registered àt the Instituto Nacional de Enfermedades Neoplásicas (I.N.E.N.), Lima, Peru between 1952-1978 are presented in this paper.

The age groupings of the patients are given in Table 1.

TABLE 1

WILMS' TUMOR I.N.E.N. (1952-1978)· 60 SELECTED PATIENTS

Age (Years)	Number of Patients
0 - 1	17
2 - 3	21
4 - 5	14
6 - 7	5
8 - 9	3
Total	60

The number of male and female patients is given in Table 2.

Table 3 indicates the incidence of tumors on the left and right sides.

Fifty-eight patients did have a complete histopathological study in accordance to Kheir and Lawler methodology (Kheir et al, 1978; Lawler et al 1975). Their distribution in accordance to the histological grading is given in Table 4.

TABLE 2

WILMS' TUMOR I.N.E.N. (1952-1978)
60 SELECTED PATIENTS

Sex	Cases
Male	36
Female	24
Total	60

TABLE 3

WILMS' TUMOR I.N.E.N. (1952-1978)
60 SELECTED PATIENTS

Side	Cases
Right	31
Left	27
Bilateral	2
Total	60

TABLE 4

WILMS' TUMOR DISTRIBUTION OF HISTOLOGICAL GRADING
(58 PATIENTS)

Histological Grade	Cases	Percent
Well Differentiated (WD)	4	6.9
Moderately Differentiated (MD)	14	24.1
Poorly Differentiated (PD)	40	69.0
Total	58	100.0

Survival and death in patients under or over 2 years of age, plotted against histological grading of tumor are shown in Table 5.

Forty-six cases are grouped in two sets in accordance to the diameter of the tumor. The first group of patients had tumors in between 10-14 cm and the second group had tumors over 15 cm in diameter. This two sets of patients are plotted against the grade of histological differentiation in order to obtain the survival rate at two years after the initial diagnosis (Table 6).

The 46 patients were also considered as a whole group bearing tumors over 10 cm in diameter, and these are tabulated according to the grade of histological differentiation and survival rate at two years after the initial diagnosis (Table 7).

TABLE 5

SURVIVAL AND DEATH OF WILMS' TUMOR PATIENTS* TWO YEARS AFTER INITIAL DIAGNOSIS

Age	Histological Grade	Alive		Death		Overall	
		Cases	Percent	Cases	Percent	Alive	Death
<2yrs.							
	WD	1/ 2	50	1/ 2	50		
	MD	0/ 2	–	2/ 2	100	4/15	11/15
	PD	3/11	27.2	8/11	72.8	26.7%	73.3%
>2yrs.							
	WD	0/ 2	–	2/ 2	100	17/43	26/43
	MD	5/12	41.7	7/12	58.3	39.6%	60.4%
	PD	12/29	41.4	17/29	58.6		

*Patients under or over two years of age are tabulated according to histologic grade (58 patients).

TABLE 6

CORRELATION BETWEEN SIZE OF WILMS' TUMOR AND HISTOLOGICAL GRADING FOR SURVIVAL RATE AT TWO
YEARS AFTER INITIAL DIAGNOSIS AND TREATMENT (46 PATIENTS)

Size	Histological Grade	Alive		Death	
		Cases	Percent	Cases	Percent
10-14 cm					
	WD	0/ 1	–	1/ 1	100
	MD	1/ 4	25.	3/ 4	75
	PD	7/13	53.8	6/13	46.2
Subtotal		8/18	44.5	10/18	55.5
>15 cm					
	WD	1/ 3	33.4	2/ 3	66.6
	MD	2/ 7	28.6	5/ 7	71.4
	PD	8/18	44.4	10/18	55.6
Subtotal		11/28	39.3	17/28	60.7
Total		19/46	41.3	27/46	58.7

TABLE 7

SIZE OF WILMS' TUMOR BEYOND 10 CM IN DIAMETER AGAINST
HISTOLOGICAL GRADING FOR SURVIVAL RATE AT TWO YEARS OF
INITIAL DIAGNOSIS AND TREATMENT; 46 PATIENTS

| Histological Grade | Size Over 10 cm in Diameter | | | |
| | Alive | | Death | |
	Cases	Percent	Cases	Percent
WD	1/ 4	25	3/ 4	75
MD	3/11	27.3	8/11	72.7
PD	15/31	48.4	16/31	51.6
Total	19/46	41.3	27/46	58.7

DISCUSSION

Children under 2 years of age bearing Wilms' tumors with
an average size diameter of 10.8 cm have a survival rate of
83-88% at two years after initial diagnosis, (D'Angio et al,
1976). When the tumor diameter averages 12.7 cm, survival
rate drops to 77-82%. Relapse of the disease at two years
has a linear correlation to the progressive increase of
tumor size. That is, there is a 12.3% relapse when the tumor
size is around 10 cm in diameter and 26% relapse when the
tumor size is around 12.8 cm in diameter.

In 1978, Leape et al found that tumor size has a significant inverse relation to the RFS (Recurrence Free Survival).
That is, tumors under 375 gm have a higher RFS. Larger
tumors get more capsule infiltration than smaller ones and
this capsule infiltration is of poor prognostic value: All
patients under this particular category have a lower RFS.

We use the criteria of follow-up at two years following initial diagnosis because most of relapses and or deaths occur during this period of time. After this 24-month period, the number of relapses and or deaths is not of statistical significance.

The consideration of advanced disease raised in this paper extends from our previous communication (Pow-Sang, Benavente 1980). Patients bearing tumors 10 to 14 cm diameter have a metastases incidence of 41.17%; this percentile average increases 54.35% when the tumor diameter is between 15 to 19 cm and when the tumor diameter is beyond 20 cm, metastases are present in an average of 60% of all diagnosed cases.

This paper deals with the correlation between tumors over 10 cm in diameter and histologic grade (well, medium and poorly differentiated tumor) as a prognostic factor. The histopathological study was done by one of us (G.R.) independent of the clinical data available. The three basic components of Wilms' tumors were taken into consideration for grouping the patients presented. These are: 1) the epithelial elements (glomeruli and tubuli); 2) the less differentiated blastic group of cells and 3) the fibroblasts, smooth muscular fibers and occasional striated muscular fibers. A progressive proportion of 25-50 and 75% undifferentiated cells in these three basic components, in serial field, establish the histological differentiation (grade) of the tumor. Only 6.9% of our patients had the well differentitated type of tumor and most of them (69%) were poorly differentiated.

Our survival rate is higher for patients over two years of age (39.53%) than for the patients under two years of age (26.67%); this is in contrast to the results of the NWTS when Stage I patients were studied (Breslow et al, 1978). Later on, the same NWTS established that there is no overall deterioration of prognosis with age beyond two years (Leape et al, 1978).

The survival rate of 44% when the patients have a tumor size of 10-14 cm correlates well to the survival rate of 39.3% when the tumor size is over 15 cm in diameter. This assertion is not in accordance with the results of Breslow et al (1978) who found no indication that increases in tumor mass beyond 250 gm are associated with progressively worse outcome; the largest diameter they measured in their cases was 12.8 cm (Table 6).

Finally, our data in Table 7 indicate that there is an inverse correlation between histological grade and the two-year survival rate. There is an increasing scale of survival rate for the well differentiated (25%), moderate differentiated (27.3%) and poorly differentiated (48.4%) histological types. Further studies are encouraged to know the explanation for these data in our patients with Wilms' tumor.

SUMMARY

The progressive proportion of 25-50 and 75% of undifferentiated cells in the Wilms' tumor mass generate three grading categories: well differentiated (WD); the moderate differentiated (MD) and the poorly differentiated (PD). The Urology Department of the Instituto Nacional de Enfermedades Neoplásicas (Lima, Peru) has studied 60 selected cases registered at its Biostatistics Department. Only 6.9% were well differentiated; 69% were of the poorly differentiated type. In 58 patients our survival rate at two years after diagnosis is higher (39.53%) when the patients are over 2 years of age; while under 2 years of age this survival rate is 26.67%. In a group of 46 patients, the survival rate at two years after initial diagnosis is 44% with a tumor size between 10-14 cm; the survival rate drops to 39.3% when the tumor size is over 15 cm in diameter. There is a linear increasing scale of survival rate for the well differentiated (25%), moderate differentiated (27.3%) and for the patients bearing poorly differentiated types of tumors (48.4%). Further studies are encouraged in order to learn the reasons for this correlation.

REFERENCES

Breslow NE, Palmer NF, Hill LR (1978). Wilms' tumor: prognostic factors for patients without metastases at diagnosis: results of the National Wilms' Tumor Study. Cancer 41:1577.
D'Angio GJ, Evans AE, Breslow N, Beckwith B, Leape LL, Sinks LF, Sutow W, Tefft M, Wolff J (1976). The treatment of Wilms' tumor. Results of the National Wilms' Tumor Study. Cancer 33:633.

Kheir S, Pritchett PS, Moreno H, Robinson A (1978). Histo-
  logic garding of Wilms' tumor as a potential prognostic
  factor: results of a retrospective study of 26 patients.
  Cancer 41:1199.
Lawler W, Marsden HB, Palmer MK (1975). Wilms' tumor.
  Histologic variation and prognosis. Cancer 36:1122.
Leape LL, Breslow NE, Bishop HC (1978). The surgical treat-
  ment of Wilms' tumor: results of the National Wilms' Tumor
  Study. Ann Surg 187:351.
Pow-Sang J, Tam G, Sebastian R (1975). Wilms' tumor:
  correlation between Garcia's and National Wilms' Group's
  clinical staging. In "Conflicts in Childhood Cancer",
  New York: Alan R. Liss, Inc., p. 249.
Pow-Sang J (1978): Tumor de Wilms' (Nefroblastoma) Estudio
  de 68 casos. Acta Cancerologica 17:39.
Pow-Sang J, Benavente V (1980). Wilms' tumor: a progressive
  study of 137 consecutive patients treated in Peru. Int
  Adv Surg Oncol 3:299.
Tefft M, D'Angio GJ, Grant W, III (1976). Review of group
  III patients in the National Wilms' Tumor Study. Cancer
  37:2768.

Renal Tumors: Proceedings of the First International Symposium on Kidney Tumors, pages 155–164
© 1982 Alan R. Liss, Inc., 150 Fifth Avenue, New York, NY 10011

SURGICAL ASPECTS OF SIMULTANEOUS BILATERAL WILMS' TUMORS

M. Gruner, B. Chaouachi, M. Bitker

Hôpital Trousseau

Paris, France

Although surgical management of non concurrent bilateral nephroblastomas, or of Wilms' tumors occurring in a solitary kidney is relatively easy, simultaneous bilateral tumors present a somewhat different problem. Various attitudes have been proposed such as surgery in one or more stages, total nephrectomy on one side associated either with radiotherapy or with nephrectomy on the other, and even bilateral total nephrectomy followed by renal transplantation. The attitude we choose is in agreement with Professor Lemerle's group at the Gustave Roussy Institute and is based on two apparently contradictory objectives:

1)   to conserve as many nephrons as possible in these children, to avoid chronic renal insufficiency, and

2)   to perform a satisfactory carcinologic surgery.

In a short series of six cases that we observed between 1972 and 1980 we always considered the possibility of performing bilateral partial nephrectomy which we discovered to be possible in three cases.

CASE REPORTS

Case Number 1

M.V., a 3-year-old girl. Abdominal pain lead to the discovery of an abdominal mass and elevation of blood pressure. Intravenous pyelography showed the existence of a bilateral nephroblastoma. Preoperative chemotherapy using Vincristine and Actinomycine gave a good diminishment of the tumors. Surgery was carried out in June, 1972. By an abdominal incision on the left side a partial nephrectomy of the upper pole was performed, removing a tumor weighing 300 gm. An IVP on the 10th postoperative day showed good function of the remaining left parenchyma. On postoperative day 21, by an abdominal incision, a right partial nephrectomy of the upper pole was performed, removing a tumor of 160 gm with some difficulties in the dissection of the venous pedicles.

Postoperative IVP showed a nonfunctional right kidney leading six months later to a right total nephrectomy. Histological examination revealed some remaining tumor and an irradiation of 30 Grays was performed on the right side associated with postoperative chemotherapy. Nine years later the child is well with normal renal function and without any recurrence of the tumor.

CASE 1

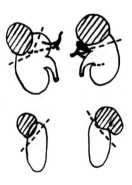

CASE N° 1

Case Number 2

    J.O., a boy 2 years old was seen for an abdominal mass
with elevation of blood pressure. The IVP suggested a
bilateral nephroblastoma. Preoperative chemotherapy lead
to a good diminishment of the volume of the tumors. The
first operation on the right side in August 1975 was by an
abdominal incision. A partial nephrectomy of the lower pole
removed a tumor of 25 gm. Postoperative histological examination indicated the need to remove more parenchyma. The
postoperative IVP was satisfactory. Three weeks later a
left total nephrectomy was performed for a central tumor of
120 gm. Postoperative chemotherapy was administered. In
October, 1980 laparotomy was performed for intestinal
occlusion. Six years after the onset of the disease no
renal insufficiency and no sign of recurrence of the tumor
has been noted.

CASE 2

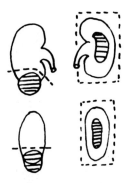

CASE N° 2

Case Number 3

H.T., a boy six years old seen for an abdominal mass. The IVP showed a nonfunctional left kidney and a tumor on the upper pole of the right kidney. Radiotherapy on the left side had been administered elsewhere. Angiography confirmed the bilaterality of the tumor. Preoperative chemotherapy of Vincristine and Actinomycine was given. A subcutaneous metastatic nodule and a carcinomatous meningitis made the diagnosis of nephroblastoma doubtful.

The first operation in February, 1977 was an abdominal incision with tumorectomies of the upper and lower pole of the right kidney. The postoperative IVP was satisfactory.

Twelve days later, by an abdominal incision, a partial nephrectomy of the lower pole of the left kidney was done. The result of histologic examination was debated but the conclusion was nephroblastoma. The postoperative chemotherapy was given and four years later the child is well without renal insufficiency or any sign of tumor recurrence.

CASE 3

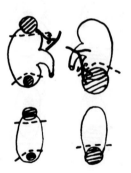

CASE N° 3

Case Number 4

K.G., a boy five years old seen for an abdominal mass.
IVP showed a bilateral nephroblastoma. The preoperative
chemotherapy with Vincristine and Actinomycin was given.
In February, 1978, by a right thoracoabdominal incision,
partial nephrectomy of the upper pole removing a small
tumor of 25 gm without pseudo capsule was completed. The
postoperative IVP was satisfactory. Ten days later, by a
left thoracoabdominal incision, partial nephrectomy of the
upper pole of the left kidney removing a tumor of 540 gm
was completed. The postoperative IVP was satisfactory.
Three years later no signs of tumor recurrence and no renal
insufficiency.

CASE 4

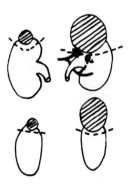

CASE N° 4

Case Number 5

G.M., a young girl 11 months old weighing 7 kg was seen for increasing volume of the abdomen. The IVP showed a bilateral nephroblastoma. Preoperative chemotherapy with Vincristine, Actinomycin and Adriamycin appeared to be unsuccessful. Irradiation of both kidneys with 15 Grays without detectable reduction of tumor volume was noted. In August, 1979, by a thoracoabdominal approach a nephroblastoma was found to have developed on the upper part of an uretero pyelic duplication. The tumorectomy removed a tumor of 500 gm. The postoperative IVP was satisfactory. Eleven days later, by a right thoracoabdominal incision, a total nephrectomy removing a tumor weighing 1000 gm was performed. Postoperative chemotherapy was given. Two years later the child is well without any recurrence of the disease.

CASE 5

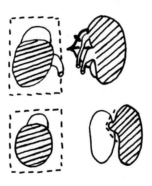

CASE N° 5

Case Number 6

A.E., a boy three years old seen for an abdominal mass.
The IVP showed right nephroblastoma. Preoperative chemotherapy with Vincristine and Actinomycin was given. In
August 1980, by an abdominal incision, two tumorlets on the
left kidney was discovered and biopsied. Right total
nephrectomy removing a central nephroblastoma extending
to the renal vein was performed. Postoperatively, histologic examination of the left biopsies showed the existence
of a nephroblastoma. Neither ultrasonography nor angiography showed any remaining tumor on the left side. Ten
days later by an abdominal approach, tumorectomies of two
small nephroblastomas on the left remaining kidney were
performed. Postoperative radiotherapy on the right side
and chemotherapy were given. One year later the child is
well with normal renal function and without any recurrence
of the tumor.

CASE 6

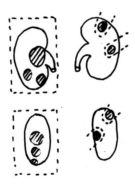

CASE N° 6

DISCUSSION

All these children were submitted to preoperative chemotherapy which was successful except in Case 5 where neither chemotherapy nor irradiation were successful. Diagnosis of bilaterality was made before operation by IVP in all cases except in Case 6 where it was necessary to open operatively the renal compartment to discover multiple tumorlets that even ultrasonography and arteriography had not revealed.

From a purely surgical point of view two questions have to be answered. What are the possibilities of performing conservative surgery and does surgery have to be carried out in one or several stages? The possibilities of conservative surgery depend on several factors. The resection of small tumors is rarely difficult. But large tumors do not exclude the possibility of partial surgery. In Cases 1, 4 and 5 we resected tumors weighing from 300 to 540 gm without special difficulties. The multiplicity of tumors does not exclude the possibility of multiple tumorectomies or of bipolar nephrectomies (Cases 3 and 6). The quantity of remaining renal parenchyma is also important to consider. In the nine kidneys on which we performed conservative surgery, we never had to sacrifice more than one-third of the kidney. It is even possible to be more conservative keeping just one-third or less of the kidney if necessary. Not only the quantity but also the quality of the remaining parenchyma is important to consider. Thus conservative management will be even more necessary if pre- or postoperative radiotherapy is indicated. The location of the tumor is important and in cases of superficial implantation, the resection will be easy whatever the location or the size of the tumor. On the contrary, in cases of central implantation only polar tomography will allow partial surgery. The vascularization of the tumor and of the healthy kidney have to be determined by preoperative angiography.

Careful dissection of all pedicles allows bloodless resection. We never had to perform total blood exclusion. In six cases out of nine partial resections and elective blood exclusions were possible. In the three remaining cases the tumors were small or polar hemostasis was performed during parenchymatosis section. Nevertheless venous blood control seemed difficult to assess preoperatively and difficult to accomplish operatively. These difficulties were responsible for the failure of the partial resection in Case 1.

Two other elements have yet to be evaluated.

1) The consistency of the tumor which, when the mass seems to be particularly soft or fragile, may lead to reject partial surgery (Case 5).

2) The absence of a pseudo capsule which may preclude any possibility of tumorectomy (Case 2).

Local extension of nephroblastoma is the last element to be considered in the decision for partial surgery. Of the twelve Wilms' tumors of this series only two were Stage II. Operatively it seems particularly difficult to know if peritumoral adherences are neoplastic or only inflammatory. If the first possibility excludes any partial resection, the doubt can be removed by multiple extemporaneous biopsies. Renal vein thrombosis leads to total radical surgery. Finally, histologic examination of a parenchymatous slice or of lymph nodes can modify the surgical approach.

Thus conservative surgery of bilateral simultaneous nephroblastoma depends on various factors. Some of them can be foreseen preoperatively.

We always performed this surgery in two stages beginning with the side for which we considered preoperatively that conservative surgery was possible. The first resection was made with the protection of contralateral kidney function. Function of the remaining renal parenchyma is evaluated on a postoperative IVP usually undertaken on the 8th day.

Thus it is possible to adopt a reasonable attitude on the other side. It can be conservative if tumoral extension allows it.

There are two other considerations for two-stage, surgery:

1) The duration of conservative surgery due to dissection and extemporaneous histologic examination.

2) The possibility of using the thoraco-abdominal approach on one or both sides.

CONCLUSIONS

The six children reported herein are alive one to nine years after the beginning of their disease. None shows any recurrence of the disease or renal insufficiency. We performed partial resection with one failure due to difficulties in venous dissection. This case was a Stage II, misdiagnosed by lack of histologic extemporaneous examination.

REFERENCES

Bischop HC, Eff TM, Evans AE, D'Angio GJ (1977). Survival in bilateral Wilms' tumor. Review of 30 National Wilms' tumor study cases. Journ Ped Surg 12:631.

Bitker MO (1981). Néphroblastomes bilatéraux: stratégie chirurgicale. Thèse, Paris.

D'Angio GJ, et al (1980). Wilms' tumor: an update. Cancer 45:1971.

Gruner M, Lemerle J, Vazquez MP. Néphroblatome. Monographies d'urologie. 109:1 Expension scientifique Francaise, Paris.

Lemerle J, Tournade MF (1980). Le traitement conservateur du néphroblastome bilateral. Journ d'Urol 86:8.

Pellerin D, Revillon Y (1980). Les néphroblastomes bilatéraux aspects chirurgicaux. Journ d'Urol 86:8.

Poisson D (1977). Nephroblastomes bilatéraux (étude retrospective de 35 cas suivis à l'Institut Gustave Roussy. Thèse médical, Paris.

Renal Tumors: Proceedings of the First International Symposium on Kidney Tumors, pages 165–166
© **1982 Alan R. Liss, Inc., 150 Fifth Avenue, New York, NY 10011**

LATE-RECURRING WILMS' TUMORS

N. Clausen

University Clinic of Paediatrics

Rigshospitalet, Copenhagen, Denmark

The increasing numbers of long-term survivors from
Wilms' tumor generate interest in the cases of late recurrence. Most authors find the risk of recurrence or
second tumors very low after two years of recurrence-free
survival. Reports on late recurrence of Wilms' tumor have
been sporadic in the literature, describing 23 cases recurring later than 36 months after surgery and believed
free of disease. The site of recurrence was reported in
nine of the cases, three being in the contralateral kidney.

We have seen two cases of Wilms' tumors recurring after
9 and 10 years, respectively. Patient A was 3 3/4 years
old when a right side Wilms' tumor and bilateral lung
metastases was disgnosed, while patient B presented at
4 1/2 years with a stage II left side Wilms' tumor. Both
patients were treated surgically and with chemotherapy.
Patient B was irradiated postoperatively. All signs of
disease disappeared, and at 10 years of age the follow-up
checks were stopped. Patient A had bilateral lung
metastases verified by biopsy at the age of 14 1/2 years.
Patient B had an acute abdominal episode at 13 1/2 years,
when an encapsulated hematoma containing nephroblastoma
was found between the intestines.

The most likely explanation for the late recurrence of
Wilms' tumors in these two patients is that the nephroblastoma
cells survived in a latent or very slowly growing state.
The growth rate of untreated Wilms' tumor is widely variable, and, as demonstrated by repeat urography, it is not
age dependent. The growth of lung metastases was not

different from the pattern of growth of primary Wilms' tumor by in vitro assay.

Although the number of late recurrences of Wilms' tumor is small, such cases demonstrate the basis of controversy which may arise when an individual is considered cured.

Renal Tumors: Proceedings of the First International Symposium on Kidney Tumors, pages 167–171
© **1982 Alan R. Liss, Inc., 150 Fifth Avenue, New York, NY 10011**

THE TREATMENT OF WILMS' TUMOR IN 1982
THE STATUS OF THE ART

Jean Lemerle, M.D.
Chief, Department of Pediatric Oncology
Institut Gustave-Roussy (I.G.R.), Villejuif,
France

At the beginning of the 1980's, the treatment policy in the case of Wilms' Tumor is governed by three considerations. First, we are treating young children with a high risk of acute complications and severe long term sequelae of treatment, mainly of radiotherapy. Figure 1 shows the age distribution in a series of 724 cases treated at Institut Gustave-Roussy.

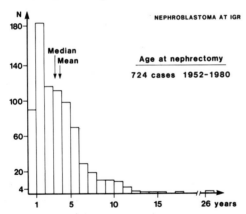

Fig. 1

The second point is that, in terms of survival, we have reached a very high level, as indicated in Figure 2 which shows actuarial survival curves of five consecutive series of non initially metastatic unilateral cases, all of which were treated in different manners from 1952 to 1980 at I.G.R (Lemerle et **al**, 1981). The last group of patients

has a survival rate of 92%. The survival of all those
cases who had metastases either at presentation (stage IV)
or subsequently during the same period has increased
from 1% to 42% (Fig. 2). The third point is that in Wilms'
Tumors, as in the majority of childhood embryonal tumors,
2-year survival without recurrence is equivalent to cure (Fig. 3)
This means that the results of a given protocol can be
rapidly assessed. Thus, we are dealing with a tumor for
which a very high cure rate has been progressively
reached, and, for which, therefore, a risk is present of
loosing what has been gained. However, on the other hand,
we are willing to improve the quality of life of the many
children who will survive, and we try to eliminate any
part of the treatment which has not proven to be necessary.

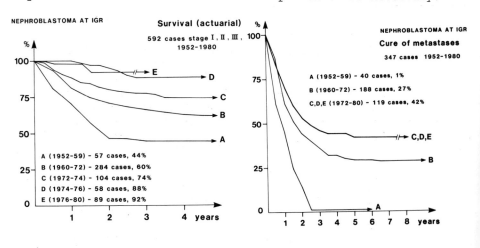

Fig. 2

Fig. 3

CURRENT TREATMENT PRACTICE

Total nephrectomy in unilateral cases is the corner-
stone of treatment. Partial nephrectomy at present is
only considered in bilateral tumors. Preoperative
chemotherapy with Vincristine (VCR) and Actinomycine D
(Act D) are now given for 3 weeks to all cases in the
current SIOP trial Number 6, since it has been shown in
SIOP study Number 5 that it is equivalent to preoperative
radiotherapy in terms of tumor shrinking and prevention
of operative tumor rupture. Another benefit derived from
preoperative chemotherapy is that it improves the
surgical pathological stage of the tumor, "creating"

more stage I tumors, which is an advantage as shown below.

Postoperative radiotherapy is now given according to
the surgical pathological stage. It has been shown by
NWTS that no radiotherapy was required in stage I tumors.
It has also been shown by SIOP trial Number 5, in which
stage I tumors had been operated on after chemotherapy,
that postoperative radiotherapy was also avoided safely.
In more advanced local stages, postoperative radiotherapy
(30 Gys in stage III, and 20 Gys in stage II) is given
systematically (1 Gy = 100 Rads). Randomized studies
are underway both in the U.S. and in Europe (NWTS 3 and
SIOP 6) which are exploring the possibility of avoiding
radiotherapy in stage II.

Chemotherapy with VCR and Act D is given to all patients.
First, in a long course split into two parts, preoperative
and postoperative therapy includes a total of 8 VCR and 10
Act D injections. Then maintenance courses of 5 Act D
and 2 VCR injections are given. This chemotherapy
schedule has been adopted according to the results of
NWTS 1 and SIOP 2 and 5, which have shown that the
incidence of metastases could be dropped from 50% to 20%
by the combined and prolonged use of VCR and Act D.

CURRENT CLINICAL TRIAL PROBLEMS

There are several unanswered questions. For example,
is radiotherapy necessary in stage II? Moreover, are
two courses of maintenance chemotherapy as good as five
courses in stage I? Can a more aggressive chemotherapy
give better results in the poor prognosis group defined
by positive nodes and stage III? Adjuvant Adriamycin
has been compared to intensive VCR. It is indeed the
belief of many investigators that cardiac toxicity of
Adriamycin precludes its use in average cases, and we hope
to be able to show that even in more severe cases increased doses of VCR may replace it. Another question
is whether cyclophosphamide, added to the three other
drugs, is active in the unfavourable histology group?
Also, are there other drugs with which VCR, Act D and
Adriamycin may be active on Wilms' tumor?

SPECIAL SITUATIONS FOR SPECIAL TREATMENTS

In bilateral tumors, simultaneous or in succession, the treatment obviously has to be individualized. Here again, we use in all cases primary chemotherapy, and we continue it as long as the tumor can be shown to diminish. Then surgery is performed, attempting at removing completely all tumor in both kidneys, if possible, by bilateral partial nephrectomy. Postoperative radiotherapy is only used when there is proven residual tumor. In our experience, we have been able to cure patients this way without any radiotherapy to the remaining kidney(s) in three-fourths of the cases.

The treatment of nephroblastomatosis associated with nephroblastoma is still a matter of controversy. The treatment of metastases is also individualized, and is preferably based on chemotherapy and surgery. Radiotherapy can only be avoided in some rare selected cases. In those cases relapsing while on a VCR-Act D maintenance regimen, excellent results can be obtained with Adriamycin. In single metastases of the lungs, the treatment of choice is wedge resection followed by chemotherapy.

Babies do not necessarily do better than older children, but they tolerate the treatment poorly. This is the main reason why their treatment should be undertaken with great care and the doses of radiotherapy and chemotherapy adjusted to the young age.

CONCLUSION

Wilms' tumor is a rare tumor of childhood. No more than 100 new cases are diagnosed every year in France, a nation with 55 million inhabitants. This means that it is not possible for a large number of doctors to acquire the practical experience necessary to treat this tumor. We wish, as stated, to achieve the difficult and ambitious project of improving the cure rate of the bad cases, and of minimizing the adverse effects of treatment in average cases, without losing the excellent results we now obtain with our current treatment in terms of overall survival.

Moreover, we must realize that all Wilms' tumors in any country should be treated by experienced specialized teams or in a close cooperation with such teams. Also,

this has to be done on the basis of cooperative research
protocols. Any surgeon can remove a kidney, but only
one who is aware of the problem will be able to give the
pathologist and the chemotherapist the complete information which will enable them to define accurately the
stage and to decide the following treatment. The same
considerations apply to the pathologist, to the radio-
therapist and to the pediatric oncologist. Finally, none
of the individuals in charge of the patient is of critical
importance, but the team overall is. The major problem
of the present and of the near future may be an excess of
optimism, reflecting a veiw that "it is now easy to treat
Wilms' tumor and anybody can do it." This statement is
wrong and may lead to, and probably already has led to,
an increasing number of failures which could be avoided.

Lemerle J, Tournade MD, Sarrazin D, et al, 1981. Progrès
   et perspectives dan le traitement du néphroblastome.
   Etude de 724 cas traités à l'Institut Gastave-Roussy
   de 1952 à 1980. Arch Franc Pédiatrie, 38:329.

KIDNEY TUMORS IN ADULTS

Renal Tumors: Proceedings of the First International Symposium on Kidney Tumors, pages 175–206
© **1982 Alan R. Liss, Inc., 150 Fifth Avenue, New York, NY 10011**

MURINE RENAL CELL CARCINOMA: A SUITABLE HUMAN MODEL

Gerald P. Murphy, M.D., D.Sc.

Roswell Park Memorial Institute
666 Elm Street
Buffalo, NY   14263

Treatment of renal cell carcinoma in the advanced state
is not **always** effective (Murphy et al. 1970 and Woodruff
et al. 1967).   The growth pattern of this tumor is not as
well understood as that of some other malignant diseases,
and animal models of this pathologic entity have been
correspondingly scarce (Soloway and Myers Jr. 1973).

The **rare** clinical observation of regression of lung and
other measurable metastases after removal of the primary
renal tumor suggested the possibility of some controlling
factors, e.g., hormonal or immunologic (Hewitt 1967).   This
has spurred the clinical investigation of hormonal therapy
of this relatively radioresistant tumor (Wagle and Murphy
1971).   Two of the few existing models of renal cell tumor
have yielded experimental evidence for the hormonal control
of renal tumor growth.   These are the male Syrian golden
hamster model, which requires high concentrations of
diethylstilbestrol for both induction and transplantation
of the tumor (Horning and Whittick 1954, Kirkman and Bacon
1952 and Kirkman 1951), and the spontaneous tumor model,
studied by Soloway and Myers, in which growth is retarded
by either diethylstilbestrol or testosterone (Soloway and
Myers Jr. 1973).   This difference in response suggests that
some of these tumors are either stimulated or suppressed by
hormone therapy.   However, the results from clinical trials
with such therapy have been disappointing (Woodruff et al.
1967).   A quantitatively well-characterized renal cell
tumor model would be useful for evaluation of the many
chemotherapeutic agents produced each year.   The present
report discusses studies undertaken to develop, describe,

and characterize a transplantable renal cell carcinoma model, which may be more closely analogous to the human renal tumor.

GENERAL CHARACTERIZATION

Six-week-old weanling BALB/cCr male mice were used. This is a closely inbred line of BALB/c mice maintained at the West Seneca Laboratories, Roswell Park Memorial Institute. Histocompatibility studies by skin grafting are routinely performed at the West Seneca Laboratories to confirm maintenance of the line. Since details of preparation and handling can be critical, these will be included in this report.

The tumor was originally sent to us in July 1970 by Dr. Sarah Stewart, National Cancer Institute, Bethesda, Maryland. It arose spontaneously as a renal cortical adenocarcinoma and was passaged subcutaneously approximately every 35 days. The first descriptive study was begun when the tumor was in its sixth transfer generation.

The tumor was aseptically excised, trimmed of excess connective tissue, placed in a small sterile petri dish, and minced with two sterile knife blades. Chilled (4°C) McCoy medium containing 5% fetal bovine serum, penicillin (100 U/ml), and streptomycin (50µg/ml) was then added in a ratio of 9 ml: 1 g tissue. The mixture was poured into a sterile, chilled tissue grinder and quickly crushed into a suspension. After the solution was passed through a sterile, 27-gauge needle, cells were counted by hemocytometer. Viability was determined by erythrosin red (Lillie 1969), which stains living cells refractile green. The viability rate was consistently 90->95%. Unless otherwise indicated, the concentration was adjusted to 1×10^5 live tumor cells) either as a single injection or the same dose as 2 concurrent injections. A 27-gauge needle and a sterile glass 0.25 cc syringe were used for all transfers. The suspension was kept at 4°C and frequently agitated to prevent the settling of cells.

A cell suspension (1×10^6 live tumor cells) was frozen and thawed 4 times to rupture the cell membranes. There were no intact cells in this suspension as determined by erythrosin red stains. The chilled suspension was diluted tenfold with McCoy's medium and initially centrifuged at approximately 1200 rpm (International Clinical Centrifuge

Model CL) for 20 minutes; the supernatant was recentrifuged at approximately 3000 rpm (International Centrifuge, Model PR-2) for 1 hour. The supernatant was passed through a 200 mμ Millipore filter and then frozen at -40°C. Warmed (37°C) CFE solution (0.1 ml) was administered to experimental animals through a 27-gauge needle. The dose was equivalent in cytoplasmic content to 1×10^4 cells capable of transforming tumors 100% of the time (vide infra). Controls received 0.1 ml of McCoy's medium.

Groups received the tumor cell suspension, CFE, or McCoy's medium (controls) through a 27-gauge needle as a single, 0.1 ml dose or 2 doses of 0.05 ml either intra-peritoneally (ip), intramuscularly (im, hind thigh muscles), subcutaneously (sc, abdominal region), intravenously (iv, jugular vein exposed), or intrarenally (ir). The last group received a split dose (0.05 ml/kidney) after exposure and delivery of the kidneys through a 5-mm incision in the flanks through both skin and muscle layers. The cells remained under the renal capsule at a distance from the insertion point of the needle. Indicated surgical procedures were aseptically performed under ether anesthesia.

Careful autopsies were done on animals from each group after they were killed at days 28 and 40, and at death. In another experiment, autopsies were done on groups with tumor beneath the renal capsule on days 7, 14, 21, 28, 35, 42, 49, and at death from tumor. The tumors were examined by light and electron microscopy. At autopsy, tumor growth was measured as to degree of local extension, tumor weight, and presence or absence of local intracavity or distant metastases.

For comparison, a rating system was devised to measure quantitatively the degree of metastasis. Different anatomic situations of tumor spread were graded and given a value from 0-3+ as follows: 0=no tumor; 1+=local growth at injection site, 2+=local growth plus intracavity or regional spread; 3+=local growth plus intracavity (regional) spread plus distant metastasis. Each animal was given a score at autopsy. Group scores were totaled and divided by the number of animals in the group to yield an average metastatic score for comparison. Unusually heavy metastases were indicated by adding pluses to the basic score to a maximum of 3 (+++).

The results of the experiments were placed in 4 categories. 1) A general or descriptive category comprised observations consistent for each experiment--gross and histologic description of the tumor. Other general statements about the tumor were placed in this section, i.e., strain specificity and sex distribution of the tumor. 2) This category covered the kinetics of tumor growth and spread, and the survival of tumor-bearing animals as influenced by several controlled variables.

The group of experiments included: a) Determination of the minimum number of live tumor cells that induced the tumor 100% and 50% of the time and the standard dose of live tumor cells. b) Detailed comparison of 5 routes of transplantation with respect to percent of transferability, metastatic pattern, and average tumor weight 28 and 40 days after cell administration. Additional comparisons included the effects of this tumor in various organs on serum chemistries, hematocrit, and erythropoietin levels (Murphy et al. 1969). Erythropoietin assays were performed in the laboratories of Dr. E.A. Mirand, Roswell Park Memorial Institute (Camiscola and Gordon 1970). c) Choice of the ir route of transplant for more detailed evaluation because of its close resemblance to clinical primary renal cell carcinoma, its consistently quick lethality, and reproducible, early, widespread metastasis. Growth measured by tumor weight and metastatic pattern was evaluated by serial autopsy on days 7, 14, 21, 28, 35, 42, and 49 after tumor implantation. The mean survival rates of large groups of animals receiving a standard tumor transfer dose (1×10^5 live cells) ir were determined. d) Testing of the tumor model for sensitivity to hormones, i.e., to determine whether growth, metastatic spread, or survival was either facilitated or retarded by exposing the host to high doses of progestational (Depo Provera, The Upjohn Co., Kalamazoo, Mich.), androgenic (delatestryl, E.R. Squibb & Sons, New York, N.Y.), and estrogenic (diethylstilbestrol, Eli Lily & Co., Indianapolis, Ind.) agents. 3) This category includes results of investigations on the etiology of the tumor. Photomicrographs of the tumor consistently revealed virus-like particles 90-110 mμ in diameter that budded from the cell membrane and were free in the intercellular spaces. To investigate the possible viral etiology of the tumor, CFE's were prepared and passaged into groups of 6-week-old BALB/c mice, and 6-week-old Swiss mice. 4) This group of experiments investigated the immunogenicity of the tumor, i.e., whether the tumor cells contained antigens.

When the tumor was first received it was tested in both male and female groups of BALB/Cr mice with a 100% transfer by 1×10^5 live tumor cells. Since no sex difference in tumor growth were observed, males were used to facilitate animal maintenance. Swiss mice were given 1×10^6 cells--ten thousand times the dose of live tumor cells that induced the tumor in >90% of BALB/cr mice. Groups of 10 animals were killed and autopsied at 40, 60 and 90 days after inoculation. Tumors were not found either by gross or microscopic inspection.

Grossly and microscopically the tumor structure was essentially the same in all experiments. Grossly, it was grey to white and fairly vascular. It was usually firm to hard and fixed to its tumor bed. Often there was a necrotic center due to rapid growth, with visible hemorrhage into the necrotic tissue. The tumor invaded surrounding tissue and did not have a grossly definable encapsulation. Often this invasion included the entire abdominal viscera, the body wall, and diaphragm. Extensive metastases to lymph nodes were detectable at autopsy, as were later metastases to lung and other distant organs, including the liver, spleen, mediastinum, bladder and serosal surfaces of all gastro-intestinal organs. Regardless of inoculation site, the tumors were microscopically similar and were described as renal cell tumors that consisted of closely packed, large cells about half as large as renal tubular cells. The nuclei were large and moderately pleomorphic with approximately a 2:1 nuclear-to-cytoplasm ratio. These nuclei had 5-10 dark-staining nucleoli and mitotic figures were frequent. The cytoplasm was fairly homogenous with a small amount of vacuolization. There were occasional giant cells and multinuclear cells within the tumor mass. There was no consistent mononuclear cell reaction at the tumor margins. The cellular arrangement was that of an anaplastic carcinoma of renal origin. Microscopically there was no capsule, though there were sheets of somewhat more closely related epithelial cells at the periphery. The surrounding tissue was invaded, displaced, and compressed by the rapidly growing malignancy. The primary tumor and metastatic lesions were structurally similar (fig. 1 and 2).

TUMOR CELL KINETICS

The kinetics of tumor growth and metastases were

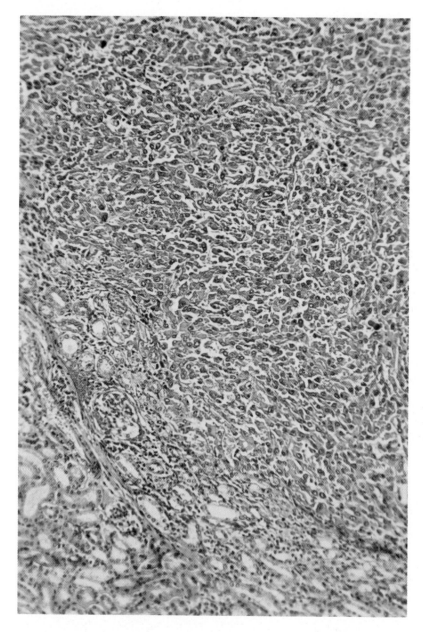

Fig. 1. Kidney inoculated with 1 X 10⁵ live tumor cells showing primary tumor lesion. Hematoxylin and eosin (H&E) X 220.

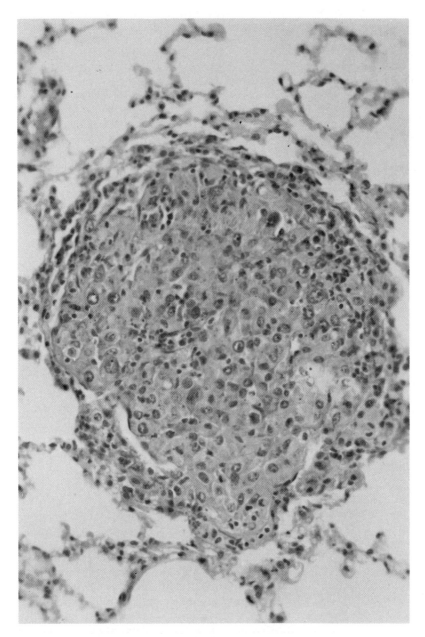

Fig. 2. Lung parenchyma with metastasis of renal cell tumor.
Note similarity to primary tumor. H&E X 400.

studied to define more clearly the growth rate of this neoplasm. Although the results might be affected by a host's immunogenic capability, as well as technical factors (e.g., cell preparation and dilution), these were minimized by randomizing the animals into groups and maintaining one known constant variable, i.e., cell dose. The tumor was transplanted by bilateral ir injection. Equal portions of cells were injected into each kidney for a total dose of $1X10^5$, $1X10^4$, $1X10^3$, $2X10^2$, $1X10^2$, or $5X10^1$ live tumor cells/animal. Thirty-five mice received each dose, and subgroups of the surviving animals were autopsied on days 40 and 60. Metastatic index, tumor weight, and tumor incidence were determined. The three highest doses transferred the tumor 100% of the time. The metastatic index and tumor weight were directly related to the number of cells transferred. The fourth and fifth highest doses transferred the tumor >90% of the time. The fourth highest dose transferred the tumor 100% in animals randomly autopsied at 40 days, but 3 of the animals autopsied on day 60 did not have tumor, giving an overall transfer rate of 92%. The metastatic index was low in this group. The incidence of tumor transfer at 40 days for the two lowest doses (100 and 50 cells) was 90 and 100%, respectively, and these animals had only small, local tumor growth. No tumor was observed in 25 control animals receiving McCoy's medium. The metastatic index and tumor weight were directly related to the number of cells transferred.

A dose of $1X10^5$ tumor cells was chosen as the standard for further experimentation because of the rapid extensive tumor growth, early metastasis, and the observation that 100% of these animals were dead before day 60, but few had died before day 40. This seemed an excellent period of survival for drug studies and other experimentation, since it would allow time for manipulation of variables and also have the advantage of obtaining results in a reasonable length of time.

To determine which method of transplant would serve best as a model of human renal cell carcinoma, 5 routes were compared in detail. Controls for this experiment consisted of an untreated group and a group that received McCoy's medium ir. These groups were compared at 28 and 40 days after transplant for tumor weight, metastatic index, survival, and anatomic resemblance to the human disease state. It was obvious that both tumor weight and metastatic index were greater at both days 28 and 40 in the animals that received the tumor cells ir. Animals receiving ir cells survived an average of 46 days, whereas in all other groups more than half the animals survived 60 days (Table 1). Animals receiving tumor cells iv developed lung tumor primarily.

The intrarenal transplantation route was the most interesting. It was chosen for further investigation for reasons previously cited. The survival of 105 animals that received $1X10^5$ live tumor cells ir was plotted. The mean was 46 days with few animals dying before 35 days or after 60 days (fig. 3). The early deaths recorded in this table were due to early, postoperative mortality which in this, the first group done, averaged 10%. In later groups this decreased markedly. This mortality range was suitable for the interposition of schedules and other variables. By day 21, 50% of the animals had palpable tumors. Thus the clinical situation was approximated in that the animals could be treated after they were symptomatic and receive several weeks of therapy before death.

Further studies were conducted on the tumor growth rate in the renal transplant site. Groups of animals were autopsied every 7 days after receiving $1X10^5$ live cells ir. Transferability, metastatic index, and tumor weight were recorded (Table 2). From these data tumor doubling time and numbers of tumor cells in the animal at various times after transfer could be estimated. Tumor doubling time was approximately 7 days.

At day 21, all animals had metastatic tumor, of which 50% were grossly palpable. An example of intermediate tumor growth in a representative animal on day 35 is shown in figure 4.

METABOLIC STUDIES

Serum chemistries were generally similar for all groups, though animals receiving tumor intrarenally had slightly elevated blood urea nitrogen and calcium, decreased alkaline phosphatase, and measurable bilirubin compared with other groups.

Some patients with renal tumor have a concurrent

TABLE 1

DISTRIBUTION, METASTASIS, INCIDENCE, AND TUMOR WEIGHT 40 DAYS AFTER IR TRANSFER

OF 1 X 10⁵ LIVE TUMOR CELLS, AND AVERAGE SURVIVAL TIME

Injection Route	Number of Animals	Index Distribution				Metastatic Index	Transfer (%)	Average Gross Primary Tumor weight (g)	Average Survival
		0	1+	2+	3+				
ir..............	105	0	0	13	92	2.9+	100	2.9 ± 0.5	46 days
ip..............	30	0	16	12	2	1.5+	100	1.1 ± 0.3	50%>60 days
iv..............	32	0	20	12	0	1.4+	100	1.8 ± 0.6	50%>60 days
im..............	29	0	29	0	0	1.0+	100	2.5 ± 0.5	50%>75 days
sc..............	30	0	30	0	0	1.0+	100	2.4 ± 0.3	50%>75 days
ir control, McCoy's medium	30	30	0	0	0	0	0	0	100%>6 months
Control.........	30	30	0	0	0	0	0	0	100%>6 months

ir: intrarenally
ip: intraperitoneally
iv: intravenously
im: intramuscularly
sc: subcutaneously

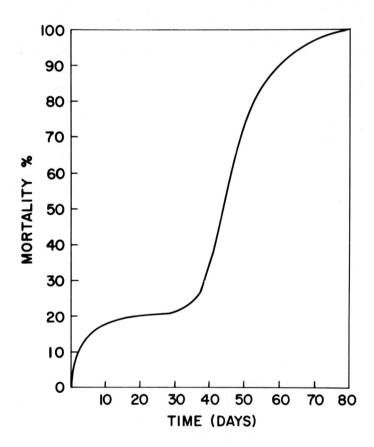

Fig. 3. Rate of mortality of mice given injections under the renal capsule of 1 X 10^5 live tumor cells.

Table 2

TUMOR GROWTH RATE AFTER IR ADMINISTRATION OF 1 x 10^5 LIVE TUMOR CELLS

Time (days	Animals Autopsied Animals Started	Transfer (%)	Metastatic Index	Average Gross Primary Tumor weight (g)
7	5/5	100	1.0+	Not measurable
14	5/5	100	2.0+	0.06 ± 0.02
21	5/5	100	2.4+	0.23 ± 0.05
28	20/25	100	2.4+	0.49 ± 0.20
35*	20/25	100	2.6+	1.04 ± 0.40
42	20/25	100	2.6+	1.35 ± 0.55
49	2/25	100	3.0+	0.66 ± 0.88

* Animals began dying of tumor.

polycythemia (Thorling and Ersback 1964, Rosse et al. 1963) and certain of these tumors produce an erythroid-stimulating factor (ESF) responsible for the secondary polycythemia (Murphy et al. 1970, Kenny et al. 1970, and Murphy et al. 1967). Measurements were therefore made to evaluate the effect of the route of tumor transplantation on the mean hematocrit of large groups of animals and the further effect of this tumor on plasma ESF levels as measured by bioassay (Murphy et al. 1969).

These values were all obtained at day 28, approximately 7 days after 50% of the animals had symptomatic or palpable tumor. The mean hematocrits of large groups of animals with ir tumor were significantly higher (p<0.05) than both untreated controls and controls which were surgically prepared to receive bilateral ir injections of McCoy's medium (54.1 vol%+3.8 as compared with 49.7 vol%+4.8, and 47.5 vol%+2.3, respectively). Groups with tumor implantation in the 4 other areas had hematocrits intermediate between ir value and the control values but not significantly above controls. Most groups with tumors had mean hematocrits greater than the control value (fig. 5).

There was suggestive evidence that the tumor was producing ESF or affecting normal ESF production and utilization. At day 28, the degree of pulmonary metastasis could not explain a systemic basis for hypoxic polycythemia (Table 1) (Fried et al. 1970). Silk reported that when inert, space-occupying glass beads were placed within the kidney, the hematocrit increased significantly. This was thought to be due to increased ESF production by the displaced, hypoxic normal kidney as measured by hematocrit level--not by ESF assay (Silk 1969).

To establish the relationship between tumor and the polycythemia in this experimental situation, the plasma ESF level of groups of animals with various routes of tumor transplant were compared with plasma obtained from controls (fig. 6a).

The only plasma with a significantly (p<0.05) elevated ESF level was that taken from animals with intrarenal tumor. This was greater than twice the control value. This result suggested that the polycythemia was caused by physical disruption and compression of the normal renal parenchyma. The observation was further evaluated by a bioassay of a

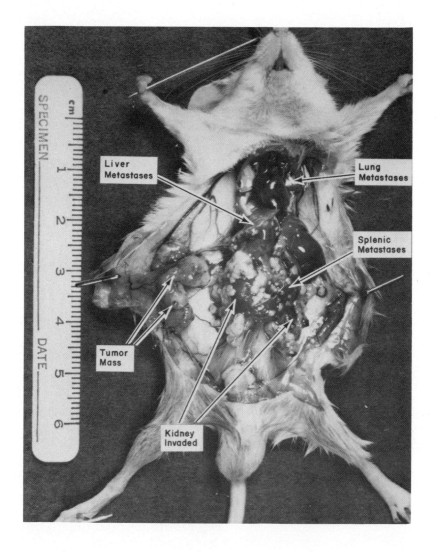

Fig. 4. Thirty-five days after bilateral ir tumor transplant. Tumor involves both kidneys and is metastatic to virtually all abdominal organs, with small metastatic nodules in the lung.

supernatant of tumor mash. The activity was the same as that found in plasma from controls (fig. 6b).

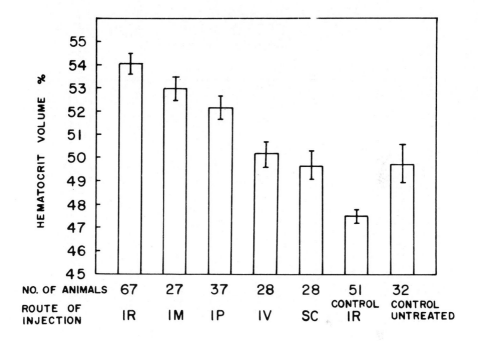

Fig. 5. Effect of tumor on hematocrit 28 days after transplantation by various routes of injection (1 x 10^5 live tumor cells).

HORMONAL STUDIES

This renal cell tumor model was studied for hormone sensitivity because of contrasting reports with other models and because of past efforts to treat renal cell tumor patients with hormonal therapy (Woodruff et al. 1967 and Kirkman 1951). Three hormones were investigated:

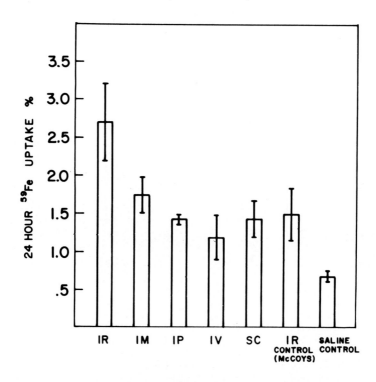

POOLED PLASMA ESF LEVELS ON
MICE INJECTED WITH TUMOR BY
VARIOUS ROUTES

Fig. 6a. Plasma levels of ESF 28 days after transplantation
by various routes of injection.

testosterone enanthate (Delatestryl), medroxyprogesterone
acetate (Depo-Provera), and a long-acting estrogen
(diethylstilbestrol in oil).

Depo-Provera: Fifty animals were given 15 mg. Depo-
Provera (DP) im on day 1. On day 2, 30 of these animals

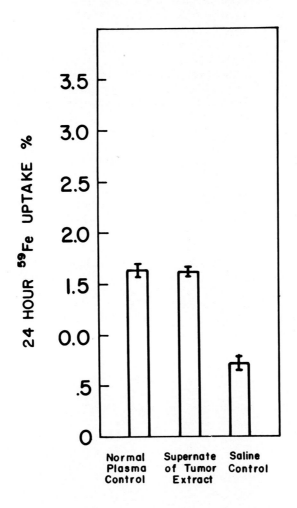

Fig. 6b. Plasma levels of ESF after injection of supernatant of tumor mash.

and 40 untreated controls received tumor by bilateral ir
transplant. Fifteen with DP and tumor and 10 with tumor
only were killed on day 40. Tumor weights were not significantly different (2.85$\pm$1.06 g) respectively, and animals
in both groups were rated 3+ for metastases. Ten DP animals
killed on day 40 were tumor free by gross and microscopic
examination. Fifteen DP and tumor and 10 tumor-control
animals lived until death by tumor. The hormone-treated
animals survived 44.9$\pm$6 days and the control animals 45$\pm$6
days. The 10 animals given hormone only, all alive at day
90, were killed and found to be tumor free. Thus DP did not
affect tumor weight, metastasis, or survival time significantly,
and high doses did not shorten life or induce renal tumors in
controls. This renal tumor model, then, is not sensitive to
progestational compounds either as inhibitors or stimulators
of tumor growth (Table 3).

Testosterone: Fifty animals were given 50 mg
testosterone-enanthate im on day 1; 30 of these received
tumor on day 2. Groups were divided as above. Forty
controls received tumor only, and twenty received only
testosterone. The hormone controls killed at 40 days had
no gross or microscopic tumor and all survived >90 days.
Animals given tumor plus hormone lived 29.4$\pm$6 days, and
controls with tumor only survived 50% longer (46$\pm$6 days)
(p<0.01). Metastases at day 40 were more extensive in the
group receiving hormone plus tumor. Tumor weight was less
at day 40 (2.34$\pm$0.4 g compared with 3.12$\pm$1.06 g in the 30
control animals). However, this weight was based on few 40-
day survivors and may not be significant.

Diethylstilbestrol: This estrogenic compound was tested
in a manner similar to the hormones outlined above. The
animals were given 0.5 mg of the compound im, every 7 days.
Animals receiving hormone only developed no tumor by day 40,
and 100% survived and were tumor free >90 days. Animals
given tumor plus hormone lived 29.4$\pm$6 days, and controls with
tumor only survived >50% longer (46$\pm$6 days) (p<0.1).
Metastases at day 40 were more extensive in the group
receiving hormone plus tumor. Tumor weight was less at day
40 (2.34$\pm$0.4 g compared with 3.12$\pm$1.06 g in the 30 control
animals). However, this weight was based on few 40-day
survivors and may not be significant. To summarize, tumor
growth was enhanced by both testosterone and synthetic
estrogen, but was not affected significantly by a progestational agent (Table 3).

Table 3

HORMONAL RESPONSE TO RENAL CELL—TREATED ANIMALS

| | Control | DP* (15 mg) | | DP* (30 mg) | | Diethylstilbestrol (0.5 mg) | |
	Tumor Only	Control	Tumor	Control	Tumor	Control	Tumor
Total number of animals.......	50	20	30	20	30	20	30
Survival (days)..............	45.00±6.00	90	44.90±6.0	90	37.00±5.0	90	20.40±6.0
Day 40							
Tumor weight (g)............	3.12±1.06	0	2.85±0.0	0	2.67±0.5	0	2.34±0.4
Metastatic Index............	3+	0	3+	0	3+++	0	3+++

*DP = Depo-Provera

TUMOR ETIOLOGY

The etiology of this tumor was investigated to a limited extent. For example, during a previous year over 1,500 mice have been processed in this laboratory and no tumors of any organ were noted, except those transplanted. However, most animals were killed before the age of 6 months, possibly before a genetic predisposition would be expressed.

Routine electron microscopy consistently revealed virus-like particles measuring 90X110 mμ in diameter in the cells, in intercellular spaces, and budding from cell membranes. To help determine if these particles could cause the tumor, several additional experiments were done. CFE was prepared as outlined and 10 hypoimmune 20-hour-old BALB/Cr mice were given ip injections of 0.1 ml warmed to 37°C. Ten control 24-hour-old mice received 0.1 ml of warmed McCoy's medium. All 20 animals were healthy and tumor free at day 90 and at a second observation 6 months after inoculation. CFE was also given by bilateral ir injection to 30 six-week-old BALB/cCr males. These animals and controls given McCoy's medium were tumor free when killed in groups of 10 at day 40, 60, and 90 after treatment. Thirty 6-week-old Swiss mice received this CFE and were also tumor free when killed and examined according to the same schedule. Another group was followed 6 months and no tumors were found. If these virus-like particles are responsible for this renal cell tumor, it was not proved by transfer of the tumor with a CFE alone. Possibly, intrauterine exposure to CFE could produce different results.

To help determine if this tumor developed a tumor-specific antigen which could provoke rejection by the host, a simple experiment was performed (Myers 1971). Thirty inbred BALB/cCr males were given $1X10^5$ live tumor cells in the left hind leg. When tumor was palpated (in 15 days) the leg was removed. The animal was then challenged in the right hind leg with a second dose of $1X10^5$ live tumor cells. Although the incidence of tumor at the first injection site was 100%, the incidence in the second leg was only 85% and tumor appeared at 21 days. These preliminary results suggested a possible host response to repeated tumor challenge.

We also used this model to study unilateral nephrectomy

performed at different stages of renal tumor growth and metastatic spread. This study resulted in a predictable and reproducible survival pattern. Early nephrectomy increased survival of the mice. While the tumor cells initially appeared confined to the kidney, the animals still died from metastatic disease later. Increased survival was not observed when the mice were nephrectomized after the tumor had spread to other organs (Williams et al. 1973).

Renal tumors often have metastasized at the time of first diagnosis. Metastases from the Wilms' tumor are usually found in regional lymph nodes, lungs, and liver but have also been found in unusual sites such as the bone marrow, parotid gland, and tonsil (Movassaghi et al. 1974). Metastases from the renal cell carcinoma can be found in practically all organs and tissues in the body but most of the metastases go to the lungs, lymph nodes, liver and bones (Mostofi 1967). The high metastatic incidence of these tumors is shared by a transplantable renal cell carcinoma in BALB/c mice (Muntzing et al. 1976).

The growth rate of metastases from various human carcinomas have been found to exceed the growth rate of their primaries in most cases (Charbit et al. 1971) Similar findings have been reported for animal tumors such as the Lewis lung carcinoma (Simpson-Herren et al. 1974) and already in 1915 Takahaski in his experimental study of metastases, found that tumor cells must be able to divide fast if they were to form metastases (Takahaski 1915). This difference in growth rate between metastasis and primary might indicate that the metastases are derived from selected cells with other metabolic characteristics than the majority of the tumor cells. This hypothesis is supported by the observation of chromosomal differences between the primary and metastases of an experimental animal tumor (Mitelman and Mark 1970).

As the tumor cells in the metastases have different growth characteristics from the tumor cells in the primary, it could be expected that transplanted metastatic cells would give rise to more rapidly growing tumors with a higher frequency of metastasis formation than in the case of transplanted tumor cells obtained from the primary. In a study we examined this hypothesis using the mouse renal cell adenocarcinoma as a model. These experimental tumors give

rise to lung metastases in a high frequency. Tumor cells
from such metastases, as well as tumor cells from primary
tumors, were transplanted to the experimental animals and
the growth and metastatic potential of the resulting tumors
were studied.

Wistar-Furth rats and BALB/c mice were implanted with
tumor cells from renal cell adenocarcinoma. In a preliminary
study the survival time, metastasis formation and growth of the
primary tumor after implantation of metastatic tumor cells did
not exceed those found after implantation of tumor cells from
the tumor primaries. It was then concluded that the higher
growth rate usually found in metastases was not necessarily
due to a selection of metastatic cells with a short cell
growth cycle but that there are other environmental factors
enhancing the growth of metastases (Muntzing et al. 1976).

METASTATIC STUDIES

Recent animal studies have indicated that metastatic
cells have different properties than the primary cells
(Muntzing et al. 1976 and Sugarbaker 1979) and may even
have a selective process which may determine the site of
metastatic growth (Poste and Fidler 1979, Fidler and Kripke
1980). Induction of this metastatic process requires these
specific cells to complete many steps before such growth
is accomplished (Fidler 1979, Fidler and Kripke 1977). In
other studies, a murine renal cell adenocarcinoma was used to
develop a more predictable model of metastatic murine renal
cell adenocarcinoma (Williams et al. and Suffrin et al. 1979).

Metastases occurred in all transfer groups at various
percentages in the animals implanted with metastatic lung
tissue (Table 4). In the first transfer, 40% of the animals
observed had gross metastatic lung growth. The first death
occurred on day 34. On day 35, ten animals were sacrificed
to harvest the lung metastases for implant of the second
transfer. Five animals from the 10 had lung metastases at
death. All animals had tumor growth at the primary implant
site in the second transfer group. On day 36 the remaining
10 animals were sacrificed and lung metastatic cells implanted
for the third transfer generation. At day 21, ten animals
were sacrificed and the lung metastatic tissue was implanted
for the next transfer. This procedure was followed for all

Table 4

SERIAL PASSAGE OF EXPERIMENTAL RENAL CELL METASTASES

Transfer Generation	Date of Implant	Day of Implant	Route of Implant	% of Metastases	Days of Survival
TG-1	1- 3-80	35	IM	40%	x̄41 ±7 n=15
TG-2	2- 8-80	36	IM	60%	x̄32 ±4 n=10
TG-3	3- 5-80	21	IM	+	x̄38 ±8 n=12
TG-4	3-26-80	21	IM	+	x̄28 ±7 n=15
TG-5	4-17-80	21	IM	+	x̄34 ±6 n=10
TG-6	5- 8-80	21	IM	+	x̄27 ±7 n=15
TG-7	5-29-80	21	IM	+	x̄31 ±3 n=12
TG-8	6-19-80	21	IM	+	x̄34 ±2 n=17
TG-9	7-10-80	21	IM	+	x̄37 ±8 n=12
TG-10	7-31-80	21	IM	+	x̄34 ±3 n=15
TG-11	8-22-80	21	IM	80%	x̄29 ±4 n=12
TG-12	9-11-80		IM	90%	x̄26 ±2 n=15

+ minimum % of metastases 25%
values are expressed as x̄± SEM
n = number of animals evaluated

the successive transfer generations. After several passages
an increase in the incidence of lung metastases was observed
from 40% in the first transfer to 90% in the twelfth transfer.
Metastases occurred in all groups in animals implanted with
grossly metastatic tissue. By the 12th transfer generations
90% of animals had developed lung metastases. Animals
receiving the tumor implants were observed to have metastases
earlier and died also as soon as 28 days. Histological
evaluation of these tumor (primary and lung) metastases
demonstrated renal cell adenocarcinoma and similar lung
metastases invading the vascular structures. These
results suggest that some tumor selection without tissue
culture can occur by renal tumor passage which will, as a
result, kill some with more widespread tumor.

CHEMOTHERAPY SCREENING

At present multiple chemotherapeutic agents are
potentially available for treating metastatic renal adenocarcinoma. However, the clinical value of some of these
agents in this tumor remains untested. Clearly, a
predictive experimental model for the testing of drugs for
possible clinical use would be of value (Schabel 1975). We
studied the kinetic aspects of the growth of this tumor and
describe the effect of drugs or of radiation on tumor
deoxyribonuclease acid (DNA) synthesis. The present status
of the model thus permits added insight into fundamental
mechanisms of tumor control and correlates well with other
important investigational end points such as tumor weight
and animal survival (Sufrin et al. 1979, Murphy and
Hrushesky 1973).

This model is based on a transplantable murine renal
adenocarcinoma whose growth follows Gompertzian kinetics,
relates to tumor RNA and DNA content, and also correlates
with the rate of tumor DNA synthesis. This model in the
current study was also evaluated for the ability of various
therapeutic agents to inhibit tumor DNA synthesis (Sufrin
et al. 1979). Such tests may be valuable for the preclinical
screening of potentially useful drugs and may provide insight
into fundamental aspects of tumor control. In this study,
CCNU, BCNU, and adriamycin were potent inhibitors of tumor
DNA synthesis whereas cytosine arabinoside, bleomycin,
and cyclophosphamide were not (Sufrin et al. 1979). These
observations were confirmed by autoradiography and correlated

with other experimental end points of tumor therapy such
as tumor weight and animal survival. This preclinical
screening model is an effective and helpful means whereby
new drugs and drug combinations can be tested for potential
use in human renal cell carcinoma (Sufrin et al. 1979).

MeCCNU (1-(2-chloroethyl)-3-(4-methylcyclohexyl)-1-
nitrosourea (NSC95441) alone and in combination with Velban
were also evaluated for therapeutic effectiveness in a
previously characterized, transplantable murine renal cell
adenocarcinoma. MeCCNU given early or late in a normal 32
day untreated survival period showed a dose-related,
significant increase in survival rate without remarkable
inhibition of the growth of the transplanted renal primary
tumor. Velban in combination with MeCCNU did not detectably
improve this state. Animals were also treated or untreated,
and were sacrificed at 28 days for various measurements.
MeCCNU given early at low doses was associated with a
significant (p<.01) decrease in the number of metastases,
and a significant decrease in the growth of the renal primary.
MeCCNU in this system appears to have significant effects,
although the mode of action is unsettled (Murphy and Williams
1974).

However, further studies using BALB/c mice with implanted
tumor cells from primary tumor in donor animals bearing
renal cell adenocarcinoma were completed. Survival time,
tumor growth and metastatic occurrance in treated animals
were not significantly improved by high dose Methyl-CCNU,
CCNU or Vincristine. It was also concluded that the dose
levels of Methyl-CCNU and CCNU used for this study were
highly toxic causing early death in the animals. Such
studies thus fail to support clinical hopes that these
agents would be effective for chemotherapy regimens in human
renal tumors (Williams et al. 1981).

An evaluation of hexamethylmelamine was attempted to
establish its therapeutic value in the treatment of renal
cell carcinoma. A murine renal cell adenocarcinoma model
was treated with three dosage levels of hexamethylmelamine
at an early and late stage of disease occurrence. From
the results observed and analyzed, it seems unlikely that
hexamethylmelamine may be of clinical benefit in the
treatment of renal carcinoma in man (Williams et al. 1974).

The potential prolongation of survival of actinomycin

D entrapped in liposomes was also examined in BALB C/Cr mice
inoculated intrarenally with renal cell adenocarcinoma.
There were five groups of animals: group A, a control group,
received phosphate-buffered saline 0.3 cm i.p.; group B
received free actinomycin D 300µg/kg i.p.; group C received
liposomes containing actinomycin D 300µg/kg i.p.; group D
received a mixture of free actinomycin D 300µg/kg and empty
liposomes i.p.; group E received empty liposomes i.p. The
best median survival was of group (free drug) -- 54 days
followed by group C (liposome entrapped actinomycin D) 45.2
days and group E (a mixture of free and entrapped actinomycin
D) - 42 days.

In vitro studies utilizing cell lines obtained from the
tumor showed no statistical difference in ID_{50} or in
cytotoxicity between the cells treated with free actinomycin
D and those treated with liposomes containing drug (Kedar
et al. 1981).

It seems, in contrast to earlier hopes that liposome
entrapment would result in selective drug delivery to
tumor (Kaye et al. 1980, Papahadjopoulos et al. 1976 and
Gregoriadis 1973), that a slow release of the drug into
the circulation (Mayhew et al. 1978, Kimelberg and Mayhew
1978) with 45-50% of the injected dose still present in
the blood 3 h later (Juliano and Stamp 1978) probably is
the explanation of liposome drug effects. Although it
has been postulated that actinomycin D resistance acquired
in vivo is a result of failure of drug retention rather than
failure of drug uptake (Kaye et al. 1980), this postulate
is not required to explain our results.

The mechanism of cytotoxicity of actinomycin D has
been shown to be different for a high and for a low dose
(Papahadjopoulos et al. 1976 and Gregoriadis 1973). For
low dose, cytotoxicity is thought to be limited to cells in
DNA synthesis similar to the action of phase-specific agents;
whereas for high dose of actinomycin D, an exponential dose-
survival relationship exists (Papahadjopoulos et al. 1976
and Gregoriadis 1973). This mechanism may well explain our
in vivo results as well as those obtained in vitro where
no difference was found in cell kill between free and
entrapped actinomycin D. Apparently, cytotoxicity in both
cases was due to free drug released from the liposomes.
Indeed, if slow release of drug is the mechanism of action
of agents entrapped in liposomes, it can be predicted that

the action of phase-specific drugs can be enhanced by entrapment in nontargeted presently available liposomes while the action of nonphase-specific agents could even be retarded. In other current pilot studies there appear to be such promising results.

OTHER MODELS

Other attempts at the induction of renal tumor have been successful and have varied. Cycasin is an example (Mayhew et al 1978, Williams and Murphy 1971). Cycasin treated young mice or rats were studied for the induction of renal or hepatic tumors. In mice, hepatomas can be induced with two doses (0.25mg each) of cycasin (Williams and Murphy 1971). In contrast, in rats renal adenomas are induced following a single dose (0.5mg) of cycasin. Prior unilateral nephrectomy or ureteral ligation and cycasin treatment does not increase renal adenoma incidence. Interruption of the renal counterbalance as performed in the present experiments, thus did not influence tumor induction. Metastasizing tumors following higher cycasin doses have been previously reported. These observations demonstrate that renal adenomas or hepatomas can be induced at lower doses, but at lower frequency. Dimethylnitrosamine is a further example of chemical induction of a renal tumor (Murphy et al. 1966, Schmidt and Murphy 1966). Unfortunately, with this tumor the incidence, as in cycasin, is not as high, the incidence of metastases is not as high nor is it reproducible as with the BALB/c model extensively described in this report. Other attempts in selection have occurred and have been recently described but are similarly unimpressive (Bannasch et al. 1979).

Other more recent studies have suggested that other compounds can and should be screened for potential effect (Iker et al. 1981, Bannasch et al. 1974, Bannasch et al. 1978, Bannasch et al. 1978 and Bannasch et al. 1980). Using the Wistar/Lewis rat, Olssen has also developed a model which appears similar to the BALB/c model described herein (White and Olsson 1980). For easy review of other spontaneous hormonal and chemically induced animal models, a recent workshop of the International Union Against Cancer provides available references (Sufrin and Beckley 1980). Hormones, aromatic amines, natural products and other natural agents can induce tumor. Viral models of renal adenocarcinoma are are available in frogs, rodents, hamsters, and chickens.

Despite this parallelity of observations, few of these models are comparable, in our opinion, to the reproducible and available BALB/c model which we have employed since 1970 at Roswell Park Memorial Institute. The tumor model has been successfully distributed to others and the results are similar to those herein described.

ABSTRACT AND SUMMARY

Many models of renal cell carcinoma are available. They have been observed in various species of animals. However, a renal adenocarcinoma which metastasizes, is available for study, and can be serially transplanted in BALB/c mice, appears to be the currently favored model. Our results reported herein describe a study on tumor kinetics, the effects of chemotherapy and other manipulations which appear relevant to the human state. A brief description of other available models is provided.

ACKNOWLEDGMENT

Much of this work was performed in collaboration with Dr. William J. Hrushesky, now at the University of Minnesota Medical Center, Dr. Gerald Sufrin, now at the Washington University Medical School, and Phyllis D. Williams at Roswell Park Memorial Institute, over the past 10 years.

Bannasch P, Mayer D, Krech R (1979). Neoplastiche und Praneoplastische Veranderungen bei ratten nach einmaliger oraler applikation von N-nitrosomorpholin. J. Cancer Res. Clin. Oncol. 94:233.

Bannasch P, Schacht U, Storch E (1974). Morphogenese und mikromorphologie epithelialer nierentumoren bei nitrosomorpholin-vergifteten ratten. I. Induktion und histologie der tumoren. Z. Krebsforsch 81:311.

Bannasch P, Krech R, Zerban H (1978). Morphogenese und mikromorphologie epithelialer nierentumoren bei nitro-somorpholin-vergifteten ratten. Z. Krebsforsch, II. Tubulare Glykogenose und die genese von klar-oder acido-philzelligen tumoren. Z. Krebsforsch 92:63.

Bannasch P, Krech R, Zerban H (1978). Morphogenese und mikromorphologie epithelialer nierentumoren bei nitro-somorpholin-vergifteten ratten. III. Onkocytentubuli und onkocytome. Z. Krebsforsch 92:87.

Bannasch P, Krech R, Zerban H (1980). Morphogenese und mikromorphologie epithelialer nierentumoren bei nitro-somorpholin-vergifteten ratten. IV. Tubulare lasionen und basophile tumoren. J. Cancer Res. Clin. Oncol. 98:243.

Camiscola JF, Gordon AS (1970). Bioassay and standardization of erythropoietin. In "Regulation of Hematopoiesis," p 369.

Charbit A, Malaise EP, Tubiana M (1971). Relation between the pathological nature and the growth rate of human tumors. Europ. J. Cancer 7:307.

Fidler IJ, Gersten DM, Hart IR (1978). The biology of cancer invasion and metastasis. Adv. Cancer Res. 28:149.

Fidler IJ, Kripke ML (1980). Biological variability within murine neoplasms. Antibiot. Chemother. 28:123.

Fidler IJ (1979). Tumor heterogeneity and the biology of cancer invasion and metastasis. Cancer Res. 37:2481.

Fidler IJ, Kripke ML (1977). Metastasis results from pre-existing variant cells within a malignant tumor. Science 197:893.

Fried W, Johnson C, Heller P (1970). Observations on regulation of erythropoiesis during prolonged period of hypoxia. Blood 36:607.

Gregoriadis G (1973). Drug entrapment in liposomes: possibility for chemotherapy. FEBS Lett. 36:292.

Hewitt CB (1967). Renal cell carcinoma: A clinical challenge. In Renal Neoplasia, Stanton King J., Jr. (ed). Boston: Little, Brown and Company, p 3.

Horning ES, Whittick JW (1954). The histogenesis of stilboestrol-induced renal tumours in the male golden hamster. Brit. J. Cancer 8:451.

Iker R, Mossige J, Johannesen JV, Aars H (1981). Hereditary renal adenomas and adenocarcinomas in rats. Diag. Histopathol. 4:99.

Juliano RL, Stamp D (1978). Pharmacokinetics of liposome-encapsulated antitumor drugs. Biochem. Pharmac. 27:21.

Kaye SB, Boden JA, Ryman BE (1980). The application of liposome entrapped cytotoxic drugs to the treatment in vivo of drug resistant solid murine tumours. Proc. ASCO/AACR 20:254.

Kedar A, Mayhew EG, Moore RH, Murphy GP (1981). Failure of Actinomycin D entrapped in liposomes to prolong survival in renal cell adenocarcinoma-bearing mice. Oncology 38:311.

Kenny GM, Mirand EA, Staubitz WJ et al. (1970). Erythropoietin levels in Wilms' tumor patients. J. Urol. 104:758.

Kimelberg H, Mayhew E. (1978). Properties and biological effects of liposomes and their uses in pharmacology and toxicology. Crit. Rev. Toxicol. 6:25.

Kirkman H, Bacon, RL (1952). Estrogen-induced tumors of the kidney. I. Incidence of renal tumors in intact and gonadectomized male golden hamsters treated with diethylstilbestrol. J. Nat'l Cancer Inst. 13:745.

Kirkman H (1951). Relation of sex hormones to the induction and control of renal tumors in the golden hamster. Anat. Rec. 109:311.

Lillie RD (1969). H.J. Conn's Biological Stains. Baltimore: The Williams & Wilkins Co., p. 248.

Mayhew E, Papahadjopoulos D, Rustum YM, Dave C (1978). Use of liposomes for the enhancement of the cytotoxic effect of cytosine arabinoside. Ann. N.Y. Acad. Sci. 308:371.

Mitelman F, Mark J (1970). Chromosomal analysis of primary and metastatic Rous sarcoma in the rat. Hereditas 65:227.

Mostofi FK (1967). Renal Neoplasm. Stanton King, J. Jr. (ed): "Pathology and spread of renal cell carcinoma." Boston: Little, Brown and Company, p. 41.

Movassaghi N, Leikin S, Chandra R (1974). Wilms' tumor metastatis to uncommon sites. J. Pediatr. 84:416.

Muntzing J, Williams PD, Murphy GP (1976). The growth characteristics of metastases from experimental renal tumors. Res. Comm. Chem. Path. and Pharm. 13:541.

Murphy GP, Moore RH, Kenny GM (1970). Current results from primary and secondary treatment of renal cell carcinoma. J. Urol. 104:523.

Murphy GP, Mirand EA, Grace JT, Jr. (1969). Erythropoietin activity in anephric or renal allotransplanted man. Ann. Surg. 170:581.

Murphy GP, Kenny GM, Mirand EA (1970). Erythropoietin levels in patients with renal tumors or cysts. Cancer 26: 191.

Murphy GP, Mirand EA, Johnston GS et al. (1967). Erythropoietin release associated with Wilms' tumor. Johns Hopkins Med. J. 120:26.

Murphy GP, Hrushesky WJ (1973). A murine renal cell carcinoma. J. Nat'l Cancer Inst. 50:1013.

Murphy GP, Williams PD (1974). Testing of chemotherapeutic agents in murine renal cell adenocarcinoma. Res. Comm. Chem. Path. and Pharm. 9:265.

Murphy GP, Mirand EA, Johnston GS, Schmidt JD, Scott WW (1966). Renal tumors induced by a single dose of Dimethylnitrosamine: Morphologic, functional, enzymatic, and hormonal characterizations. Invest. Urol. 4:39.

Myers GH, Jr. (1971). Detection of tumor-specific transplantation antigens in a murine renal cortical carcinoma. Surg.
Forum 22:517.

Papahadjopoulos D, Poste G, Vail WJ, Biedler JL (1976). Use
of lipid vesicles as carriers to introduce actinomycin D
into resistant tumor cells. Cancer Res. 36:2988.

Poste G, Fidler IJ (1979). The pathogenesis of cancer
metastasis. Nature 283:139.

Rosse WF, Waldmann TA, Cohen P (1963). Renal cysts, erythropoietin and polycythemia. Am. J. Med. 34:76.

Schabel FM, Jr. (1975). Animal models as predictive systems.
"Cancer Chemotherapy - Fundamental Concepts and Recent
Advances," Chicago: Year Book Medical Publishers, Inc.
p. 323.

Schmidt JD, Murphy GP (1966). Urinary lactic dehydrogenase
activity in rats with Dimethylnitrosamine induced renal
tumors. Invest. Urol. 4:57.

Silk M (1969). Erythrocythemic response to a nonfunctioning
renal "mass" lesion. Surgery 65:943.

Simpson-Herren L, Sanford AH, Holmquist JP (1974). Cell
population kinetics of transplanted and metastatic Lewis
lung carcinoma. Cell Tissue Kinet. 7:349.

Soloway MS, Myers GH, Jr. (1973). The effect of hormonal
therapy on a transplantable renal cortical adenocarcinoma
in the syngenic mice. J. Urol. 109:356.

Sufrin G, Tritsch GL, Moore RH, Murphy GP (1979). Adenosine
deaminase activity in a transplantable murine renal
adenocarcinoma. Invest. Urol. 16:321.

Sufrin G, Beckley SA (1980). A series of workshops on the
biology of human cancer, report no. 10. "Renal
Adenocarcinoma", Geneva: International Union Against
Cancer, vol. 49.

Sugarbaker EV (1979). Cancer Metastasis: A product of
tumor-host interactions. Curr. Probl. Cancer 7:3.

Takahaski M (1915). An experimental study of metastases.
J. Path. Bact. 20:1.

Thorling EB, Ersbak J (1964). Erythrocytosis and hypernephroma. Scand. J. Haematol. 1:38.

Wagle D, Murphy GP (1971). Hormonal therapy in advanced
renal cell carcinoma. Cancer 28:318.

White RD, Olsson CA (1980). Renal adenocarcinoma in the
rat. A new tumor model. Invest. Urol. 17:405.

Williams PD, Bhanalaph T, and Murphy GP (1973). Unilateral
nephrectomy. Its effect on primary murine renal adenocarcinoma.
Urology 2:619-622.

Williams PD, Pontes JE, Murphy GP. Studies on the growth of
a murine renal cell carcinoma and its metastatic patterns.
Res. Comm. in Chem. Pathol. & Pharm. (in press)

Williams PD, Burdick J, Murphy GP (1974). Evaluation of
Hexamethylmelamine in murine renal cell carcinoma model.
Res. Comm. in Chem. Path. and Pharm. 7:399.

Williams PD, Murphy GP (1971). Dose related effects of
Cycasin induced renal and hepatic tumors. Res. Comm. in
Chem. Path. and Pharm. 2:627.

Williams PD, Kantor P, Murphy GP (1981). Evaluation of
Vincristine, CCNU, and Methyl-CCNU at high level doses in
an experimental murine renal adenocarcinoma model. Res.
Comm. in Chem. Path. and Pharm. 31:529.

Woodruff MW, Wagle D, Gailani SD et al. (1967). The
current status of chemotherapy for advanced renal carcinoma.
J. Urol. 97:611.

Renal Tumors: Proceedings of the First International Symposium on Kidney Tumors, pages 207–208
© 1982 Alan R. Liss, Inc., 150 Fifth Avenue, New York, NY 10011

THE CLINICAL SIGNIFICANCE OF NMRI NU/NU MICE TUMOR MODEL

Ullrich Otto, Hartwig Huland

Wissenschaftlicher Assistent, Oberarzt
Urologische Klinik der Universität Hamburg
2000 Hamburg 20, W. Germany

There is a need for a tumor model for renal adenocarcinoma. Five-year survival results have been almost
stable during the last 20 years at the level of deprimating
(50%) (Flocks, Kadesky 1958; Skinner et al. 1972). Clinical
data are difficult to obtain since adenocarcinoma of the
kidney is relatively rare, presents with different staging
morphology and sometimes unpredictable clinical course
develops. So, reliable prognostic parameters are not yet
available in our opinion.

In this study we present data of 20 transplantations
of renal adenocarcinoma to nu/nu mice taken from 20 consecutive patients seen and operated during a period of 2
years in our department. To prove the significance of the
nu/nu mice tumor model we were interested in the identity
of the transplanted and primary tumor and the correlation
of the clinical course of the 20 patients with the growing
rate of the transplant in the mice.

Thymus-aplastic NMRI nu/nu mice (Hannover) were used.
At the time of transplantation the animals were 7 weeks old.
From each patient a tissue sample (3 x 3 x 1 cm) was taken
immediately after nephrectomy under sterile conditions
and transplanted to the neck of at least four animals
subcutaneously. At the time of operation all but one
patient was free from metastases on the basis of chest X-ray
and whole body computer tomogram. The following observations
were made.

a) In almost all cases the morphology comparing the

primary and the transplanted tumors was identical, except
in one case of a mixed granular cell and sarcomatoid tumor
in which the latter was identified in the test mouse. Cellular proliferation, according to the flowcytometric analysis,
was also identical before and after transplantation. Chromosomal analysis was compatable with human tissue in two
transplanted tumors that were examined.

b) Calculation of the growing rate in the nu/nu mice
after transplantation was based on weekly measurements of
the tumor size. All transplanted tumors were accepted
except in 6 out of 7 animals which received tumors that
had received preoperative radiation therapy. In the other
cases we found a close correlation between the growth rate
of the transplanted tumors in the nu/nu mice and the
clinical course of the patients in the first one or two
years after tumor nephrectomy. According to the growth
rate in the nu/nu mice, we had 3 groups, with either a
fast, a moderate or a slow growth rate. Three out of four
patients whose tumors belonged to fast group died 3, 4 and
5 months after operation. The fourth who had metastases
at the time of operation had a temporary decrease of
pulmonary metastases. This was considered to be either the
result of chemotherapy or as spontaneous remission. The
one corresponding patient of the moderate group died 14
months after his tumor nephrectomy. Nine tumors transplanted belong to the slow group. All corresponding
patients are still alive. Eight are clinically tumor free.
The only one in this group who developed metastases had
the fastest growth rate in the nu/nu mice in this group.
In contrast to the patients in the fast and moderate groups,
his metastases developed 15 months after operation.

It is our impression that this model may give reliable
information about the expected prognosis of some renal
tumor patients. The initial good but limited clinical
correlation also suggests that the transplanted tumor in
the nu/nu mice may be a relevant model for further investigation.

Flocks RH, Kadesky MC (1958). Malignant neoplasma of the
   kidney: an analysis of 353 patients followed five years
   or more. J Urol 79:196.
Skinner DG, Vermillion CD, Colvin RB (1972). The surgical
   management of renal cell carcinoma. J Urol 107:705.

Renal Tumors: Proceedings of the First International Symposium on Kidney Tumors, page 209
© 1982 Alan R. Liss, Inc., 150 Fifth Avenue, New York, NY 10011

EVALUATION OF EFFECTIVE VINBLASTINE-SULFATE DOSAGE IN DIFFERENT RENAL CELL CARCINOMAS AFTER TRANSPLANTATION TO THE NU/NU MICE

U. Otto, H. Huland, H. Klosterhalfen

Department of Urology

University of Hamburg
West Germany

Four different human renal cell carcinomas, successfully transplanted to the NMRI nu/nu mice, were treated for six weeks in four different groups receiving 0.6, 1.2, 1.8 µg/kg vinblastine-sulfate or NaCl to obtain objective data about tumor response. Results of this study indicate that vinblastinetherapy was effective in all groups. Tumors with fast growing-rates and high rates of proliferation, as judged by flowcytometry, showed a significantly better response to vinblastinetherapy. Tumor response correlated well with the vinblastine dosage, particularly those with high proliferation rates.

We, therefore, conclude that our experimental data suggest that vinblastine therapy might be useful only in highly proliferating renal cell carcinomas.

Renal Tumors: Proceedings of the First International Symposium on Kidney Tumors, pages 211–244
© **1982 Alan R. Liss, Inc., 150 Fifth Avenue, New York, NY 10011**

RECEPTOR PROFILES IN RENAL CELL CARCINOMA

James P. Karr, Sarah Schneider, Hanna Rosenthal, Avery A. Sandberg and Gerald P. Murphy
Roswell Park Memorial Institute
666 Elm Street
Buffalo, New York   14263

INTRODUCTION

The role of steroid receptors in carcinomatous tissue was the subject of a recent review (Sandberg and Karr, 1980) which pointed to the growing number of reports on human organs and glands in which cytosolic and nuclear receptors have been detected. Even though some tissues are not considered, in a very strict sense, to be target tissues of hormonal action, the presence of specific hormone receptors in such "non-target" organs suggests that primary malignancies known to occur in such tissues could be hormonally dependent. Human renal cancer represents such a possibility.

Current interest in steroid receptors in renal tissue and the use of hormonal therapy in renal cell carcinoma stems in part from 1) an early report (Mathews et al, 1947) on the occurrence of renal damage in golden hamsters following chronic administration of diethylstilbestrol (DES) and 2) the subsequent observations (Kirkman and Bacon, 1950, 1952; Kirkman and Robbins, 1959) of estrogen induced transformation of the proximal convoluted tubules of the kidney to adeno-carcinoma in this species. Other endocrine related traits of the Syrian hamster renal carcinoma including the presence of steroid receptors and a dependency on estrogen have since been documented (Li et al, 1977, 1979). These and other studies (Steggles and King, 1972) have, in fact, characterized the presence of significant concentrations of (7 to 8S) cytosolic receptors for progesterone, estradiol (E_2), 5α-dihydrotestosterone (DHT), dexamethasone and aldosterone, the steroid receptor complexes of which all undergo nuclear translocation. While there is no apparent cross reactivity of estrogen and progesterone receptors for their respective hormones, progesterone does compete for both androgen and adrenocorticord binding. Expressed in femtomoles per mg of cytosol protein, the most prevalent specific receptor protein in the hamster renal cancer model is that for progesterone (1946), followed by E_2 (218), DHT (154), dexamethasone (138) and aldosterone (40).[2] Relative concentrations similar to those of primary tumors persist following three or more intraperitoneal serial tumor transfers to estrogenized hamsters, as do other characteristics including cross compe- tition, binding affinity constants and sedimentation coefficients (Li and Li, 1980). Estrogen binding levels of normal hamster kidney cytosol (6.48 fmol/mg protein) increased to 9.23 fmol over a 6-month period of estrogen treatment and the development of renal tumors is associated with even higher levels (13.7fmols) of estrogen binding (Andersson et al, 1979). Similarly, the concentration of progesterone binding sites increases within two months of the initiation of estrogen induced tumorigenesis in the hamster kidney, and this change is detectable prior to the formation of tumors at six months (Lin et al, 1978).

The presence of estrogen receptors in kidney tissue of other species, including the rat, mouse, and guinea pig,have been described (Murono et al, 1979; DeVries et al, 1972; Pasqualini et al, 1973), but these rodents are not known to be susceptible to estrogen induced renal cell carcinoma. Interestingly, the cytosol concentration of estrogen receptor in normal rat kidney is over twice that of normal hamster kidney (Andersson et al, 1979).

Tumor models of renal adenocarcinoma in the mouse (Murphy and Hrushesky, 1973) and rat (deVere White and Olsson, 1980) have been reported to have features suitable for comparison to human renal cancer, including the sponta- neous origin of both tumors and their predictable patterns of metastases and hormonal independence. In contrast to the estrogenic induction of renal tumors in hamsters,which can be inhibited by the antiestrogen nafoxidine (Antonio et al, 1974), the prolactin inhibitor bromocriptine (Hamilton et al, 1975) and desoxycorticosterone and progesterone (Kirkman, 1959), renal tumor growth in the murine model was enhanced with a determined effect on animal survival and increased metastases by exogenous testosterone or DES. Growth of the murine tumor model was unaffected by Depo-Provera, a progestational agent (Murphy and Hruskesky, 1973); however, the tumor is successfully transferred with as few as 1000 live cells in untreated animals. Recent analyses in our laboratory indicate that there is no detectable progestin binding in cytosols of pooled specimens of this tumor, and that while there is a small amount (<3fmol/mg cytosol protein) of strong, displaceable R1881 binding in the cytosol, there is none in the nuclear extract. There is, however, a measurable estrogen cytosol receptor in this tumor, which ranges in concentration from 10-15fmoles/mg of cytosol protein, and has a K_d of 3-7 x 10^{-9}M. On sucrose density gradient centrifugation analysis, an 8S binding component for (^{3}H)-estradiol is readily displaced by nafoxidine (Figure 1).

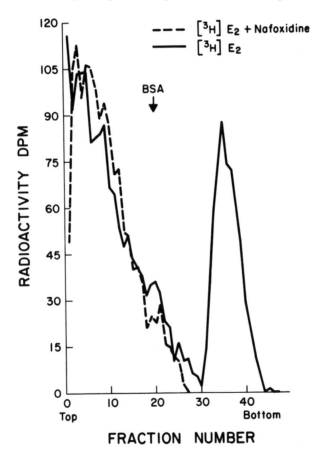

Fig. 1. Estrogen cytosol receptor in murine renal cell carcinoma.

Hormonal therapy was also ineffective against the rat renal cancer model described by deVere White and Olsson (1980); such findings are in sharp distinction to the estrogen induced Syrian hamster renal adenocarcinoma which can be treated successfully with progestins and androgens (Kirkman and Bacon, 1952; Shefner and Marlow, 1975; Bloom et al, 1967; Bloom et al, 1963).

The various animal studies cited above, as well as a number of clinical and epidemiological observations, have led to the suggestion that an endocrine imbalance may accompany human renal cell carcinoma and to the hypothesis that this cancer may be hormonally dependent. These views are based, in part, on statistics which show that the incidence of renal carcinoma is significantly greater in men than women, the male to female ratio being greatest in the child bearing ages of women (~4:1), and dropping to 2:1 during the early- to mid-forties and remaining unchanged following menopause (Matsuda et al, 1976). In the United States, an estimated 17,000 new cases of renal carcinoma will be diagnosed in 1981, with approximately an incidence twice as high in men than in women (Whitehead, 1981). Men, however, are favored in terms of having a higher frequency of reported spontaneous regression of renal cell carcinoma than in women (Bloom, 1973). There are also some data which suggest that adrenal hormones play a role in the primary growth and metastatic spread of renal tumors. One clinical case reported over thirty years ago concerned an extensive metastasizing renal cell carcinoma associated with massive adrenal adenomas (Taylor, 1948); a later report described regression of primary renal cell carcinomas in patients with adrenal tumors (Bartley and Hultquist, 1950). Similar relationships have been reported in animals, with cortisone, for example, having an inhibitory effect on primary renal tumors in hamsters (Bloom, et al, 1963), whereas administration of the same hormone is associated with an increased incidence of metastases in this model (Kirkman, 1959). Studies of a murine renal cell carcinoma model at Roswell Park Memorial Institute led to the conclusion that the higher rate of metastases in this model is not necessarily due to a selection of cells with a short cell growth cycle (Muntzing et al, 1976), thereby pointing to the possibility of adrenal secretion and/or other factors as being involved with enhanced growth of metastases.

In spite of the varied reports which suggest a hormonal causality of renal cell carcinoma, the fact remains that the

etiology of this disease in humans is obscure. Moreover,
two arguments which do not strongly support the "hormonal
hypothesis" have been advanced by Kantor (1977), who noted
that if hormones were directly related to induction of this
cancer, then there would be a higher frequency of bilateral
renal carcinoma; instead this is a rare occurrence. Kantor
(1977) also observed that the disease almost always occurs
in patients over 40 years of age when gonadal hormone production is on the decline; the ratio of estrogens to androgens,
however, may begin to increase in some men at about this
period in life (Karr and Murphy, 1980).

During the early 1960's, the use of hormonal therapy
for patients with metastatic renal carcinoma was not uncommon,
and varying degrees of success were reported. The response
rates of patients treated with progestins and/or androgens
ranged from 7 to 33%, as reported in the literature prior to
1971 (Hrushesky and Murphy, 1977); the average objective
response rate for most studies was about 17%. However,
response criteria were not uniform among the various reports.
Morales reported no objective responses to androgen or
progesterone therapy in his series of patients and suggested
that objective responses (20%) to hormonal therapy probably
were, in fact, spontaneous remissions (Morales et al, 1975);
other studies on the incidence of this phenomenon indicate
that spontaneous regression of primary tumors or metastatic
lesions is extremely rare (Freed et al, 1977), thus supporting other estimates of less than 1% (Montie et al, 1977;
Bloom, 1973a,b). As previously mentioned, spontaneous
regression is more frequent in men than in women. Through
1973, only 40 cases of spontaneous regression were known
(Bloom, 1973a) and 80% of these occurred in males; survival
rate, however, at 10 years is higher for female patients
(Mostofi, 1967). In one study responses to progestational
therapy occurred only in some men versus no responses in
women (Pavine et al, 1970). Others have explained differences in response to hormonal therapy on the basis of the
amount of drug administered (Alberto and Senn, 1974). When
tabulated, objective response rates to hormonal therapy
reported in the literature after 1971 were markedly lower;
out of a total of 416 patients evaluated, only 8 (<2%)
showed objective evidence of response (Hruskesky and Murphy,
1977), and this difference from the pre-1971 literature
could reflect the application of more rigorous and specifically defined objective versus subjective response criteria.

Renal Steroid Receptors

The selection of hormonal therapy for renal cancer has been an empirical practice in many instances, rather than one based on a diagnostic rationale or some positive means of identifying potential responders. In fact, hormonal therapy has generally followed resection of the primary tumor and subsequent metastatic spread. Since the response of advanced renal carcinoma to hormonal therapy had been favorable in some patients, the search for steroid hormone receptors in normal and malignant kidney tissue was a logical sequel to the accumulated clinical experience. Indeed, the value of profile analyses of steroid receptors in other cancers is well known and has been recently reviewed (Sandberg and Karr, 1980).

The presence of high affinity, low capacity binding sites for progesterone, androgens, estradiol and mineralo- and glucocorticoids has been described in normal human kidney and in human renal adenocarcinoma (Table 1). Localization studies of fluoresceinated estrogens, progesterone and testosterone ligand-conjugates revealed the binding of these steroids predominantly at the glomerular level in various animal species, including men and women (Pertschuk et al, 1980). The function and significance of steroid receptors in renal tumor have not been fully elucidated, and whether they are involved in metabolic processes of any or all of the cells, or if they are related to tumor grade or cell types is not known. Biochemical and kinetic values reported for human renal receptors vary greatly, and probably reflect different receptor methodologies, tissue handling procedures, and clinical factors (previous and ongoing therapy, tumor grade, sex and age of the patient, and primary versus metastatic lesions). Table 1 illustrates the wide range of steroid receptor values and quantitative charactertistics which have been reported from different laboratories. The extreme ranges in some cases reflect the conflicting reports which have characterized the literature on this subject. Generally, the binding capacity and affinities reported for these receptors have been reasonably consistent with those values accepted as characteristic of specific steroid hormone receptors in other tissues (Karr and Sandberg, 1979). In most instances, when reported, the sedimentation coefficients were in the 4S range, with one study showing an 8S androgen binder in cytosol from renal carcinoma (Bojar et al, 1980) and another reporting 7 - 8S values for glucocorticoid and

TABLE 1

CYTOSOL RECEPTORS IN HUMAN KIDNEY AND RENAL CELL CARCINOMA

	Normal Kidney		Renal Carcinoma	
	Fmol/mg Cytosol Protein	K_d	Fmol/mg Cytosol Protein	K_d
Androgen	7-12	$1 - 5 \times 10^{-9}$ M	1-27	$1 \times 10^{-9} - 50 \times 10^{-10}$ M
Estrogen	1-60	$2 - 7 \times 10^{-9}$ M	1-10	$1 - 9 \times 10^{-9}$ M
Progestin	8-40	$2 - 64 \times 10^{-9}$ M	<3-50	$3 \times 10^{-8} - 9 \times 10^{-9}$ M
Glucocorticoid	18	$7 - 10 \times 10^{-9}$ M	7-31	$2 \times 10^{-8} - 7 \times 10^{-9}$ M
Aldosterone	1-110	$3 \times 10^{-7} - 3 \times 10^{-9}$ M	1- 7	1×10^{-8} M

Condensed from data emanating from the Laboratories of Bojar, Chem, Concolino, Hemstreet, Pasqualini, Rafestin-Oblin, and Tobin.

androgen receptors (Chen et al, 1980). In the latter study, these proteins were significant and readily determined by the dextran coated charcoal technique, but none of the human hypernephroma specimens contained detectable estrogen receptor and in only a few instances were progestin binders demonstrable (Chen et al, 1980). In ten primary tumor specimens, dexamethasone binding ranged from 0 - 62.5 fmol/mg cytosol protein ($\bar{x}$=23.3±21.1); corresponding values for androgen and progestin binding were 1.4 to 26.7 fmol ($\bar{x}$=13.5±8.4) and 0 to 3.7 fmol ($\bar{x}$=1.3±1.2), respectively. These authors concluded that the response of some patients to hormonal therapy is mediated directly at the intracellular level, with exogenous progesterone or androgen blocking glucocorticoid receptor activity. The affinity of glucocorticoid receptors for progesterone is known and both progesterone and aldosterone are moderate competitors for dexamethasone binding (Bojar et al, 1979b). Medroxyprogesterone acetate inhibited an average of 87% of the specific dexamethasone binding, suggesting that this widely used compound for treating metastatic renal cancer may cause tumor regression by binding to glucocorticoid receptors, thereby eliminating the growth promoting action of endogenous glucocorticoids (Bojar et al, 1979b). Other studies have reported an elevated concentration (approximately 2-fold) of a dexamethasone binder in neoplastic versus normal kidney tissue (Rafestin-Oblin et al, 1979).

The concentration of aldosterone receptors is significantly greater in tumor-free versus malignant renal tissue (Pasqualini et al, 1977). These authors suggest that as renal adenocarcinoma advances in Stage (I-IV), aldosterone receptors diminish, a view similar to that reported by Rafestin-Oblin et al (1979). Indeed, cytosol aldosterone binding in the latter study was six to seven-fold lower (p<0.001) in neoplastic than normal human renal tissue. This low binding of (^{3}H)-aldosterone suggests that mineralocorticoid receptors are absent in renal adenocarcinoma, an hypothesis in concert with the epithelial cell proximal convoluted tubule origin of these tumors (Rafestin-Oblin et al, 1979).

In a study primarily designed to determine whether there is a correlation between estrogen receptors in renal tissue from renal carcinoma patients and clinical response to therapy, Fronzo et al (1980) concluded that estrogen receptors are not detectable in significant concentrations in kidney carcinoma. Thirty-one cases were studied, using the charcoal absorption technique, and in 17 normal and 19 neoplasia samples estrogen receptors were not detected; the other specimens had very low content, i.e. 13 fmol/mg protein or less. These authors point out the discrepancies between their data and those of other studies, and suggest that methodological differences could account for the wide range of values reported in the literature for estrogen and other steroid hormone receptors. It should be noted that Ferrazzi et al (1980) reported a prospective study of 12 patients with advanced renal cell cancer who received tamoxifen (30mg/day for at least two months) and concluded that this agent is of questionable value in the treatment of this disease. As part of the series reported by Fronzo et al (1980) progestin or DHT receptor assays in four cases (both normal and malignant tissue) were negative by use of a gel filtration technique.

The role of progestin in treatment of advanced renal carcinoma is controversial and there is little recent evidence to support the empirical use of this mode of therapy. Nevertheless, a rationale is found by some for progestin therapy, which has been developed from indirect evidence of renal cancer being androgen dependent, this being derived from the male predominance of patients suffering from this disease. Progestins may act on tumor tissue by inhibiting the secretion of gonadotropins, thereby lowering the levels of growth promoting androgens. In a retrospective study of 88 patients with renal cell carcinoma, no statistical difference in actual survival rates was detected between homogeneous groups treated with either progesterone caproate (250mg, 3 times/week) or other therapeutic regimens (Bono et al, 1979). Detection of cytosolic androgen receptors in normal or carcinomatous human renal tissue, however, is not always achieved (Bojar et al, 1975). Nevertheless, progestins have been the most widely used steroids in the treatment of metastatic renal cancer, and thus, the search for specific progestin receptors in normal and tumor specimens has been extensive, in the hope of defining a logical basis for this treatment. Concolino et al (1976) demonstrated progestin binding in all 3 normal specimens and in 9 out of 10 renal cell cancers studied; estrogen receptors were detected in only 1 of the 3 normal and in 5 of the 10 tumor specimens. On a quantitative basis, though based on a limited number of samples, the number of binding sites and K_d's were found to be higher in tumors than in normal tissues. These data also suggested a lower binding affinity for the progestins than the estrogen receptor in renal cell cancer; no correlation between degree of tumor differentiation and progesterone binding capacity was noted. In a later report (Concolino, 1979b), cytosolic estrogen and progesterone receptors were each detected in 59% of 27 renal carcinomas assayed; 37% of the tumors were positive for both receptors versus 19% which were negative (Table 2). Eighteen

TABLE 2

ESTROGEN AND PROGESTIN CYTOSOL RECEPTORS IN HUMAN RENAL CARCINOMA

	PR^+	PR^-	Total
ER^+	10	6	16
ER^-	6	5	11
Total	16	11	27

Concolino et al, 1979.

of the 23 patients without metastases at nephectomy were given progestin therapy; 14 were reported to have had a partial remission or disease stabilization. The authors concluded that progestin therapy could be indicated for those tumors characterized by having both progestin and estrogen receptors, as well as in those with a transient dependency on hormones, as characterized by having either one of the two receptors. Thus, according to these studies, the election of a particular hormone therapy for a renal cell cancer patient need not be arbitrary, because progesterone therapy may be indicated for PR^+, ER^- tumors, and when progesterone therapy fails, androgen or antiandrogen therapy may be attempted. Antiandrogen may be indicated for PR^-, ER^+ tumors.

Other studies conflict with the preceding data. For example, progestin binding components in human renal cell cancer were found to be negligible, i.e., the concentration of the progestin receptor in tumor cytosol of 30 women never exceeded 4 fmol/mg cytosol protein (Bojar et al, 1979a). In an attempt to explain these low levels, Bojar et al (1979b) investigated nine human renal cell carcinomas for progestin binding inhibitors, such as enzymes which are released and degrade receptors upon tissue homogenization. Although the source or biochemical nature of inhibitors of progestin receptor binding were not elucidated, these investigators concluded that failure to demonstrate high receptor levels in kidney tissue could be related to inhibitory interactions in certain preparations. However, they concluded that human kidney carcinomas do not contain significant amounts of progestin receptors, based on their analyses of cell-free systems undisturbed by inhibitors (Bojar et al, 1979b). Low levels of progestin receptor in such tumors may explain the limited value of progesterone in the treatment of metastatic renal carcinoma (Hruskesky and Murphy, 1977).

Recently, Hemstreet et al (1980) reported on the measurement of estrogen, progestin and glucocorticoid receptors in 47 autologous pairs of normal and malignant tissue from patients with renal cell carcinoma. A significant difference in progestin receptor concentrations was found between normal ($\sim$18 fmol/mg cytosol protein) and malignant ($\sim$10 fmol/mg cytosol protein) specimens. A receptor concentration of >10 fmol/mg protein and an affinity of $<9.9 \times 10^{-9}$ M were arbitrarily selected for establishing tissue positivity for progestin receptor. While 17% of the tumor and 45% of the normal tissue contained high affinity progestin receptors in concentrations >10 fmol, no differences were detected using the same criteria for glucocorticoid or estrogen receptors (Table 3).

Hemstreet's studies point to heterogeneity of renal tumor and the significantly reduced concentration of progestin receptors in malignant tissues (Hemstreet et al, 1980). The criteria which identified progesterone receptors in 17% of the tumors suggested to these authors an adjuvant approach to selecting patients for hormonal therapy. Indeed, these studies raise the obvious question as to whether the tumors of the 17% responders to hormonal therapy reported in early (pre-1971) studies could also have been positive for progestin receptors according to these criteria. Clearly, such receptor assays and rigorous criteria may identify a larger proportion of potential responders to hormonal therapy.

Taken in total, the preceding review suggests that there may be a potential diagnostic utility of steroid hormone

TABLE 3

POSITIVE RECEPTOR PROFILE (% POSITIVE)[1] IN NORMAL AND
MALIGNANT RENAL TISSUE[2]

	Receptor		
	Progestin	Estradiol	Glucocorticoid
Cancer	17	30	48
Normal	45	38	40

[1]Affinity $<9.9 \times 10^{-9}$ M with $\geq$10fmol/mg cytosol
protein
[2]Hemstreet et al, Internat. J. Cancer, 26:769,
1980.

receptor analyses of renal specimens and that the field has
been sufficiently documented to warrant further exploration.
Presented in the remaining pages of this chapter are the
procedures we use for such receptor assays and preliminary
results on human and animal renal specimens.

Progestin Receptor Assay and Human Renal Tumors

Materials and Methods. Trizma (free base) was purchased
from Sigma Chemical Co.; sucrose (RNase free) from Schwartz-
Mann; monothioglycerol from Aldrich Chemical Co.; activated
charcoal (NoritA) from Matheson, Coleman and Bell; and (^{3}H)-
R5020 (17α-methyl-^{3}H-promegestone, 87mCi/μmole) was purchased
from New England Nuclear. The labeled steroids were checked
for radioactive purity by thin layer chromatography in
heptane:ethyl acetate (60:40, v/v). The buffer used was
comprised of 50mM sodium phosphate, 1.5mM EDTA, 12mM monothioglycerol, 15mM sodium molybdate, pH7.6 (MoPOSH) and contained
10% glycerol. Scintillation fluid was Omnifluor (New England
Nuclear) in toluene.

Preparation of Cytosols. Specimens were surgically
removed and placed intact into liquid nitrogen. The frozen

tissue was pulverized to a fine powder with an automatic
frozen tissue pulverizer and stored at -70° until assayed.
Weighed aliquots of powder (300 to 600mg) were thawed in
MoPOSH -10% glycerol buffer (w/v, 1g/2ml) at 0°. Homogenization was done with a Polytron-PT10 using two 10-seconds
bursts which were interrupted with 2-3 minutes cooling on
ice. The homogenate was centrifuged at 200,000 x g; the
protein content of the supernatant was estimated spectro-
photometrically (Layne, 1957) and by the biuret method
(Zamenhof and Chargraff, 1957). The protein concentrations
of cytosols were then adjusted to 4-6mg/ml.

Sucrose Density Gradient Analysis. Specific isotopic
binding patterns in sucrose gradients were determined by a
modification of the method of Jordan and Prestwich (1977).
Linear gradients were 20-35% sucrose in 5mM sodium phosphate
buffer containing 15mM sodium molybdate. Aliquots (300µl)
of cytosol were incubated with (17α-methyl-^{3}H)-promegestone
(15nM) in the presence and absence of a 100-fold molar
excess of unlabeled R5020 or progesterone. Labeled cytosol
was incubated for 18 hours at 0°C and then treated with a
dextran charcoal pellet as described by McGuire (1975). The
gradients were centrifuged for three hours in a Beckman
VTi65 rotor at 65,000 rpm (371,700 x g). After centrifugation,
each gradient was fractionated from the top by displacement
from the bottom with 55% sucrose (w/v) with the use of an
Isco sucrose gradient fractionator. Sixty fractions of 70µl
each were collected into scintillation vials to which 10ml
of scintillation cocktail were added. ^{14}C-labeled bovine
serum albumin was prepared according to the procedure of
Rice and Means (1971) and sedimentation coefficients were
estimated using albumin (4.6S) and alkaline phosphatase
(6.1S) as references according to the method of Martin and
Ames (1961).

Quantitation of Progestin-Binding Capacity. The specific
(^{3}H)-R5020 binding was estimated at 4°C by the dextran-
charcoal assay described for estrogen receptors by McGuire
(1975), with minor modifications. Cytosols were incubated
with R5020 (0.1nM to 10nM) in the presence and absence of
200-fold excess of unlabeled R5020 in microtiter plates
(Cooke Microtiter Plates). Dexamethasone ($\sim10^{-7}$M) was included
in all incubations to ensure that R5020 did not bind to
glucocorticoid receptor, as has been observed by others
(Lippmann et al, 1977). Aliquots of cytosol (100µl) were
incubated for 18 hours at 0°. The unbound ligand was removed

TABLE 4

PROTEIN AND DNA CONTENT OF HUMAN RENAL TUMORS

Patient	mg Cytosol Protein per g Tissue	mg DNA per g Tissue
1	16	2.8
2	12	2.7
3	22	0.8
4	25	2.2
5	19	1.7
6	25	1.0
7	30	n.d.*
8	19	0.9
9	23	4.1
10	16	2.5
11	18	0.8
12	32	1.3
13	21	2.6

*n.d. = not detected

by the addition of 150µl of 0.5% charcoal in MoPOSH-10%
glycerol buffer. Ligand bound in the presence of excess
unlabeled R5020 and dexamethasone was classed as non-specific
binding, and this value was subtracted from the total steroid
bound to give the amount of R5020 bound specifically.
Calculations of the total binding capacity and K_d were
derived graphically from Scatchard plots of the saturation
analysis data (Scatchard, 1949). Results were expressed as
fmoles bound per mg cytosol protein, fmoles bound per µg
DNA, and fmoles bound per g of tissue. DNA was determined
by the method of Burton (1956) as modified by Richards (1974).

Progestin Binding Results. Consistently high yields of
cytosol protein/g tissue were recovered from the human renal
tumors analyzed in this series (Table 4). Since the cytosols
contained high, but unknown levels of plasma contamination,
the amount of DNA/g tissue was also determined. The wide
range of DNA recovered indicates a significant inconsistency
in the number of tumor cells in the different samples. Such
a difference in tissue sampling can seriously affect accurate
measurement of receptor binding sites. Samples containing
very low amounts of DNA (Table 4) may yield erroneous results
due to the low number of cells. For example, in human breast
tumor samples, the heterogeneity within any one tumor has
been shown to have a profound effect on the estrogen receptor
assay. In contrast to renal tumors, the normal kidney
samples used in the present study gave a consistent recovery
of DNA/g tissue (Table 5).

TABLE 5

PROTEIN AND DNA CONTENT OF NORMAL HUMAN KIDNEY

Patient	mg Cytosol Protein per g Tissue	mg DNA per g Tissue
3	27	1.9
8	18	1.9
10	14	1.8

Progestin specific binding was determined in 13 human renal tumor samples. When dexamethasone was included in all assays, three (23%) were found to obtain saturable, high affinity progestin binding elements. The addition of dexamethasone to all incubations apparently prevented the binding of R5020 to glucocorticoid receptor as reported by Lippman et al, (1977). Table 6 compares the apparent specific binding of R5020 to renal tumor cytosols in the absence and presence of dexamethasone. Dexamethasone reduced the binding of (^{3}H)-R5020 in most samples and in some cases (^{3}H)-R5020 binding could not be detected in its presence. These data extend and confirm the observation of Lippman et al, (1977) and, therefore, dexamethasone was added to all subsequent progestin binding assays of human renal cell tumors and normal renal tissue.

TABLE 6

EFFECT OF DEXAMETHASONE ON (^{3}H)-R5020 SPECIFIC BINDING

Patient	Unlabeled Ligand	fmoles per mg Cytosol Protein
1	R5020	36
	R5020 + Dexamethasone	23
3	R5020	17
	R5020 + Dexamethasone	n.d.*
4	R5020	20
	R5020 + Dexamethasone	19
2	R5020	68
	R5020 + Dexamethasone	38

*n.d. = not detected

Saturation analysis of progestin binding in both normal kidney (Figure 2) and tumor (Figure 3) showed the presence of very high amounts of non-specific binding. As a result, specific binding was measured as a small difference between

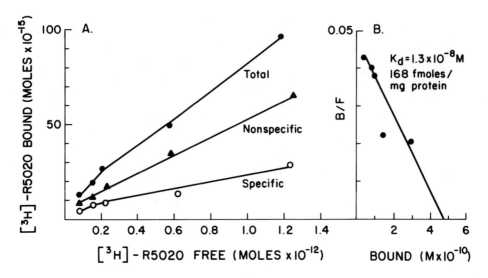

Fig. 2. Saturation binding analysis (A) and specific R5020 binding (B) in normal human kidney cytosol.

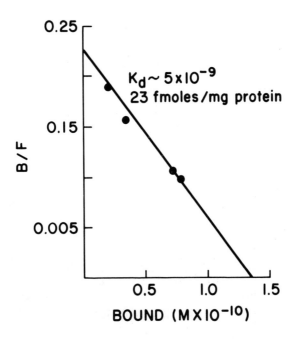

Fig. 3. Specific R5020 binding in cytosol of human renal cell carcinoma.

saturable high affinity binding and non-saturable binding. In this situation the sensitivity of the dextran charcoal assay becomes a limiting factor in assays performed at a single saturating dose of ligand. Therefore, binding at different concentrations of ligand was considered preferable so as to permit the application of Scatchard plot analysis for quantitation of the data. Scatchard analysis (Figures 2B and 3) of the binding data yielded K_d estimates of 10^{-8} M and 10^{-9} M for R5020 binding in normal kidney and tumor, respectively, thereby supporting the conclusion that high affinity progestin binding receptor was present in these specimens.

Sucrose gradient centrifugation was used to further characterize the high affinity progestin binding. Figure 4 illustrates the clear separation of ~7.6S progestin specific

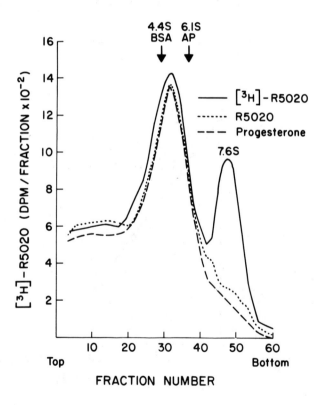

Fig. 4. Progestin specific binding in cytosol of human renal cell carcinoma.

saturable binding in cytosol from a human renal tumor. The binding of (^{3}H)-R5020 to the 7.6S peak is suppressed by a 100-fold molar excess of either progesterone or R5020, thereby adding further evidence in support of the contention that the binding is progestin specific. In contrast, the material sedimenting in the 4-5S region of the gradient is not affected by excess progesterone or R5020, adding further distinction between this non-specific and non-saturable binding, and the presence of specific progesterone receptors in certain renal specimens.

Table 7 presents the results of the assay for progestin specific binding in 13 human renal tumors. When the data are expressed as fmoles bound/µg DNA, the specimen from patient #3 appears to have a high content of progestin bind-ing compared to the other two samples (see Table 4). However, this resulted in part from the calculation which was based on the very low DNA content of that sample (see Table 4) and, therefore, may not reflect the true amount of specific binding present.

Table 8 presents the progestin binding assay results of three normal kidney tissues. Normal tissue and tumor from patient #3 produced mixed results, in that the tumor was PR$^+$ (Table 6) while no binding was detected in the normal tissue. The reverse situation was seen in specimens from patient #10, with normal tissue having high levels of progestin binding (Table 8) and virtually nondetectable progestin binding in the tumor specimen (Table 7).

Quantitative values for progesterone receptor in normal human kidney cytosols have been reported in the range from 11-45 fmoles/cytosol protein (Concolino et al, 1978). These data indicate that renal tumors contain from 0.1-2 pmoles binding per µg DNA (our data is in fmoles/µg DNA). Concolino et al (1978), whose data were not reported in terms of fmoles/ mg cytosol protein, stated that their quantitative results were lower than those for normal kidney, suggesting that perhaps the samples assayed may have had a very high protein to DNA ratio. For example, if the binding had been approxi-mately 10 fmoles per mg cytosol protein, then in order to have 0.13 pmoles to 1.46 pmoles per µg DNA would require a calculation based on at least 13mg to 146mg protein per µg DNA. In the samples we analyzed, the protein DNA ratio was approximately 10mg protein/mg DNA. Although not necessarily related, these yields are consistent with literature values

TABLE 7

PROGESTIN SPECIFIC BINDING IN HUMAN RENAL TUMORS

Patient	fmoles Bound per mg Cytosol Protein	fmoles Bound per μg DNA	fmoles Bound per g Wet Wt. Tissue
1	23	0.17	0.46
2	38	0.16	0.48
3	19.6	1.14	0.45
4	n.d.	-	-
5	n.d.	-	-
6	n.d.	-	-
7	n.d.	-	-
8	n.d.	-	-
9	n.d.	-	-
10	n.d.	-	-
11	n.d.	-	-
12	n.d.	-	-
13	n.d.	-	-

TABLE 8

PROGESTIN SPECIFIC BINDING IN NORMAL KIDNEY

Patient	fmoles per mg Cytosol Protein	fmoles per μg DNA	fmoles per g Tissue Wt.
3	n.d.	-	-
8	n.d.	-	-
10	168	1.33	2361

for breast tumors. Such differences in protein to DNA ratios may account for our values being in the range of fmoles per μg DNA while others have reported picomoles per μg DNA (Concolino et al, 1978). This clearly reflects the problems in reporting which could be resolved with standardization among laboratories.

Androgen Receptor Assay and Human Renal Tumors

Radioactive methyltrienolone (^{3}H-R1881), 87 μCi/nmole, and nonradioactive R1881 were purchased from New England Nuclear. Triamcinolone acetonide was obtained from Sigma Chemical Co.

Androgen receptors were measured with a dextran coated charcoal method (Hicks and Walsh, 1979). Large pieces of tissue were pre-cooled in liquid nitrogen and shattered with a tissue pulverizer prior to homogenization. Most samples were small enough to be homogenized directly. All procedures were carried out at $-4°$ C. Tissues were homogenized in TED buffer (10mM Tris-HCl, 1.5mM EDTA, 1mM dithiothreitol, pH 7.4) containing 10% (wt./vol.) glycerol by three to four intermittent 10-second bursts with a polytron interrupted by two-minute cooling periods. The proportion of sample weight (in grams) to ml TED-glycerol varied over a wide range (1:10 to 1:180) according to available sample size. A crude nuclear pellet was obtained by centrifugation at 800 x g.

for 20 minutes. The supernatant was centrifuged at 105,000 x g for 60 minutes and a clear cytosol was collected for analysis. The nuclear pellet was resuspended and centrifuged twice in TED (g tissue/ml buffer in a ratio of 1:2). The pellet was then homogenized in TED buffer containing 0.6M KCl (g tissue/ml TED-KCl buffer varied from 1:6 to 1:180) by a two-second burst with the polytron; the homogenized pellet was left standing for 60 minutes and then centrifuged at 105,000 x g for 60 minutes, leaving the supernatant crude nuclear extract for analysis.

Radioactive steroid solutions were prepared in TED buffer at six concentrations. Fifty µg of steroid solution were incubated with 200µl of cytosol or nuclear extract for about 22 hours at 0-4°C. The steroid concentrations in the incubate were 0.2, 0.4, 0.8, 1.6, 3.2 and 100nM. In addition, for the assay of cytosol, the mixtures contained a 1,000-fold excess of triamcinolone acetonide except for the cytosolic incubates with 100nM R1881 to which only a 16-fold excess was added. Samples were prepared in duplicate when sufficient material was available. Dextran-coated charcoal solutions contained either 0.5% Norit A charcoal and 0.005% dextran or, for very dilute samples, 0.25% charcoal and 0.0075% dextran in TED buffer. Five hundred µl of the dextran coated charcoal solution was added to 250µl of the incubated samples and vortexed. Vortexing was repeated after five and ten minutes, and after exactly 15 minutes, the mixtures were centrifuged at about 10,000 x g for 15 minutes. The supernatants were transferred to scintillation vials and counted at about 30% efficiency.

Analysis of 10 tumor and two normal kidney specimens revealed displaceable binding in each case, but the specific values were so low (1-4.5 fmol/mg cytosol protein) compared to the high amount of non-specific binding that is typical of such specimens, that the Scatchard analyses were generally non-quantifiable. In several instances, reliable K_d estimates were obtained which registered in the 10^{-8} M range. Cytosols of only two of the 12 specimens had quantifiable androgen receptor concentrations greater than 3 fmol, and these were in tumor specimens from a man (7.3 fmol) and a woman (4.5 fmol). Specific binding was determined in the nuclear extract from both normal specimens (7-8 fmol/mg protein) and in 6 of the 10 tumor specimens (2.9-4.8 fmoles).

Estradiol Receptor Assay and Human Renal Tumors

Frozen specimens are pulverized to a fine powder and thawed in TESH buffer (pH 7.8) comprised of .02M TRis-HCl, .0015M EDTA, 15nM sodium molybdate, 12mM monothioglycerol and 5% glycerol. 2, 4, 6, 7-(^{3}H)-17β-Estradiol (90 Ci/mmole) was purchased from New England Nuclear. Cytosol and nuclear pellets (for DNA determinations) were prepared as described in the preceding sections. For sucrose density gradient analysis, the aliquots of cytosol were incubated for 4 hours at 4°C with (^{3}H)-estradiol (10nM) in the presence or absence of a 1000-fold molar excess of nafoxidine. Unbound steroid was removed from the cytosol-steroid mixture with the dextran coated charcoal solution (McGuire, 1975) prior to layering the incubated cytosol steroid solution (150μl) on the top of 10-30% linear sucrose gradients. Using a Beckman SW 60 rotor, the gradients were spun at 50,000rpm for 16-18 hrs. Fractions were then collected for liquid scintillation counting as described in the section on progestin binding.

Dextran coated charcoal assays for Scatchard plot analyses were performed on aliquots of cytosol (50μl) incubated with (^{3}H)-estradiol (0.2nM-10nM) in the presence and absence of nafoxidine (1000-fold molar excess). The solutions were incubated in micro-titer plates for 18 hrs. at 4°C. The cytosol-steroid solutions were then mixed with dextran coated charcoal solution (125μl) for a 20-minute period with vortexing every 5 minutes, followed by centrifuging the micro-titer plates at 1500rpm for 20 minutes. Aliquots (50μl) of DCC free cytosol mixture were counted for radioactivity in duplicate; binding curves were calculated and plotted using a Wang computer and software system (Kirdani, et al, 1979).

The results of the current series of patient specimens which have been studied with these methods are shown in Table 9a and 9b. Clearly, these data indicate that specific 8S binding for estradiol in tumor from both male and female patients is not detectable, whereas a 4S component was identified in eight of the 18 specimens analyzed. In three cases (one male patient and two female patients) autologous tumor and normal specimens were clearly positive for 4S cytosolic estrogen binding. Normal kidney tissue removed with the renal cell carcinoma only contained a barely detectable 8S binding component for estradiol, whereas 6 of the 18 specimens contained a measureable 4S binder. The K_d for the

TABLE 9a

CYTOSOL RECEPTORS[1] IN HUMAN RENAL CARCINOMA AND NORMAL KIDNEY

| | Estrogen Receptors | | | | | |
| | Tumor | | | Normal | | |
	4S	8S	DCC	4S	8S	DCC
Male Patients						
1	19.5	n.d.	n.d.	1.4	n.d.	n.d.
2	4.5	n.d.	n.d.	7.1	n.d.	n.d.
3	3.9	n.d.	n.d.	n.d.	n.d.	n.d.
4	n.d.	n.d.	n.d.	n.d.	n.d.	n.d.
5	n.d.	n.d.	n.d.	n.d.	n.d.	n.d.
6	24.2	n.d.	1.9			
7	n.d.	n.d.	2.0			
8	n.d.	n.d.	n.d.			
9	n.d.	n.d.	n.d.			
10	n.d.	n.d.	n.d.			
11				n.d.	1.2	2.6
12				1.7	1.4	n.d.
13				3.8	n.d.	n.d.
14				3.0	3.9	n.d.

RPMI series
[1] fmoles/mg cytosol protein
n.d. = not detectable

TABLE 9b

CYTOSOL RECEPTORS[1] IN HUMAN RENAL CARCINOMA AND NORMAL KIDNEY

	Estrogen Receptors					
	Tumor			Normal		
	4S	8S	DCC	4S	8S	DCC
Female Patients						
1	5.7	n.d.	n.d.	7.0	n.d.	10.4
2	2.6	n.d.	0.7	n.d.	n.d.	n.d.
3	14.2	n.d.	n.d.	n.d.	n.d.	n.d.
4	3.7	n.d.	n.d.	20.1	1.7	2.2
5	n.d.	n.d.	n.d.	n.d.	1.1	1.7
6	n.d.	n.d.	n.d.	n.d.	n.d.	n.d.
7	n.d.	n.d.	n.d.	n.d.	n.d.	n.d.
8	n.d.	n.d.	n.d.			
9				21.5	n.d.	2.4
10				n.d.	1.34	n.d.

RPMI series
[1] fmoles/mg cytosol protein
n.d. = not detectable

TABLE 10

HUMAN RENAL ADENOCARCINOMA AND NORMAL KIDNEY CYTOSOL RECEPTORS

Pt. #	Tissue	Sex	Receptors (fmol/mg Cytosol Protein)		
			E_2Rc	PrgRc	DexRc
1	Normal Kidney	M	n.d.*	n.d.	n.d.
	Tumor		n.d.	n.d.	n.d.
2	Normal Kidney	M	n.d.	n.d.	
	Tumor		n.d.	n.d.	
3	Normal Kidney	M	8.2 $(k_d = 2.4 \times 10^{-9} M)$	n.d.	
	Tumor			n.d.	
4	Tumor	F	n.d.	n.d.	
5	Tumor	F	n.d.	n.d.	
6	Normal Kidney	F	n.d.	n.d.	n.d.
	Tumor		4.2 $(k_d = 4.3 \times 10^{-9} M)$	n.d.	118.5 $(k_d = 9.5 \times 10^{-9} M)$

*n.d. = not detected (<3fmoles/mg protein)
E_2Rc = estrogen receptor
PrgRc = progestin (R5020) receptor
DexRc = glucocorticoid receptor

estrogen receptor, as determined in an earlier pilot study (Table 10) was 2 to 4 x 10^{-9} M, a value which falls within the range of binding affinity known to be characteristic for this receptor.

A summary of the combined receptor analyses on human renal cell cancer analyzed at Roswell Park Memorial Institute is given in Table 11. Even though the total number of

TABLE 11

ESTROGEN, PROGESTIN AND ANDROGEN RECEPTORS IN HUMAN
RENAL TUMOR CYTOSOL

	Estrogen		Progesterone		Androgen	
	Male	Female	Male	Female	Male	Female
	4+	5+	2+	2+	1+	1+
	2±	1±				1±
	10-	7-	10-	5-	4-	3-
% +	25	38	17	29	20	20

RPMI Oct., 1981
± <3fmol/mg cytosol protein

specimens analyzed is not large, the trend suggested by these data indicates that there is a small number of tumors which contain detectable levels of steroid hormone receptors. When our data are analyzed separately according to sex, or if the patient data are combined to give total values for specimens that are positive for estrogen (31%) and progesterone (23%) receptors, they are in general agreement with those reported by Hemstreet et al (1980), in that a higher percentage of the tumors contain estradiol as compared to progestin receptors. The opposite was evident in a group of specimens from 23 patients reported by Concolino et al (1979b), (Table 2).

While we are not able to conclude from our data that steroid hormone receptor analyses are of predictive value for identifying renal cell carcinoma patients in whom hormone therapy could be beneficial (or detrimental), there is sufficient evidence to warrant the effort to determine, retrospectively, whether the steroid receptor content of renal cell carcinomas treated hormonally correlate with carefully defined response criteria and survival. The diagnostic utility of steroid receptor analyses in human renal cell carcinoma may be appropriately determined through studies of a large population of patients, perhaps through a multi-institutional study.

REFERENCES

Alberto P, Senn HJ (1974). Hormonal therapy of renal carcinoma alone and in association with metastatic drugs. Cancer 33:1226.
Anderson NS, David Y, Fanestil DD (1979). Estrogen receptor in hamster kidney during estrogen-induced renal tumorigenesis. J Steroid Biochem 10:123.
Antonio P, Gabaldon M, Lacomba T, Juan A (1974). Effect of the anti-estrogen nafoxidine on the occurrence of estrogen-dependent renal carcinoma. Horm Metab Res 6:522.
Bartley O, Hultquist GT (1950). Spontaneous regression of hypernephromas. Acta Path Microbiol Scand 27:448.
Bloom HJG (1971). Medroxyprogesterone acetate (provera) in the treatment of metastatic renal cancer. Brit J Cancer 25:250.
Bloom HJG (1973a). Hormone-induced and spontaneous regression of metastatic renal cancer. Cancer 32:1066.
Bloom HJG (1973b). Adjuvant therapy for adenocarcinoma of the kidney: present position and prospects. Brit J Urol 45:237.
Bloom HJG, Baker WH, Dukes CE, Mitchley BCV (1963). Hormone dependent tumours of the kidney-II. Effect of endocrine ablation procedures on the transplanted oestrogen-induced renal tumour of the Syrian hamster. Brit J Cancer 17:646.
Bloom HJG, Dukes CE, Mitchley BCV (1963). Hormone-dependent tumours of the kidney. I. The oestrogen-induced renal tumour of the Syrian hamster; hormone treatment and possible relationship to carcinoma of the kidney in man. Brit J Cancer 17:611.
Bloom HJG, Roe FJC, Mitchley BCV (1967). Sex hormones and renal neoplasia-inhibition of tumour of hamster kidney by

an oestrogen-antagonist, an agent of possible therapeutic value in man. Cancer 20:2118.

Bojar H, Balzer K, Dreyfürst R, Staib W, Wittliff JL (1976). Identification and partial characterization of oestrogen-binding components in human kidney. J Clin Chem Biochem 14:515.

Bojar H, Dreyfürst R, Balzer K, Doscher D, Staib W (1975). Investigations on specific steroid binding components from human kidney and renal cell carcinoma. Acta Endocrinol (Kbh), Suppl 199:130.

Bojar H, Dreyfürst R, Balzer K, Staib W (1976). Oestrogen-binding components in human renal cell carcinoma. J Clin Chem Clin Biochem 14:521.

Bojar H, Maar K, Staib W (1979a). The endocrine background of human renal cell carcinoma. I. Binding of the highly potent progestin R5020 by tumor cytosol. Urol Internat 34:302.

Bojar H, Maar K, Staib W (1979b). The endocrine background of human renal cell carcinoma. III. Role of inhibitors of R5020 binding tumor cytosol. Urol Internat 34:321.

Bojar H, Maar K, Staib W (1980a). The endocrine background of human renal cell carcinoma. V. Binding of highly potent androgen methyltrienoline (R 1881) by tumour cytosol. Urol Internat 35:154.

Bojar H, Maar K, Staib W (1980b). The role of steroid hormones in human renal cell carcinoma. The Prostate 1:139.

Bojar H, Maar K, Staib W (1980c). R-5020 binding components in human renal cell carcinoma. In Wittliff JL, Dapunt O (eds.): "Steroid Receptors and Hormone-Dependent Neoplasia," New York: Mason Publishing USA, Inc., p. 193.

Bojar H, Wittliff JL, Balzer K, Dreyfürst R, Staib W (1974): Properties of specific estrogen-binding components in immature rat kidney. Hoppe Seylers Z Physiol Chem 355:1181.

Bono AV, Benvenuti C, Gianneo E, Comeri GC, Roggia A (1979). Progestogens in renal carcinoma. A retrospective study. Eur Urol 5:94.

Brown TR, Bullock L, Bardin CW (1979). In vitro and in vivo binding of progestins to the androgen receptor of mouse kidney: correlation with biological activities. Endocrinology 105:1281.

Bullock PL, Bardin CW (1975). The presence of estrogen receptor in kidneys from normal and androgen-insensitive tfm/y mice. Endocrinology 97:1106.

Burton K (1956). A study of the conditions and mechanism of the diphenylamine reaction for the colorimetric estimation of deoxyribonucleic acid. Biochem J 62:315.

Chen L, Weiss FR, Chaichik S, Keydar I (1980). Steroid receptors in human renal carcinoma. Israel J Med Sc 16:756.

Concolino G (1979a). Renal cancer: steroid receptors as a biochemical basis for endocrine therapy. In Thompson EB, Lippman ME (eds.): "Steroid Receptors and the Management of Cancer," Boca Raton: CRC Press, Inc., volume I, p. 174.

Concolino G, DiSilverio F, Marocchi A, Bracci U (1979b). Renal cancer steroid receptors: biochemical basis for endocrine therapy. Eur Urol 5:90.

Concolino G, DiSilverio A, Marocchi R, Tenaglia R, Bracci U (1977). Steroid receptors in normal human kidney and in human renal adenocarcinoma. Proc X Eur Congr Int Coll Surg Milan, June 26-29, 1977.

Concolino G, Marocchi A, Concolino F, Sciarra F, DiSilverio F, Conti C (1976a). Human kidney steroid receptors. J Steroid Biochem 7:831.

Concolino G, Marocchi A, Conti C, Liberti M, Tenaglia R, DiSilverio F (1980). Endocrine treatment and steroid receptors in urological malignancies. In Iacobelli S, et al. (eds.): "Hormones and Cancer," New York: Raven Press, p. 403.

Concolino G, Marocchi A, Conti C, Tenaglia R, DiSilverio F, Bracci U (1978). Human renal cell carcinoma as a hormone-dependent tumor. Cancer Res 38:4340.

Concolino G, Marocchi A, DiSilverio F, Conti C (1976b): Progestational therapy in human renal carcinoma and steroid receptors. J Steroid Biochem 7:923.

Concolino G, Marocchi A, DiSilverio F, Ricci G, D'Attoma C, Tenaglia R (1980). Androgen receptor and endocrine treatment of renal cell carcinoma. The Prostate 1:138.

Concolino G, Marocchi A, Tenaglia R, DiSilverio F, Sparano F (1978). Specific progesterone receptor in human renal cancer. J Steroid Biochem 9:399.

DeVries JR, Ludens JH, Fanestil DD (1972). Estradiol renal receptor molecules and estradiol-dependent antinatriuresis. Kidney Internat 2:95.

deVere White R, Olsson CA (1980). Renal adenocarcinoma in the rat. A new tumor model. Invest Urol 17:405.

DiFranzo G, Ranchi E, Bertuzzi A, Vezzoni P, Pizzocaro G (1980). Estrogen receptors in renal carcinoma. Eur Urol 6:307.

Fanestil DD, Vaughn DA, Ludens JH (1974). Steroid hormone receptors in human renal carcinoma. J Steroid Biochem 5:338.

Ferrazzi E, Salvagno L, Fornasiero A, Cartei G, Fiorentino M (1980). Tamoxifen treatment for advanced renal cell carcinoma. Tumori 66:601.

Freed SZ, Halperin JP, Gordon MI (1977). Idiopathic regression of metastases from renal cell carcinoma. J Urol 118:538.

Hamilton JM, Flaks A, Saluja PG, Maguire S (1975). Hormonally induced renal neoplasia in the male Golden Syrian hamster and the inhibitory effect of 3-bromo-α-ergocryptine methanesulfonate. J Nat Cancer Inst 54:1385.

Hemstreet GP III, Wittliff JL, Sariff AM, Hall ML III, McRae LJ, Durant JR (1980). Comparison of steroid receptor levels in renal-cell carcinoma and autologous normal kidney. Internat J Cancer 26:769.

Hicks LL, Walsh PC (1979). A microassay for the measurement of androgen receptors in human prostatic tissue. Steroids 33:389.

Hrushesky WJ, Murphy GP (1977). Current status of the therapy of advanced renal carcinoma. J Surg Oncol 9:277.

Jordan VC, Prestwich G (1977). Binding of (^{3}H)-tamoxifen in rat uterine cytosols. A comparison of swinging bucket and vertical tube rotor sucrose density gradient analysis. Mol Cell Endocrinol 8:179.

Kantor AF (1977). Current concepts in the epidemiology and etiology of primary renal cell carcinoma. J Urol 117:415.

Karr JP, Murphy GP (1980). Hormone manipulation in prostate cancer. In Harris JE, Taylor SG IV (eds.): "Reviews on Endocrine Related Cancer," Delaware: Stuart Pharmaceuticals, supplement 6, p. 93.

Karr JP, Sandberg AA (1979). Steroid receptors and prostatic cancer. In Murphy GP (ed.): "Prostatic Cancer," Littleton: PSG Publishing Co., Inc., p. 49.

Kirdani RY, Priore RL, Murphy GP, Sandberg AA (1979): Systemization of Scatchard or Lineweaver-Burk Plot linearization: application to receptor analysis. In Murphy GP, Sandberg AA (eds.): "Progress in Clinical and Biological Research: Prostate Cancer and Hormone Receptors," New York: Alan R. Liss, Inc., volume 33, p. 145.

Kirkman H (1959). Estrogen-induced tumors of the kidney in the Syrian hamster. J Nat Cancer Inst Monog 1:1.

Kirkman H (1972). Hormone-related tumors in Syrian hamsters. Prog Exp Tumor Res 16:201.

Kirkham H, Bacon RL (1950). Malignant renal tumors in male hamsters (Cricetus auratus) treated with estrogen. Cancer Res 10:122.

Kirkham H, Bacon RL (1952). Estrogen-induced tumors of the kidney. I. Incidence of renal tumors in intact and gonadectomized male golden hamsters treated with diethylstilbestrol. II. Effect of dose, administration, type of estrogen and age on the induction of renal tumors in intact male golden hamsters. J Nat Cancer Inst 13:745.

Layne E (1957). Spectrophotometric and turbimetric methods for measuring proteins. Meth Enzymol 3:447.

Li JJ, Cuthbertson TL, Li SA((1977). Specific androgen binding in the kidney and estrogen-dependent renal carcinoma of the Syrian hamster. Endocrinology 101:1006.

Li JJ, Li SA (1980). High yield of primary serially transplanted hamster renal carcinoma: steroid receptor and morphologic characteristics. Eur J Cancer 16:1119.

Li JJ, Li SA, Cuthberston TL (1979). Nuclear retention of all steroid hormone receptor classes in the hamster renal carcinoma. Cancer Res 39:2647.

Li JJ, Talley DJ, Li SA, Villee CA (1974). An estrogen binding protein in the renal cytosol of intact, castrated and estrogenized golden hamsters. Endocrinology 95:1134.

Lin YC, Talley DJ, Villee CA (1978). Progesterone receptor levels in estrogen-induced renal carcinomas after serial passage beneath the renal capsule of Syrian hamsters. Cancer Res 38:1286.

Lippman ME, Huff K, Bolan G, Neifeld JU (1977). Interaction of R5020 with progesterone and glucocorticoid receptors in human breast cancer and peripheral blood lymphocytes in vitro. In Baulieu EE, McGuire WL, Raynaud JP (eds.): "Roussel Workshop on Application of R5020 to the Detection of Progesterone Receptors," New York: Raven Press, p. 193.

Martin RG, Ames BN (1961). Method for determining the sedimentation behavior of enzymes: application to protein mixtures. J Biol Chem 236:1372.

Mathews VS, Kirkham H, Bacon RL (1947). Kidney damage in the golden hamster following chronic administration of diethylstilbestrol and sesame oil. Proc Soc Exper Biol & Med 66:195.

Matsuda M, Osafune M, Kotake T, Sonoda T (1976). A clinical study on renal cell carcinoma. Jap J Urol 67:635.

McGuire WL (1975). Quantitation of estrogen receptor in mammary carcinoma. Meth Enzymol 28:248.

Montie JE, Stewart BH, Straffon RA, Bonowsky LH, Hewitt CB, Montague DK (1977). The role of adjunctive nephrectomy in patients with metastatic renal cell carcinoma. J Urol 117:272.

Morales A, Kiruluta G, Lott S (1975). Hormones in the treatment of metastatic renal cancer. J Urol 114:692.

Mostofi FK (1967). Pathology and spread of renal cell carcinoma. In Stanten, KJ, Jr. (ed.): "Renal Neoplasia,"

London: J and A Churchill, Ltd., p. 63.

Müntzing JA, Williams PD, Murphy GP (1976). The growth characteristics of metastases from experimental renal tumors. Res Comm Chem Path Pharm 13:541.

Murono EP, Kirdani RY, Sandberg AA (1979). Specific estradiol-17β binding component in adult rat kidney.   J Steroid Biochem 11:1347.

Murphy GP, Hrushesky WJ (1973). A murine renal cell carcinoma. J Nat Cancer Inst 50:1013.

Paine LH, Wright FW, Ellis F (1970). The use of progesterone in the treatment of metastatic carcinoma of the kidney and the uterine body. Brit J Cancer 24:277.

Pasqualini JR, Portois MC, Küss R, Khoury S, Petit J, Degennes JL, Dairou F (1977). Aldosterone and estradiol specific binding in normal and carcinomatous human renal tissues. Proc X Europ Congr Int Coll Surg Milan, June 26-29, 1977.

Pasqualini JR, Sumida C, Gelly C (1974). Steroid hormone receptors in fetal guinea pig kidney. J Steroid Biochem 5:977.

Pasqualini JR, Sumida C, Gelly C, Nguyen BL (1973). Formation de complexes (^{3}H)-oestradiol-macromolécules dans les fractions cytosoliques et nucleaires du tissu rénal du foetus de cobaye. CR Acad Sci Paris, Srie D 276:3359.

Pasqualini JR, Sumida C, Gelly C, Nguyen BL, Tardy J (1978). Specific binding of estrogens in different fetal tissues of guinea-pig during fetal development. Cancer Res 38:4246.

Pertschuk LP, Carvounis EE, Tobin EH, Gaetjens E (1980). Renal glomerular steroid hormone binding. Detection by fluorescent microscopy. J Steroid Biochem 13:1115.

Rafestin-Oblin, ME, Michaud A, Claire M, Corvol P (1977). Dramatic protective effect of ligand against thermal degradation on mineralo and glucocorticoid receptors of rat kidney. J Steroid Biochem 8:19.

Rafestin-Oblin, ME, Roth-Meyer C, Claire M, Michaud A, Baviera E, Brisset JM, Corvol P (1979). Are minerolocorticoid receptors present in human renal adenocarcinoma? Clin Sci 57:421.

Richards GM (1974). Modifications of the diphenylamine reaction giving increased sensitivity and simplicity in the estimation of DNA. Anal Biochem 57:369.

Rice RN, Means GE (1971). Radioactive labeling of proteins in vitro. J Biol Chem 246:831.

Sandberg AA, Karr JP (1980). Hormonal receptors in human neoplasia. In Murphy GP (ed.): "International Advances in Surgical Oncology," New York: Alan R. Liss, Inc., volume 3, p. 311.

Scatchard G (1949). The attraction of proteins for small molecules and ions. Ann New York Acad Sc 51:660.

Shefner AM, Marlow M (1975). Preliminary drug trials in a renal cell carcinoma animal model. Cancer Chemother Rep 5:514.

Steggles AW, King RJB (1972). Oestrogen receptors in hamster tumours. Eur J Cancer 8:323.

Sufrin G, Alvarez J, Swaneck GE (1981). Nuclear estrogen-binding sites in the hamster renal carcinoma. Proc AACR 22:8, abstract #31.

Taylor JA (1948). Extensive metastasizing hypernephroma associated with massive bilateral adenoma of the adrenal. J Urol 59:557.

Tobin EH, Mouhaddeb I, Bloom ND (1980). Analysis of specific progesterone receptor proteins in human kidney and renal cell carcinoma. In Wittliff JL, Dapunt O (eds.): "Steroid Receptors and Hormone-Dependent Neoplasia," New York: Mason Publishing USA, Inc., p. 171.

Whitehead DE (1981). Management of renal cancer. New York State J Med 81:911.

Zamenhof S, Chargraff E (1957). Microbiuret procedure for protein determination. Enzymes 3:702.

Renal Tumors: Proceedings of the First International Symposium on Kidney Tumors, pages 245-254
© 1982 Alan R. Liss, Inc., 150 Fifth Avenue, New York, NY 10011

Steroid Receptors in Kidney Tumours

R. Ghanadian, Ph.D., G. Auf, M.Sc.,
G. Williams, FRCS and A.P.M. Coleman, B.Sc.
Royal Postgraduate Medical School, Hammersmith
Hospital, Ducane Road, London W.12 OHS, England.

INTRODUCTION

It has been reported that both androgens and oestrogens may be involved in mediating some of the functional activities of the kidney. Dihydrotestosterone has been shown to promote prolonged enzyme induction and hypertrophy in rat kidney (Ohno and Lyon, 1970, Ohno, 1971), whereas, oestrogens are capable of reducing kidney weight in the mouse (Shimkin et al. 1963) as well as reducing the daily sodium excretion in the human (Johnson et al. 1970). Earlier studies (Bloom et al. 1963) have demonstrated that steroids can induce abnormalities in the growth of the kidney. Furthermore, the presence of receptor proteins for progesterone and oestrogens in normal and malignant human kidneys have been reported by a number of investigators, (Bojar et al. 1975, Concolino et al. 1976). However, the presence of receptor proteins for androgens in these tissues has not been investigated, despite the ability of androgens to induce hypertrophy of the kidney in some animal species. In this comunication we wish to report the presence of an androgen binding component as well as an oestrogenic one in normal and malignant human kidneys.

MATERIALS AND METHODS

Steroids

$[17\alpha\text{-methyl-}^3\text{H}]$ Methyltrienolone (17α-methyl 4, 9, 11-estratrien-3-one) (^{3}H R1881) with specific activity of 78 Ci/mmol was purchased from New England Nuclear (Southampton, UK).

[2,4,6,7,-^{3}H] oestradiol-17β, specific activity 109 Ci/mmol
was purchased from the Radiochemical Centre, Amersham. 5α-
dihydrotestosterone (DHT), testosterone, progesterone, triamcinolone acetonide (TMA), oestradiol-17β, and diethylstilboestrol were purchased from Sigma Chemicals, Dorset, UK.
Stock solutions of steroids were made in ethanol and stored
at -20°C.

Buffers

    Two buffers were used through out these investigations.
Buffer A: This contained tris (10 mM) EDTA (1.5 mM) and
sodium molybdate (10 mM),
Buffer B: This was the same as buffer A, but also contained
10% v/v glycerol.
All buffers were adjusted to pH 7.4 at 4°C with HCl.

Chromatographic material

    Polyacrylamide gel plates 245 X 110 X 2 mm (PAG-plates)
containing 2.4% (w/v) Ampholine, pH range 3.5-9.5 were purchased from L.K.B. Instruments, South Croydon, Surrey, UK.
Electrode solutions were prepared in distilled water and
contained 1M sodium hydroxide (cathode) and 1M orthophosphoric
acid (anode).

preparation of cytosol

    Normal and malignant kidneys were frozen in liquid
nitrogen and stored at -35°C. Samples of frozen kidney
tissues were cut into 2-4 mm^3 cubes and pulverized in a
microdismembrator (Braun Melsungen, F.T., Scientific Instruments, Gloucester, UK) for two periods of 30 sec at full
speed with a cooling interval of 2 min. in liquid nitrogen.
The pulverized tissue was transferred to a precooled homo-
genisation vessel and 3 vol. (v/w) of buffer B added. The
mixture was homogenised with a motor driven pestle at 0-4°C
using three bursts of 10 sec. with a 30 sec. cooling interval.
The homogenate was then centrifuged at 105,000 g for 1 h. at
4°C to yield a supernatant which was referred to as cytosol.

Labelling of cytosol with tritiated steroids

    Tritiated steroids (10 nM of ^{3}H R1881 or oestradiol)
were dried down in vacuo at 40°C. When required, an excess
of radioinert competitors were also included. The tubes

were transferred to an ice-water bath and aliquots of cytosol added. At the end of the incubation period, the tubes were placed in ice and the free steroids separated from the bound by the addition of half vol. of dextran-coated charcoal (DCC) suspension (0.625%) dextran T-70 and 1.25% water washed Norit GSX charcoal prepared in buffer A). The tubes were incubated at 4°C for 10 min. and then centrifuged at 1000 g for 15 min. at 4°C. Aliquots of the resulting supernatant were then taken for further processing.

Glycerol density gradient centrifugation

Glycerol density gradient centrifugation was performed on 4.4 ml, 5-35% (v/v) linear gradients using the general principles as outlined by Martin and Ames (1961). The glycerol solutions were all prepared in buffer A and the pH was re-adjusted to 7.4 with HCl. Aliquots of labelled and DCC treated samples were diluted 1:1 with buffer A and 400 µl aliquots were applied to the surface of the gradients which were then loaded in an MSE. 6 X 5.5 ml, aluminium swing-out rotor and centrifuged at 40,000 r.p.m. in an MSE 65 MK.II ultra-centrifuge for 17 h. at 2°C. Gradients were fractionated into 24 equal portions, each of 200 µl collected from the bottom of the tube.

Isoelectric focusing

Isoelectric focusing was performed with the LKB 2117 Multiphor tank and an LKB 2103 power pack. The instruments were set in a cold room at 4-6°C and coolant from a cooling Circulator (Churchill Instruments, Middlesex, UK) set at 2°C was continually circulated through the cooling plate of the multiphor. Isoelectrophoresis was carried out in preformed polyacrylamide gel plates 245 X 110 X 2 mm. containing 2.4% w/v Ampholine, pH range 3.5-9.5 (L.K.B. Instruments, South Croydon, Surrey, UK). Aliquots (100 µl) of the labelled and DCC treated cytoplasmic preparations were analysed in accordance with the general procedure described by Auf and Ghanadian, (1981).

Quantitation of the cytoplasmic androgen receptor

Aliquots (200 µl) of cytosol or nuclear extract were incubated at 4°C for 20 h. with dried residues of [3]H R1881 solution to give final concentrations of 0.125 - 5 nM. A similar set of tubes, which also contained 100-fold excess of radioinert R1881 were used in order to correct for non-specific binding. All tubes contained 700-fold excess of triamcinolone acetonide (Zava et al, 1978) to inhibit the binding of ^{3}H R1881 to putative progesterone receptors which may be present in some kidney specimens. Following incubation, the free steroid was separated from the bound by incubating the samples at 4°C for 10 min. with half volume of DCC and centrifuging the mixture at 1000 g for 15 min. at 4°C. Aliquots (200 µl) of the resulting supernatants were then transferred to plastic vials and the radioactivity counted in 6 ml of liquid scintillation fluid (Packard 299). Specific binding of tritiated R1881 was calculated by subtracting non-specific binding (c.p.m. in presence of R1881) from total binding (c.p.m. in absence of R1881) and the results analysed by Scatchard plots as described by Chamnes and McGuire (1975).

RESULTS

Androgen Receptors

Partial characterization of the cytoplasmic androgen receptors was established by glycerol density centrifugation and isoelectric focusing on polyacrylamide gel. In all these experiments the labelling of the receptor was carried out at 0-4°C for 20 h. in buffer media containing 10 mM sodium molybdate in order to stabilize the receptor.

Analysis of the R1881 labelled cytosol by glycerol density gradient centrifugation revealed a peak of radioactivity associated with material which sedimented at the 7-8s regions. Specificity studies to establish the nature of this binding moeity showed that the inclusion of 100-fold excess of either radioinert R1881 or DHT could completely abolish the binding in this region. The addition of 100-fold excess of testosterone also caused substantial inhibition of this peak. However, neither the inclusion of 100-fold excess of progesterone or 700-fold excess of TMA were capable of producing a significant inhibition. This specificity pattern was consistent in the 4 tumours that contained a ^{3}H R1881 binding peak. Similar results were also obtained in cytosol prepared from the normal human kidney. A representative of these results is shown in fig. 1. In 9 tumours analysed by gradient centrifugation only 4 revealed a binding peak for R1881, whilst the other 5 tumours did not display any binding in this region. From 7 normal kidneys, only 3 showed a saturable binding peak at the 7-8s region. The results from the specificity studies clearly shows that the binding of R1881 in the 7-8s region is to a saturable androgen binding component and not to a progestogenic one.

Having established the presence of androgen binding component by glycerol gradient centrifugation, further characterization of this binding entity was carried out to determine its isoelectric point. The results which are displayed in fig. 2, shows a sharp peak of radioactivity with a pI of 6.2 which was completely abolished with 100-fold excess of radioinert R1881. The second peak of radioactivity having a pI of 4.5 was not affected by the inclusion of R1881 and is probably associated with albumin. The peak with pI of 6.2 is consistent with that of androgen receptors from target tissues.

Quantitation of the cytoplasmic androgen receptor was carried out by a 7 point corrected Scatchard plot analysis as described in materials and methods. A representative of a typical Scatchard plot is shown in fig. 3. Analysis of the receptor was performed on 7 normal and 9 malignant tumours. In the normal tissue, receptor analysis was carried out in the separated cortex and medulla. Four malignant kidneys and 3 normals were receptor positive whereas, androgen receptors were not detectable in the remaining tissues. The results are shown in table I. The dissociation constant (Kd) in all tissues was in the order of 10^{-9} M which is an indication of the high affinity binding nature of this protein binding component. The content of cytoplasmic receptors in the tumours was generally higher than in the normal kidneys (see table 1).However, it was not possible to confirm this observation statistically due to the limited number of tissues.

Oestrogen Receptor

The presence of an oestrogen binding component was also investigated in 9 tumours and 7 normal kidneys by glycerol density gradient centrifugation. All analyses were carried out in the presence of 10 mM sodium molybdate. In 8 tumours and only one normal kidney an 8s oestradiol-17β binding peak was observed. The activity associated with this binding peak was completely abolished when 100-fold excess of either radioinert oestradiol or diethylstilboestrol were included in the incubation media. Neither DHT nor R1881 were effective in displacing radioactivity from this binding peak. In most tissues the concentration of the oestrogenic binding component was extremely low and for this reason no attempt was made to quantitate it.

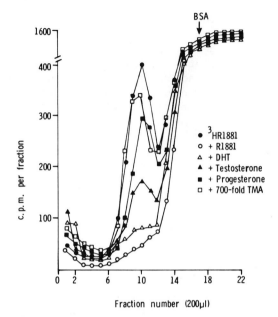

Fig.1 Glycerol density gradient profile of kidney tumour cytosol labelled at 0 C for 20 h. with 10 nM ^{3}HR1881. All buffers contained 10 mM sodium molybdate.

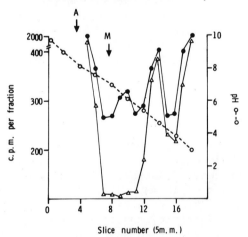

Fig. 2 Isoelectric focusing of cytosol from human kidney tumours. Cytosol is labelled with 20 nm ^{3}HR1881 (●) in the presence of 100-fold excess radioinert R1881 (△).
A=application point, M=myoglobin standard

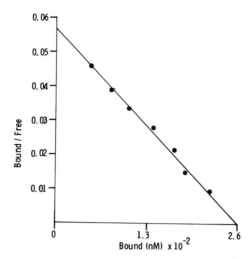

Fig. 3 Scatchard plot analysis for the binding of [3]HR1881 in the cytosol of human kidney tumour. Incubations were made in the presence of 700-fold excess TMA at 0 C for 16h. All media contained 10 mM sodium molybdate.

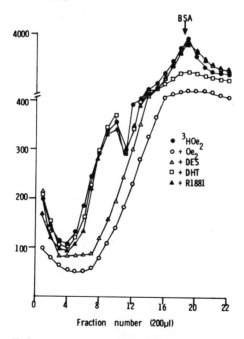

Fig. 4 Glycerol density gradient profile of kidney tumour cytosol labelled at 0 C for 20h. with 10nM [3]HOe$_2$. All buffers contained 10mM sodium molybdate.

Table I. The concentrations and dissociation constant of the cytoplasmic androgen receptors in normal and malignant human kidneys.

Normal Male	Dissociation constant (nM)		Receptor concentration (fmol/g tissue)	
	Cortex	Medulla	Cortex	Medulla
1	0.29	0.75	79	44
2	0.4	0.35	238	165
3	-	0.56	ND	88

Kidney tumours (Male)	Dissociation constant (nM)	Receptor concentration (fmol/g tissue)
1	0.63	298
2	0.45	91
3	1.2	255
4	0.8	670

DISCUSSION

The results presented clearly demonstrate the presence of an androgen binding component with characteristics of androgen receptors. The 7-8s binding peak obtained by gradient centrifugation was only detectable when the stabilizing agent sodium molybdate, was included in the incubation media. A similar stabilizing effect has been reported for both glucocorticoid (Nielson et al. 1977) and progesterone (Bevin and Bashirelahi, 1980) receptors. Despite this, androgen receptors were detectable only in about 40% of the normal or malignant kidneys. The receptor concentration appeared to be higher in the malignant kidneys. However, due to the limited number of tissues analysed, this difference could not be proven statistically.

Although the conditions of incubation in this study $(0-4°C)$ allows the binding of R1881 to both androgen and progesterone receptors, the results of the characterization study by gradient centrifugation revealed that progesterone and TMA were ineffective in suppressing the R1881 binding peak. This therefore, suggests that none of the specimens examined in our study possessed a progesterone binding component, which is in contrast with reports by others (Bojar et al. 1980 and Tobin et al. 1980).

Steroid Receptors

The analysis of oestrogen binding components in kidney tumours revealed that 8 out of 9 (89%) samples contained this binding component. However, the concentration of this receptor was very low and we were unable to quantitate it by Scatchard plot analysis. Furthermore, in the normal kidney one out of 7 tissues possessed this binding component. Although more kidney tumours contained oestrogen binding proteins it would be inappropriate to comment on these findings until further studies especially on the nuclear binding of oestrogens have been carried out. This also applies to the significance of the presence of a relatively higher concentration of androgen receptors in the kidney tumours.

SUMMARY

The presence of androgen and oestrogen receptors in normal and malignant human kidneys is reported. Characterization of these receptors was performed by glycerol gradient centrifugation and isoelectric focusing. Androgen receptors were detected in 40% of the tissues and its concentration was higher in the malignant kidneys. Oestrogen receptors were demonstrable in 8 out of 9 tumours, but only one out of 7 normal kidneys. The level of this receptor was extremely low.

Auf G, Ghanadian R (1981). Analysis of androgen receptors in the human prostate by isoelectric focusing in polyacrylamide gel. J Steroid Biochem. In press.

Bevins CL, Bashirelahi N (1980). Stabilization of 8s progesterone receptor from human prostate in the presence of molybdate ion: Cancer Research 40:2234.

Bojar H, Wittliff JL, Balzar E, Dreyfurst R, Beninghaus F, Stails W (1975). Properties of specific estrogen-binding components in human kidney and renal carcinoma. Acta endocr Copenh Suppl 193:51.

Bojar H, Maar K, Staib W (1980). R5020 Binding Components in Human Renal Cell Carcinoma. In Wittliff JL, Dapunt O (eds.): "Steroid receptors and hormone-dependent neoplasia" New York: Mason Publishing, p. 193.

Bloom HJG (1963). Hormone treatment of renal tumours:
Experimental and clinical observations. In: Riches EW
(ed.): "Tumours of the kidney and ureter" London:
Livingstone, p. 311.

Chamness CG, McGuire WL (1975). Scatchard plots:
Common errors in correction and interpretation:
Steroids 26:538.

Concolino G, Marocchi A, Concolino F, Sciarra F,
DiSilverio F, Conti C (1976). Human kidney steroid
receptors. J Steroid Biochem 7:831.

Martin RG, Ames BNA (1961). A method for determining the
sedimentation behaviour of enzymes: application to
protein mixtures. J Biol Chem 263: 1372.

Nielson CJ, Vogel WM, Pratt WB (1977). Glucocorticoid
receptor inactivation under cell-free conditions. J
Biol Chem 252:7568.

Ohno S, Lyon NF (1970). X-linked testicular feminization
in the mouse as a non-inducible regulatory mutation of
the Jacab-Monod type. Clin Genetics 1:121.

Ohno S (1971). Simplicity of Mammalian regulatory
systems inferred by single gene determination of sex
phenotypes. Nature 234:134.

Shimkin MB, Shimkin PM, Andervant HB (1963). Effect of
oestrogens on kidney weight in mice. J Nat Cancer
Inst 30:135.

Tobin EH, Mouhaddeb I, Bloom ND (1980). Analysis of
specific progesterone receptor proteins in human
kidney and renal cell carcinoma. In: Wittliff JL,
Dapunt O (eds.): "Steroid receptors and hormone
dependent neoplasia" New York: Mason Publishing,
p. 197.

Zava DT, Landrum B, Horowitz KB, McGuire WL (1978).
Androgen receptor assay with (^{3}H) methyltrienolone
(R1881) in the presence of progesterone receptors.
Endocrinology 104:1007.

Renal Tumors: Proceedings of the First International Symposium on
Kidney Tumors, pages 255–271
© 1982 Alan R. Liss, Inc., 150 Fifth Avenue, New York, NY 10011

AETIOLOGY OF RENAL CANCER*

Michele Pavone-Macaluso, Giovanni B. Ingargiola
and Marcello Lamartina
Institute of Urology, University of Palermo
Palermo, Italy

Surveys of possible aetiological factors were made in
1963 and in 1967 by Pavone-Macaluso who reviewed 44
articles hoping to find some clues to the causes of tumours
of kidney.

It is apparent that from the aetiological standpoint
renal cell carcinoma must be considered separately from
nephroblastoma, transitional cell carcinoma, sarcoma and
other types of renal neoplasia, although in rare instances
the same cause was experimentally found to be responsible
for the occurrence of renal tumours of different histotypes.
For instance, benzpyrene was found to produce either renal
cell carcinoma, kidney sacroma or squamous cell carcinoma
of the renal pelvis, depending on the experimental animal
and route of administration.

Apart from this and other exceptions, it appeared that
adenoma and adenocarcinoma (renal cell carcinoma) were
often caused by the same factors, whereas Wilms' tumours
and the other neoplasias were related to different aetiological factors.

1. NEPHROBLASTOMA
Nephroblastoma is not infrequently congenital and bilateral. It can be associated with various congenital mal-

* By kind permission of Plenum Publishing Company and the
editors of "Cancer of kidney and prostate", New York and
London: Plenum Press, in press.

formations especially with hemihypertrophy and aniridia.
It has been suggested that the presence of aberrant embryonal germs, or the abnormal growth of multipotent cells during foetal life, might be responsible for their formation.
Heredity may represent a predisposing factor, whereas geographic and environmental conditions, including chemical
carcinogens and hormones, do not appear to play a significant role in their aetiology. It is extremely difficult
to produce Wilms' tumours experimentally although a nephroblastoma could be induced in fowl by the myeloblastosis
avian tumour virus.

2. SQUAMOUS CELL CARCINOMA
    Squamous cell carcinoma has been described in patients
as a late complication of retrograde pyelography with a
radioactive compound, thorotrast. Squamous cell carcinomas
have also been produced experimentally by the intrarenal
administration of chemical carcinogens. Renal stones,
infection and other factors producing "chronic irritation"
are likely to play a role in the development of both
squamous cell carcinoma and mucus secreting adenocarcinoma
of the renal pelvis.

3. TRANSITIONAL CELL CARCINOMA OF THE RENAL PELVIS
    Transitional cell carcinoma of the renal pelvis can be
produced by the same exogenous or endogenous carcinogens
that are held responsible for the induction of bladder
tumour. Papillary tumours of the renal pelvis have been
produced experimentally using 2 naphtylamine and have been
detected in workers exposed to industrial carcinogens.
Urothelial carcinoma of the renal pelvis has often been
found in association with two conditions which lead to two
types of chronic interstial nephritis, namely Balkan nephropathy and nephritis due to prolonged use of analgesics
containing phenacetin.

4. RENAL ADENOMA AND ADENOCARCINOMA
    As this presentation deals with renal cell carcinoma, a
more detailed discussion will be devoted to the spontaneous
occurrence of renal adenocarcinoma in various animals, as
well as to the various aetiolgical factors that have been
investigated in different animal species.

    Adenoma and adenocarcinoma will be considered together,
as we believe that there is no clear distinction between
the two conditions and that the traditional differentiation

based only on the size of the tumours is arbitrary. In addition, both adenoma and carcinoma can be produced by the same carcinogen in various animal models and serial transplantation of adenoma may give rise to frankly malignant carcinoma. In the following sections only the term adenocarcinoma will be employed; its definition in this text includes adenoma and is considered synonymous to "renal cell carcinoma."

A. SPONTANEOUS RENAL TUMOURS IN ANIMALS
    Spontaneous renal tumours are relatively rare, both in wild and domestic animals. Among the latter, poultry, horses and swine are affected most frequently.

    Although mixed tumours, similar to Wilms nephroblastoma and renal urotheliomas have been occasionally found, only adenocarcinoma will be considered here.

    The incidence of renal adenocarcinoma in rats ranges between 0.0004 to 0.2% in various strains.

    Genetic as well as hormonal factors seem to play a role in a strain of Wistar rats in which 24% of males and 51% of females were affected (Eker 1954).

    Similarly, in mice, the overall incidence is 0.02% (Horn, Stewart 1952) but one strain was found to be affected in about one half of animals (Claude 1958).

    Spontaneous adenocarcinoma has been found in 0.5% of hamsters (Fortner et al. 1961). The occurrence of renal adenocarcinoma in frogs will be discussed apropos of viral aetiology.

B. ASSOCIATION OF RENAL TUMOURS WITH OTHER PATHOLOGICAL
    CONDITIONS

    Horseshoe kidney and other congenital malformations are occasionally associated not only with nephroblastoma but also with renal cell carcinoma. According to Patoir (1959), who collected 30 such cases from the medical literature up 1959, the incidence of renal tumours in horseshoe kidneys is higher than in the average population. Unilateral or bilateral renal cancer has also been observed in association with polycystic disease of the kidney (Tallarigo 1950; Puigvert 1958), multilocular cystic disease (Beckwith 1981), diabetes mellitus (Chawalla 1953), and a variety of other diseases (Pignalosa, Fernandez 1938).

It has also been suggested that adenomas are more likely to arise in atrophic kidneys with focal tubular hyperplasia than in normal organs. It is difficult to be certain that such associations are due to a cause-effect relationship, rather than merely being coincidental.

There are, however, two conditions in which renal tumours, often bilateral, are significantly more frequent than in non-affected population: 1) renal hamartomas in Bourneville's tuberous sclerosis; 2) renal adenocarcinomas in von Hippel-Lindau's haemangioblastoma. For an extensive bibliography concerning these pathological associations, see Pavone-Macaluso (1963, 1967).

C. POSSIBLE AETIOLOGICAL FACTORS FOR RENAL ADENOCARCINOMA
Such factors include race, heredity, viruses, alterations in the host's immunological reactivity (renal transplantation), irradiation, hormones, endogenous and exogenous carcinogens, as well as smoking habits, beverages, food and other environmental factors.

A detailed discussion of these various factors will be beyond the scope of the present article. For detailed information and bibliography the reader is referred not only to our previous reviews (Pavone-Macaluso 1963, 1967), but also to more recent papers on closely related topics (Kanton 1977, Sufrin 1980). Only brief comments and recent references will be given here.

C1. Race, Epidemiology and other Environmental Factors
Epidemiological studies of renal cancer are relatively scarse (Berrino 1981).

It does not seem, however, that racial factors play a major role. In the United States, no significant difference in the frequence of renal tumours was observed among Caucasian, Negro and Mexican ethnic groups, although the incidence in the Japanese population has been reported to be slightly higher. As far as geographic distribution is concerned, only minor fluctuations have been described. Comparison of mortality rates from renal malignancies in selected countries permitted a distinction among three different groups (Case 1964): 1) countries showing low rates (Ireland, Italy, Japan, Spain, Venezuela); 2) countries showing high rates (Denmark, Norway, Scotland, New Zealand); 3) countries with an intermediate incidence rate (Belgium, Holland, France, England, Wales, Australia, U.S.A). It can be inferred that the highest frequency of carcinoma of the kidney is found in the industrialized countries of western Europe, especially in the northern areas (Scandinavia and Scotland) and, to a lesser degree, in U.S.A. Urbanization and high social class appear to be associated with a comparatively high incidence of renal cancer. This does not appear to be related to animal protein, but rather to fat intake. A positive correlation with obesity has been found. The role of smoke is still controversial, although some reports show a greater incidence of renal tumours not only in cigarette but especially in cigar and pipe smokers. This may depend, at least in part, on the fact that tobacco smoking leads to increased inhalation and absorption of 'renal carcinogens', such as methylnitrosamine and cadmium, as well as to enhanced urinary excretion of 3 - hydroxyanthranilic acid and other abnormal tryptophan metabolites. Occupational hazards should also be considered. Coke oven workers appear to be especially at risk (Redmond 1965).

C2 Heredity

Heredity is not usually considered of primary importance in this context, although genetic factors have been shown to play a definite role not only in rats and mice but also in Rhesus monkeys. In the latter species a family has been described in which four animals were affected by renal adenocarcinoma (Ratcliffe 1940). In humans there also have been several observations of renal adenocarcinoma in members of the same family. Brinton (1960) described a family in which at least four persons died from kidney carcinoma in two different generations. Ten people in three generations were found to be affected in a more recent report (Goldman 1979).

The role of genetic factors is stressed by the higher incidence in subjects with blood group A, as well as by reports of cases of hereditary renal cell carcinoma associated with chromosome translocations (Cohen et al. 1979) and with colour blindness (Griffin et al. 1967). Reddy (1981), in addition to his own observation of bilateral renal cell carcinoma in a father and his two sons, noted 14 reports of familiar renal cancer in the English literature up to 1981. The association of heredity to renal cancer should be investigated with greater emphasis in the future, especially with regard to cases of bilateral tumours.

C3. Irradiation
    Whole body irradiation induced renal adenocarcinoma in 30% of intact mice and in 53% of animals with single kidneys (Rosen, Cole 1962). Fast neutrons lead to similar results.

    A case of renal adenocarcinoma following retrograde pyelography with thorotrast, a colloidal suspension of radioactive thorium dioxide, has also been described (Freidrich 1960) in addition to the more numerous cases of squamous cell carcinoma, which can be ascribed to the same aetiological factor. Radioactive compounds, such as Polonium 210 and Strontium 90, have also been incriminated in renal cancerogenesis.

C4. Viruses
    The viral aetiology of a spontaneous renal carcinoma (Lucké's tumor) occurring in the North American leopard frog (Rana pipiens) has been demonstrated beyond doubt. The lesions are well differentiated adenocarcinomas which, under favourable conditions, metastisize in 80% of cases. When adult frogs are kept in the laboratory for 8 months, the incidence is between 3 and 9%.

    An updated review was presented in 1980 by Beckley (1980). As early as 1938, Lucké had demonstrated that this tumour is strictly species specific. If its cells or their extracts are injected into green frogs (Rana clamitans), bull frogs (Rana catesbiana) or even into a different subspecies of Rana pipiens, none of the frogs of foreign species develop renal cancer. The aetiological agent has been identified as a herpes simplex virus (Granoff 1973). Interestingly enough, in a recent investigation herpes simplex virus (HSV) specific antigens were identified in a human adenocarcinoma of the kidney (Cocchiara et al. 1980).

    As the presence of HSV tumour associated antigens has been found in other human tumours, it remains uncertain whether or not this really represents demonstration of their viral aetiology.

    Renal tumours can also be produced in hamsters and in other rodents by the polyoma virus, the simian virus SV 40

and by the adenovirus 7. Such tumors are usually different
from adenocarcinoma, a sarcomotous pattern being the most
frequent histotype.

C5. Hormones

It has been known for many years that renal adenomas
and adenocarcinomas can be induced by prolonged administration of both natural and synthetic estrogens in the male
golden Syrian hamster. A recent report suggests that renal
tumours also can be consistently induced in the European
hamster (Reznick, Schuller 1979). It appears that the male
hamster is the only animal species in which renal tumours
are caused by estrogens. If administration of hormones is
stopped even after long periods of time, regression of the
tumours will take place. These tumours are similar to
adenocarcinoma of the renal kidney, including the high
lipid content of the tumour cells; they are often multiple
and bilateral. Their growth is initially expansive and
eventually becomes infiltrative. True metastases are rare.
If the estrogenic treatment is extended for at least 250
days, kidney tumours develop in about 97% of treated males.
No tumours appear in organs other than the kidneys.
Estrogen induced renal adenocarcinoma may develop not only
in intact male hamsters but also in castrated males. In
females, estrogens can induce renal tumours only before
the onset or after the cessation of sexual activity. The
tumours can be serially transplanted into other male hamsters
provided the recipient animals are also treated with estrogens. Such hormone dependence, however, can be lost after
several passages in animals, so that after many transfers,
takes can be obtained even if the recipient animals are
not given estrogens.

This animal model lends itself to attempts at treatment
with a variety of hormone manipulations. Thus, it has been
shown that deoxycorticosterone inhibits the growth of renal
carcinoma in estrogen treated male hamsters (Rivière et al.
1960). By transplantation of an estrogen independent
tumour into animals treated with various hormones or submitted to endocrine ablation procedures (Bloom et al. 1963),
it appeared that: a) cortisone produced marked tumour inhibition; b) a progestational agent, if used without concurrent administration of cortisone, had comparatively
little effect upon the tumour growth rate; c) adrenalectomy
procuded growth reduction; d) orchidectomy was followed by
inhibition of tumour development and by prevention of

further growth in established transplants; e) the effect
of orchidectomy was abolished by the administration of
testosterone or estrogens; f) bromocryptine inhibited
primary renal tumours induced by DES.

The previously mentioned experiments have been followed
by many attempts to treat human renal adenocarcinoma with
hormones. Medroxyprogesterone acetate, testosterone and
cortisone or related steroids have been used for this purpose. Human renal adenocarcinoma has long been considered
to be responsive to hormonal treatment and even to be a
hormone dependent tumour. This view was recently supported
by the finding of hormone receptors in normal kidney tissue and in renal cancer (Concolino et al. 1978). It has,
however, been challenged in the last few years, due to
conflicting clinical and experimental results (DiFronzo 1980).
This topic will receive a more thorough discussion elsewhere in this symposium. (See chapters by Haanadian et al.
and Karr et al.)

There seems to be little doubt that human renal adenocarcinoma is under some sort of hormonal influence. There
is a significant difference in incidence between sexes,
the tumour being more frequent in males than in females.
In the series of Pignalosa and Fernandez (1938), 69.9% of
renal tumours were found in males. This difference tends
to increase after menopause, reaching a male to female
ratio of 4:1. The dependence of "hypernephromas" on
endocrine disturbances has often been postulated. It was
claimed, for instance, that renal adenocarcinoma is more
frequent in patients with hypercorticism or other states
of hormonal imbalance than in the average population. It
has also been hypothesized that spontaneous regression of
renal tumours may be under the influence of endocrine
changes (Bartely, Hultquist 1950). The relationship
between hormones and renal cancer remains a controversial
issue. Estrogen-induced renal carcinoma in the male
hamster is an important experimental model but this animal
is unique in showing this particular behaviour. The gap
still remains to be filled between laboratory animals and
human beings and, in our view, it is doubtful whether
conclusion drawn from investigations performed in the
hamster can be safely applied to renal tumours in man.

C6. Chemicals
Endogenous carcinogens may be involved not only in the

production of urothelial tumours but also in that of renal
parenchymal cancer. A case of adenocarcinoma associated
with increased urinary excretion of tryptophan metabolites
was described (Kerr et al. 1963), but to the best of our
knowledge, this finding has not been confirmed in subsequent years. This remains, however, a very interesting
avenue for future research. A larger number of observations has been obtained with regard to exogenous chemical
carcinogens. A table, with a long list of substances
which have been tested for renal carcinogenic activity,
was presented in our review of 1967 (Pavone-Macaluso, 1967).
Further data from the current literature were reviewed by
Sufrin in 1980.

It has been shown that several exogenous chemical carcinogens are able to produce renal tumours in various
laboratory animals. There are also some interesting
clinical observations which suggest that this may also be
true in humans.

Among the substances that are carcinogenic to the kidney,
nitroso compounds, aromatic amines, hydrazines, alkylating
agents, anticancer chemotherapeutic agents, metals and
natural compounds deserve special attention. A few miscellaneous agents will also be considered.

NITROSO COMPOUNDS
Nitrosamines are currently employed in rubber vulcanization and textile fiber industries.

Dimethylnitrosamine (DMN) has been known for a number
of years to be a potent oncogenic agent. Chronic administration of DMN to the rat gives rise to degenerative
changes and to neoplasms in the liver and lungs. In acute
experiments with high doses of DMN, the liver undergoes
marked regression without secondary tumour formation.
Instead, renal adenoma or adenocarcinoma appear in about
one half of the surviving animals. Even a single dose of
DMN will produce renal tumours in 63% of female rats, in
spite of the fact that DMN is rapidly excreted and meta-
bolized.

With regard to other animal species, DMN feeding induced renal adenocarcinoma in 72% of Swiss mice, but was
ineffective in European hamsters. The renal tumours induced by DMN and related compounds are of two main

histological types: an adenocarcinoma arising from the
renal tubules and an anaplastic mesenchymal tumour.

Diethylnitrosamine, if given as a single intravenous bolus
to Sprague-Dawley rats, induces bilateral and multifocal
renal tumours in 30% of males and 80% of females. Tumours
tend to be present in other organs too. The same compound
is also effective in inducing renal adenocarcinoma in
either sex of the golden Syrian hamster.

Nitrosomethylurea gives rise to anaplastic or sarcomatous
renal tumours if administered to adult rats, whereas
adenocarcinoma can be obtained in 25% of Wistar rats
treated at birth or within the first days of life. Similar
results were obtained in mice.

Nitrosethylurea. Following treatment with this compound
rats develop nephroblastoma, but mice develop adenocarcinoma. This is another interesting confirmation that
the same oncogenic agent can produce various tumour
histotypes if employed under different experimental
conditions and in different animal species.

AROMATIC ANIMES
4' fluoro - 4 animodiphenyl. This anime induces renal
adenocarcinoma in 80% of treated male Wistar rats. They
are often bilateral and multifocal and are usually associated with tumours of liver, colon, pancreas and testis.
Renal carcinomas that can be serially transplanted are
induced in rats by a closely related compound, N - (4' -
fluoro - 4 biphenyl) acetamide.

Acetylaminofluorene. This compound is a well known carcinogen which is responsible for the induction of
transitional cell carcinoma in the urothelium of bladder
and renal pelvis. It can also induce renal adenocarcinoma
in 10% of treated rats.

HYDRAZINES
    Renal adenocarcinomas were obtained in 80% of Sprague-
Dawley rats treated with formic acid - nitrofuryl -
thiazolyl hydrazide (FNT). The other hydrazines tested
so far appear to be less effective.

ALKYLATING AGENTS
    An alkylating agent, the flame retardant tris (2,3 -

dibromopropyl) phosphate (TBP), if given in high doses, is
capable of inducing renal adenocarcinoma in 39% of rats
and in 21% of mice.

As recently pointed out by Reznick et al. (1979), the
use of flame retardants has greatly increased in current
years, following the introduction of U.S. federal regu-
lations concerned with fabric flammability, particularly
those requiring treatment of all children's sleepwear.
In addition, TBP is used in carpets, plastics, house
furnishings and in building materials. The oncogenic
effects of TBP in rodents occur not only after oral
administration, but also if painted on the skin of experimental animals. This has created great concern in
the United States. In the fear that a carcinogenic
substance might enter the bodies of children by being
absorbed through the skin or by being ingested by children
"mouthing" their clothing, TPB was banned from commercial
use in April, 1977.

Interestingly enough, large numbers of pajamas for
children, treated with flame retardants, are now being
exported from the USA to Europe. This fact has even led
to an official interrogation in March, 1981 by a member
of the European Parliament. Flame retardants are certainly toxic. They cause testicular atrophy and chronic
interstitial nephritis in rabbits. If traces of TPB
(1 ppm) are added to the water containing goldfish, all
fish die within 5 days. There is, however, no current
proof that TBP and related compound are responsible for
the induction of renal cancer in man.

ANTICANCER AGENTS
Streptozotocin administered by a single intravenous dose,
induces diabetes mellitus immediately and causes delayed
renal adenocarcinoma in 50% of treated male Holzman rats.
Only 7% of Wistar rats are affected, suggesting an
important strain difference.

Daunorubicin, an anthracycline antitumour antibiotic
closely related to doxorubicin (adriamycin), if administered
to Sprague - Dawley rats, has been reported to produce
chronic glomerulonephritis in nearly all animals as well
as renal adenocarcinoma in 21% of treated rats (Sternberg
et al. 1972).

METALS

Lead. In 1962 Kilham and associates reported that a high prevalence of renal tumours had been observed in wild rats living in a suburban industrial area in the vicinity of burning refuse dumps containing substantial amounts of lead. The lead content of various tissues was abnormally high and typical lead inclusions were discovered in the renal tubular cells of these animals. Furthermore, it was demonstrated that prolonged administration of lead acetate or phosphate results in the development of kidney adenocarcinomas in the rat. Hyperplastic and cystic lesions occur after short treatment periods. Such tumours can be obtained only in rats and mice, probably because of their tolerance of high doses which would be lethal to other animals. Attempts to ascertain if chronic lead intoxication is a factor in the development of renal tumours in man have yielded negative results so far. Despite marked reduction of acute saturnism in the typographic industry, chronic lead poisoning is still possible. Work involving soldering, painting, battery charging and insecticide spraying are particularly hazardous from this standpoint. Heavy air pollution in most cities, especially since lead tetraethyl is used as an additive to some petrol fuels, is a factor to be kept in mind. This may be a possible explanation for the higher incidence of renal cancer in urban than in rural areas. However, follow-up studies of workers exposed to lead vapour inhalation have failed to demonstrate any greater incidence of renal tumours among those workers than in the general population.

Cadmium. A relatively high incidence of renal cancer has been described in workers exposed to cadmium poisoning (Berrino 1981). This metal is also viewed as a possible oncogenic factor for prostatic adenocarcinoma. It is of interest that the incidence of both cancers is especially high in Sweden, where chronic cadmium poisoning represents a very severe problem. Exposure to this substance may occur in workers during manufacture of almost all industrial products, including cameras, aircrafts breaks, semi-artificial agricultural fertilizers, dyes and washing machines. It has been reported that Sweden is actually exposed to 80-100 tons of cadmium yearly, often giving rise to highly toxic clouds. It has also been calculated that its concentration in the ground increases yearly by a factor of 0.5%. It has more than doubled within the last 40 years. A similar trend has also been observed in

other countries. This should lead to a more careful search
for a correlation between exposure to cadmium and renal
oncogenesis, so that timely preventive measures can be
taken, if this correlation can be confirmed.

NATURAL PRODUCTS
Cycas circinalis is a palm-like plant which is used as a
source of starch among the Chamorro, the indigen population
of Guam, Mariana Islands. There is evidence to indicate
that the seed of this plant can induce a high yield of
kidney and liver tumours. Renal tumours correspond even
ultrastructurally to human adenocarcinomas (Gusek 1975).
The responsible substance is a glycoside, named cycasin.
Its hydrolysis liberates the active aglycone, methyl-
azoxy-methanol (MAM). Intraperitoneal MAM induces renal
adenocarcinoma or less frequently a renal sarcoma, in
78% of rats. The tumours are bilateral in 57% of cases.
The incidence of MAM or cycasin induced tumours is much
lower in mice ahd hamsters. There is not yet any clear-
cut evidence that the population of Guam presents a
strikingly high incidence of renal cancer. However, the
frequently held view that normal unadulterated foodstuff
is always free from carcinogenic hazards is no longer
tenable.

MISCELLANEOUS COMPOUNDS
A list of substances experimentally found to be capable
of inducing renal cancer would not be complete without
mention of ochratoxin A, safrole, niridazole, urethane,
and elaiomycin. The potent and almost ubiquitous polycyclic aromatic hydrocarbon carcinogens, benzpyrene,
20-methylcholanthrone and dibenzanthracene are rather ineffective as renal oncogens, since less than 10% of
treated animals develop kidney adenocarcinomas. Finally,
a recent WHO report, quoted in the Bulletin of Italian
Ministry of Health (Poggiolini 1980), suggests that
chloroform is also a relatively potent agent responsible
for experimental induction of renal adenocarcinoma in rats
and mice. In the rat, renal cancer was obtained in 8% and
24% of animals treated with daily doses of 90 and 180mg/kg,
respectively. Higher doses induced liver carcinoma. In
the mouse, renal adenocarcinoma developed in 10-25% of
males treated with 60 mg/kg/day. Chloroform has therefore been considered a potential carcinogenic agent in
man and the U.I.C.C. has suggested that all pharmaceutical products containing chloroform should be withdrawn

from free commercial distribution. This recommendation
has been put in practice in Canada, the USA, Japan, Norway,
Poland, Sweden and Switzerland. The European community
has, however, not restricted the use of tooth paste containing 4% chloroform, postponing final decision until
January, 1981. In the United Kingdom a maximum chloroform
concentration of 0.5% is still allowed in pharmaceutical
products pending more definitive information about its
actual carcinogenic risk in man. Again, as noted with
regard to flame retardants, no controls or restrictions
are requested in European countries belonging to the Common
Market with regard to products imported from abroad.

In conclusion, a few interesting animal models have
emerged from the study of spontaneous and experimental
animal tumours. They are appealing, in spite of obvious
reservations and limits, for the investigation of potential
forms of treatment (De Vere White 1981). They have, however, given us relatively little insight into the unsolved
problem of aetiology of renal cancer in man. Important
information on the early events in renal carcinogens has
resulted. It is of interest that damage to the tubular
cells appears to be the first recognizable event and that
the appearance of cystic lesions often precedes that of
adenoma and adenocarcinoma in a few experimental renal
tumours. Species or strain specificity and sex also
appear to play a significant role. In man, it is likely
that heredity, coexistence of other diseases, smoking,
food habits and irradiation represent possible aetiological
factors. It also appears that hormonal, chemical and
other environmental factors can play a role. The importance of herpes virus in renal adenocarcinoma needs
to be elucidated. Many suspects are at hand, but a major
villain still remains to be identified. It is hoped that
further research will be continued, so that data obtained from experimental work can lead to a better understanding of the aetiology of renal cancer in man.

Bartely O, Hultquist GT (1950). Spontaneous regression of
 hypernephromas. Acta Pathol Microbiol Scand 27:448.
Beckley S (1980). Viral models of renal adenocarcinoma.
 In Sufrin G, Beckley SA (eds): "Renal adenocarcinoma"
 Geneva: UICC, p. 28.
Beckwith JB (1981). Multilocular renal cysts and cystic
 renal tumors. Amer J Roentgenol 136:435.

Berrino F (1981). Epidemiologia e patogenesi dei tumori maligni del rene. Presented at the 22nd Course of the Istituto Nazionale Tumori, Milano (to be published).

Bloom HJG, Dukes CE, Nitchley BCV (1963). Hormone - dependent tumours of the kidney: I. The oestrogen-induced renal tumor of Syrian hamster; Hormone treatment and possible relationship to carcinoma of the kidney in man. Brit J Cancer 17:611.

Brinton LF (1960). Hyperneproma: familiar occurrence in one family. J Amer Med Assoc 173:889.

Case RAM (1964). Mortality from cancer of the kidney in England and Wales with data from other countries for comparison. In E Riches (ed): "Tumours of the kidney and ureter." Edinburgh: Livingstone p. 1.

Chwalla R (1953). Fenomeni endocrini nell'ipernefroma del rene. Urologia 20:9.

Claude A (1958). Adénocarcinome rénal endémique chez une souche de souris. Rev Franc Etudes Clin Biol 3:261.

Cocchiara R, Tarro G, Flaminio G, Di Gioia M, Smeraglia R, Geraci D (1980). Purification of herpes simplex virus tumor associated antigen from human kidney carcinoma. Cancer 46:1594.

Cohen AJ, Li FB, Berg S, Marchetto DJ, Tsai S, Jacobs SC, Brown RS (1979). Hereditary renal-cell carcinoma associated with a chromosome translocation. New Engl J Med 301:592.

Concolino G et al. (1978). Human renal carcinoma as a hormone-dependent tumor. Cancer Res 38:4340.

De Vere White R (1981). A spontaneously arising renal cancer in the rat. A model for drug sensitivity studies. Presented at the 4th Course of the International School of Urology and Nephrology. Erice (Sicily) 2-12 July 1981. Plenum Publ Co. In press.

Di Fronzo G (1980). Estrogen receptors in renal carcinoma. Eur Urol 6:307.

Eker R (1954). Familial renal adenoma in Wistar rats. Acta Path Microbiol Scand 34:554.

Fortner JA, Mahy AG, Contron RS (1961). Transplantable tumours of the Syrian golden hamster. Part II: Tumors of hematopoietic tissues, genito-urinary organs, mammary glands and sarcomas. Cancer Res 21:199.

Freidrich W (1960). Hypernephroides Carcinom nach Thorotrastanwendung und eosinophyles Adenom der Hypophyse. Z Krebsforsch 63:456.

Goldman SM (1979). Renal cell carcinoma diagnosed in three generations of a single family. South Med J 72:1457.

Granoff A (1973). Herpes virus and the Lucké tumor. Cancer Res 33:1431.

Griffin JP, Hughes GV, Peeling WB (1967). A survey of the familial incidence of adenocarcinoma of the kidney. Brit J Urol 39:63.

Gusek W (1975). Die Ultrastruktur Cycasin induzierter Nierenadenome. Virchow Arch Abt A Pathol 365:221.

Horn HA, Stewart JM (1952). A review of some spontaneous tumors in non-inbred mice. J Nat Cancer Inst 13:591.

Ishiguro H, Beard D, Sommer JR, Heine U, de Thé G, Beard JW (1962). Multiplicity of cell response to the BAI strain A (myeloblastosis) avian tumor virus. I: Nephroblastoma (Wilms' tumor), gross and microscopic pathology. J Nat Cancer Inst 29:1.

Kantor AF (1977). Current concepts of epidemiology and etiology of primary renal cell carcinoma. J Urol 117: 415.

Kerr WK, Barkin M, TODD, JAD, Menczyk Z (1963). Hypernephroma associated with elevated levels of bladder carcinogens in the urine: case report. Brit J Urol 35: 263.

Kilham L, Low RJ, Conti SF, Dallenback FD (1962). Intranuclear inclusions and neoplasms in the kidney of wild rats. J Nat Cancer Inst 29:863.

Lucké B (1938). Carcinoma in the leopard frog. Its probable causation by a virus. J Exp Med 68:457.

Patoir G (1959). Les tumeurs du rein en fer à cheval. J Urol méd chir 65:799.

Pavone-Macaluso M (1963). L'etiologie et la pathogènie des tumeurs du rein. Les tumeurs expérimentales. Gacette médicale de France 70:1143.

Pavone-Macaluso M (1967). Etiology of kidney tumors. In King JS (ed): "Renal Neoplasia", Boston: Little Brown and Co, p. 247.

Pignalosa M, Fernandez (1938), "Tumori del rene", Bologna: Cappelli.

Poggiolini D (1980). "Cloroformio". Bollettino d'informazione sui farmaci. Roma: Ministero della Santa. 4(11): 5.

Puigvert A (1958). Polykystose rénale et cancer bilatéral. J Urol méd chir. 64:30.

Ratcliffe HL (1940). Familiar occurrence of renal carcinoma in Rhesus monkey (macaca mulatta). Amer J Pathol 16:619.

Reddy ER (1981). Bilateral renal cell carcinoma. Unusual occurrence in three members of one family. Brit J Radiol 54:8.

Redmond (1965). J Occ Med 9:227, quoted by F. Berrino (1981).

Reznick G, Schuller H (1979). Carcinogenic effect of diethylstilbestrol in male Syrian golden hamster and European hamsters. J Nat Cancer Inst 62:1083.

Reznick G, Ward JM, Hardisty JF, Russfield A (1979). Renal carcinogenic and nephrotoxic effects of the flame retardant Tris (2, 3 - dibromopropyl) phosphate in F344 rats and (C57BL/6N x C3H/HeN)F_1 mice. J Nat Cancer Inst 63:205.

Rivière MC, Chouroulinkov I, Guérin M (1960). Action inhibitante de la désoxycorticostérone sur la production de tumeurs rénales chez le hamster mâle traité par un oestrogène. C R Soc Biol 154:1415.

Rosen VJ, Cole LJ (1962). Accelerated induction of kidney neoplasms in mice after x-radiation and unilateral nephrectomy. J Nat Cancer Inst 28:1031.

Sternberg SS, Philips FS, Croni AP (1972). Renal tumors and other lesions in rats following a single intravenous injection of daunomycin. Cancer Res 32:1029.

Sufrin G (1980). Spontaneous, hormonal and chemically induced animal models of renal adenocarcinoma. In Sufrin G, Beckley SA (eds): "Renal adenocarcinoma". Geneva: UICC, p 2.

Tallarigo A (1950). Su un raro caso di associazione tra rene policistico e tumore ipernefriode. Riv Anat Patol Oncol 3:510.

Renal Tumors: Proceedings of the First International Symposium on
Kidney Tumors, pages 273–275
© 1982 Alan R. Liss, Inc., 150 Fifth Avenue, New York, NY 10011

CLINICALLY UNRECOGNIZED RENAL CELL CARCINOMA.
AN AUTOPSY STUDY

Sverker Hellsten, M.D.*
Thorbjörn Berge, M.D.**
Folke Linell, M.D.**
Lennart Wehlin, M.D.***
*Dept of Urology, **Pathology and
***Diagn Radiology
Malmö General Hospital
S-214 01   MALMÖ, Sweden

In an autopsy series comprising 16,294 autopsies performed during a 12-year period of time,350
cases of renal cell carcinoma were found. In 115
cases the diagnosis of a renal cell carcinoma was
made ante mortem whereas 235 tumours were clinically unrecognized, the latter ones being the subject of the present study. Metastases were found
in 24 % of the patients with a clinically unrecognized renal cell carcinoma and was the main cause
of death in 21 %. The frequency and distribution
of the metastases were similar to that observed in
patients with a clinically recognized renal cell
carcinoma except for liver metastases that were
twice as common in the latter group.

Metastatic site	No and % of cases with metastases	
	Unrecognized r.c.c. (56 cases)	Recognized r.c.c. (103 cases)
Lungs	46 (82 %)	74 (72 %)
Lymph nodes	37 (66 %)	67 (65 %)
Bone	27 (48 %)	50 (49 %)
Adrenals	16 (29 %)	33 (32 %)
Liver	13 (23 %)	49 (48 %)

Table 1. The five most common metastatic sites in
159 cases of metastasizing renal cell carcinoma
(r.c.c.)

The symptomatology was generally poor as to the renal tumour in patients with a clinically unrecognized renal cell carcinoma. Cardiovascular disease was predominating and caused the death in 44 % while one or more malignant tumours other than the renal cell carcinoma were recognized in 33 % and was the main cause of death in 20 %.

The number of metastasizing tumours increased significantly with the size of the primary tumour.

Size (cm)	Number	Metastatic spread (no and %)
< 3	82	3 (3.7)
3 - 8	126	36 (29)
> 8	27	17 (63)

Table 2. Size of the primary tumour in relation to frequency of metastatic spread in 235 cases of clinically unrecognized renal cell carcinoma.

Local aggressiveness of the primary tumour in terms of vascular ingrowth or pericapsular growth was more common for large tumours but was much more closely correlated to metastatic spread than to size. Tumour ingrowth in the renal vein was significantly more common in metastasizing tumours as compared with non-metastasizing tumours.

235 r.c.c.
⟋ With metastatic spread = 56 r.c.c.
   (V - PC = 75 %)
⟍ Without metastatic spread = 179 r.c.c.
   (V - PC = 31 %)

Table 3. Vascular and/or pericapsular growth (V - PC) in 235 cases of clinically unrecognized renal cell carcinoma (r.c.c.).

Lymphatic spread was revealed in 66 % of patients with metastases. In 97 % of these patients additional, non-lymphatic metastatic spread was

seen. The most common sites of lymph node metastases were the retroperitoneal space (45 %), the
pulmonary hilum (44 %) and the supraclavicular
fossa (30 %). With involvement of these lymph node
stations a high incidence of concomitant metastases in the lungs was seen (86 %).

The present study confirmed that an analysis
of the local aggressiveness of the primary tumour
in the kidney and of the extent of the lymphatic
spread was prognostically valuable and might be
useful to define the group of patients that may
benefit from adjuvant treatment such as radiation
therapy, chemotherapy and immunotherapy.

Renal Tumors: Proceedings of the First International Symposium on Kidney Tumors, pages 277–282
© **1982 Alan R. Liss, Inc., 150 Fifth Avenue, New York, NY 10011**

PARANEOPLASTIC SYNDROMES: INTRODUCTION

Geoffrey D. Chisholm, Ch.M., F.R.C.S.

University Department of Surgery/Urology
Western General Hospital
Edinburgh, Scotland, U.K.

The traditional presentations for renal tumours in adults are loin pain, haematuria and a palpable mass.

Less commonly, this tumour may present with symptoms and signs that are unrelated to the urinary system. A solitary metastasis in a long bone may result in a pathological fracture; a metastasis can occur in almost any organ and may cause symptoms that range from visual defects to priapism.

Paraneoplastic syndromes are the third group of presentations and these have an incidence that is greater than the more traditional types of presentation (Chisholm, Roy 1971). However, some of the abnormalities are not always recognised as tumour - associated and others are missed because they may not be included amongst the screening tests.

The paraneoplastic syndromes associated with renal tumours include both clinical and laboratory abnormalities. It is convenient to classify these abnormalities in order to appreciate the range of these that has been linked with renal tumours (Chisholm 1980).

I NON SPECIFIC PARANEOPLASTIC SYNDROMES

The classification within this group is empirical and describes either the principal abnormality or the aetiology. It is recognised that many of these abnormalities are commonly associated with other malignancies but it is their high incidence with renal tumours and their disappearance after nephrectomy that suggests that they can be used as markers for the tumour. In addition, these are almost always early signs and symptoms of the tumour.

a) Haematological Syndromes

Anaemia. This occurs in approximately 33% of patients and resembles the anaemia seen in a chronic illness such as prolonged inflammation. It is not related to haematuria, tumour angiopathy or haemolysis. It is likely that erythropoietin deficiency and/or marrow depression are part of a tumour-toxic effect which results in anaemia.

Erythrocyte sedimentation rate (ESR). A raised ESR is the most frequent of systemic abnormalities - approximately 60% (Chisholm 1974). It has been stated that clear cell tumours have a higher mean ESR in addition to a lower mean haemoglobin level than granular cell tumours (Böttiger, Blanck, von Schreeb 1966).

Thrombocytosis, Thrombocytopenia, Leukaemoid reaction and Disorders of coagulation have all been associated specifically with renal carcinoma.

b) Biochemical Syndromes

Abnormalities of liver function. The specific association between abnormal liver function and non metastatic renal tumours is attributed to Stauffer (1961). The abnormalities consist of increased bromsulphalein retention, hypoprothrombinaemia, raised alpha-2 globulin and raised serum alkaline phosphatase. Liver biopsy in these patients shows no specific abnormality but lysosomal enzyme activity may be increased (Scherstén, Wahlquist, Jilderos 1971).

Alkaline phosphatase may be elevated as an isolated abnormality.

Plasma proteins. Albumin levels may be raised, alpha-2 globulin may be dramatically raised and a variety of changes in gamma globulins have been recorded.

c) Metabolic Syndromes

Pyrexia. A fever in association with a renal tumour is well known; it does not correlate with tumour size, necrosis, metastases, cell type, or age or sex of the patient. However an endogenous pyrogen has been identified in renal tumour extracts from patients with a fever (Rawlins, Luff, Cranston 1970).

Cachexia, Anorexia, Fatigue and Weight Loss are features common to all tumours. It has been suggested that renal tumours may liberate a "factor" which depresses the desire for food.

d) Immunological Syndromes

Amyloid disease may occur in patients with renal carcinoma and both clinical and experimental studies suggest an immunological basis to this association.

Neuromyopathy. An IgM paraproteinaemia has been detected in a patient with renal carcinoma and neuropathy (Thrush 1970).

II SPECIFIC ENDOCRINE SYNDROMES OR PARANEOPLASTIC ENDOCRINOPATHIES

These are abnormalities associated with hypersecretion by a renal tumour of a hormone or substance indistinguishable from a hormone. An increasing number of endocrine abnormalities have been reported so that this tumour now has one of the highest incidence of paraneoplastic endocrinopathies. In some, the evidence for an endocrine abnormality is weak and further reports are awaited; in others the availability of radioimmunoassays has enabled specific studies of the incidence of the abnormality in a group of patients. These endocrinopathies form 2 groups:

a) Hypersecretion of a Substance Normally Associated with the Kidney

Renin. Hypertension is a relatively common finding in patients with renal tumours. Circumstantial evidence for a pressor-secreting renal tumour was presented in 1969 (Ram, Chisholm) and more recently there have been reports of renin hypersecretion in both adults and children with renal carcinoma. Renin elevation was found in one-third of the patients studied by Sufrin, Mirand, Moore, Chu, Murphy(1977); it was unrelated to blood pressure but was associated with high grade, high stage lesions of mixed cell type and predicted a poor response. This tumour should not be confused with the renin-secreting tumour (haemangiopericytoma, or juxta-glomerular tumour) reported by Robertson, Klidjian, Harding, Walters in 1967.

Erythropoietin. A raised serum erythropoietin occurs in association with hydronephrosis, renal cysts and renal carcinoma. In one study of renal carcinoma, erythropoietin was raised in 36 of 51 patients (Sufrin et al 1977).

Prostaglandins (E & A). Hypercalcaemia is a common complication of renal carcinoma. Evidence that prostaglandins might be involved was reported by Brereton, Halushka, Alexander, Mason, Keiser, DeVita (1974). It has since been shown that renal carcinoma has bone-resorbing activity due to the presence of PGE.

In a single report, Prostaglandin A, a potent vaso-dilator was raised in a patient who had been hypertensive but then developed a renal tumour; there was a dramatic drop in PGA levels after nephrectomy and the blood pressure returned to hypertensive levels (Zusman, Snider, Cline, Caldwell, Speroff 1974).

b) Hypersecretion of Substances not Normally Associated with the Kidney

Parathormone. The reported incidence of hypercalcaemia in renal carcinoma varies from 3-13%. Evidence that a parathormone-like substance is responsible for hypercalcaemia was first provided by Goldberg, Tashjian, Order, Dammin (1964). It is relevant to note that coexisting primary hyperparathyroidism and renal carcinoma has been reported (Ackerman, Winer 1975).

Gonadotrophins. Ectopic human chorionic gonadotrophin by a renal carcinoma has been reported in 3 cases. In the male, gynaecomastia, feminisation or loss of libido may occur; in the female, hirsutism and amenorrhoea have been reported.

Placental Lactogen, Prolactin, Enteroglucogon and insulin-like activity have been noted in isolated cases and reviewed by Altaffer and Chenault (1979).

ACTH. Ectopic ACTH production is a common humoral syndrome associated with malignancy, especially oat cell carcinoma of the lung. A possible association with renal carcinoma has been reported (Rigg, Sprague 1961).

Conclusion. Paraneoplastic syndromes are an important clinical feature of renal tumours. They represent early manifestations of the tumour, and their disappearance with nephrectomy confirms that the tumour has been responsible for the abnormality. There is no unified explanation for these syndromes. However, the incidence of endocrine abnormalities supports the view that some tumours have poly-hormonal potential and may secrete excessive appropriate hormones as well as ectopic hormones. It is probable that hormone and enzyme production by these tumours is common but abnormal secretion is rare. It is already evident that the abnormal secretion by kidney tumours may be multiple and it is suggested that future studies may reveal an even wider range of polypeptides and amines associated with renal carcinoma.

Ackerman NB, Winer N (1975). The differentiation of primary hyperparathyroidism from the bypercalcemia of malignancy. Ann Surg 181:226.

Altaffer LF, Chenault OW Jr (1979). Paraneoplastic endocrinopathies associated with renal tumors. J Urol 122:573.

Böttiger LE, Blanck C, von Schreeb T (1966). Renal carcinoma: an attempt to correlate symptoms and findings with the histopathologic picture. Acta Med Scand 180:329.

Brereton HD, Halushka PV, Alexander RW, Mason DM, Keiser HR, DeVita VT Jr (1974). Indomethacin-responsive hypercalcemia in a patient with renal-cell adenocarcinoma. New Engl J Med 291:83.

Chisholm GD (1974). Nephrogenic ridge tumors and their syndromes. Ann NY Acad Sci 230:403.

Chisholm GD (1980). Clinical and biochemical markers in renal carcinoma. In Sufrin G, Beckley SA (eds): "Renal Adenocarcinoma", UICC Report No. 10, Geneva: WHO, pp 182-198.

Chisholm GD, Roy RR (1971). The systemic effects of
malignant renal tumours. Brit J Urol 43:687.
Goldberg MF, Tashjian AH Jr, Order SE, Dammin GJ (1964).
Renal adenocarcinoma containing a parathyroid hormone-
like substance and associated with marked hypercalcemia.
Amer J Med 36:805.
Ram MD, Chisholm GD (1969). Hypertension due to hypernephroma.
Brit Med J 4:87.
Rawlins MD, Luff RH, Cranston WI (1970). Pyrexia in renal
carcinoma. Lancet 1:1371.
Riggs BL Jr, Sprague RG (1961). Association of Cushing's
syndrome and neoplastic disease. Arch Intern Med 108: 841.
Robertson PW, Klidjian A, Harding LK, Walters G (1967).
Hypertension due to renin-secreting renal tumour. Amer J
Med 43:963.
Scherstén T, Wahlquist L, Jilderos B (1971). Lysosomal
enzyme activity in liver tissue, kidney tissue and tumor
tissue from patients with renal carcinoma. Cancer 27:278.
Stauffer MH (1961). Nephrogenic hepatosplenomegaly.
Gastroenterology 40:694.
Sufrin G, Mirand EA, Moore RH, Chu TM, Murphy GP (1977).
Hormones in renal cancer. Trans Amer Ass gen-urin Surg
68:115.
Thrush DC (1970). Neuropathy, IgM paraproteinaemia, and
autoantibodies in hypernephroma. Brit Med J 4:474.
Zusman RM, Snider JJ, Cline A, Caldwell BV, Speroff L (1974).
Antihypertensive function of a renal-cell carcinoma.
New Engl J Med 290:843.

Renal Tumors: Proceedings of the First International Symposium on Kidney Tumors, pages 283–291
© **1982 Alan R. Liss, Inc., 150 Fifth Avenue, New York, NY 10011**

FEVER IN ADULT RENAL CANCER

Friocourt L, J. Jouquan, S. Khoury, R. Richard,
G. Chomette, P. Godeau
Service de Médecine Interne
Hôpital de la Pitié, Paris

Since 1896, fever has been recognized as a classical
sign of renal cancer (Israel (1896). It is considered as
the third symptom in frequency after haematuria and flank
pain (Bottiger 1958). Generally regarded as neoplastic,
its meaning is actually more complex. A retrospective
multidisciplinary study has been done in order to establish
the significance of fever in neoplasm of kidney.

PATIENTS AND METHODS

All cancers included in this study were proven by
histologic findings. The material surveyed consisted of
three groups (Table 1): 204 patients operated for renal
cancer in an urology department (group A), 204 patients
admitted in a department of internal medicine for fever
of unknown origin (group B) and 51 records of post-
mortem examination of hypernephromas performed in a
department of anatomy and pathology (group C).

RESULTS

The general frequency of fever is 19.7% in renal cancer
and is higher in autopsy studies (27.4%) than in the clinical
ones (17.8%), whereas in patients with pyrexia of unknown
origin, only 2.5% have later proven to have a renal tumor.

In 93% of the subjects, there is generally a regular
temperature below 39°C; in the remaining files it was
described as an irregular fever, with peaks as high as
40°C.

TABLE 1

PATIENTS SURVEYED IN THE STUDY

	Group A n=204	Group B n=204	Group C n=51
Males	120(58.8%)	109(53.4%)	36(70.5%)
Females	84(41.2%)	95(46.6%)	15(29.5%)
Mean Age (Years)	60	56	67
(Extremes)	(15 - 81)	(15 - 92)	(40 - 92)

Group A: Surgical patients with renal cancer

Group B: Medical patients with fever of unknown origin

Group C: Post-mortem examinations

Fever was the occasional initial symptom in 41.6% of the cases, the sole sign in 8.3% and had developed for an average of 126 days when the diagnosis is made. In 83.3% of the patients, the fever was associated with the urological symptoms and in 52.2% the patients had experienced weight loss and fatigue.

Renal neoplasms are more often accompanied with hyperthermia in women (61.2%) than in men.

The diagnosis of hyperpyretic cancer was more difficult and delayed since there were lapses of time of over six months between the first symptom and the excretory urography in 27% of pyretic cancers versus 16% in apyretic forms.

Their symptomology was slightly different (Table 2). Weight loss, palpable flank mass and biochemical inflammatory syndrom were more often seen, whereas haematuria was less frequent.

But, on the other hand, there was no significant difference in the prognosis of the febrile group and of the apyretic one (average survival time of 26 months in both groups). Besides, the local, regional or metastatic extension was similar in both groups, and other para endocrine cancer syndromes were similar in either group.

The postoperative outcome of the fever varied. In 27.7% of the cases, pyrexia disappeared completely in the 48 hours following the removal of the tumor, which suggested its neoplastic origin. In 55.5% of the cases, fever remained unchanged but in 2.7% of the cases, the tumor could not be removed; in 11.1% of the cases, the surgery of cancerous adenopathies was not complete because of technical difficulties; in 19.4% of the cases there were infectious complications, among them one parietal abcess, two septicemias, one pneumopathy and three cases of peritumoral pyelonephrites. In 2.7% of the cases there was a colic fistula. In only 16.7% of the cases, fever persisted after the operation without a plausible explanation.

As to the fever reported in autopsy studies, in 50% of the cases it appeared only a few days before death and was probably due to infection or to thromboembolic complications. In the other 50% of the cases, it was a fever

TABLE 2

CLINICAL AND BIOLOGICAL FEATURES IN 204 SURGICAL PATIENTS
WITH RENAL CANCER

	Pyretic Forms n=36 (17.8%)		Apyretic Forms n=168 (82.2%)
Males	14(38.8%)		106
Females	22(61.2%)	..	62(37.0%)
Mean Age (years)	59.3		60.4
Weight Loss	19(52.8%)	...	37(22.1%)
Urologic Signs	30(83.3%)		122(73.0%)
Palpable Flank Mass	15(41.7%)	..	29(17.4%)
Flank Pain	6(16.6%)	N.S.	22(13.1%)
Hematuria	9(25.0%)	.	71(42.5%)
Metastases	8(22.2%)	N.S.	61(36.3%)
Vein Thrombosis	10(27.7%)	N.S.	59(35.1%)
Tumor Mecrosis	5(13.9%)	N.S.	16(9.6%)
Tumor Mass			
Unique	20(55.6%)	N.S.	106(63.4%)
Multiple	4(11.1%)	N.S.	10(6.0%)
Whole Kidney	7(19.4%)	N.S.	23(13.8%)
E S R 25mm	30(83.3%)	...	86(51.5%)
Polycythemia	1(2.8%)	N.S.	4(2.3%)
Hypercalcemia	4(11.1%)	N.S.	18(10.8%)
Average Survival Time (months)	26		26

. = $p < 0.05$
.. = $p < 0.01$
... = $p < 0.001$
N.S. = Not Significant

that had been developing for more than three weeks, of unknown origin in 2.1% of the subjects, and due partly, at least, to infection or thrombosis in 2.8% of the subjects.

COMMENTS

This study confirms some data already given in the literature. The overall frequency of renal cancer fever was generally between 11% and 41%; fever was the sole sign in 2% to 12% of the patients by earlier publications (Berger, Sinkoff 1957; Chisholn, Roy 1971; Ewert 1963; Godeau, Ghazlan 1972; Lange 1972; Warren et al. 1970; Weinstein et al. 1961).

Pyrexia was more often seen in women during renal cancer, although this cancer was generally more common in men (Bottiger 1958). Mean age, local, regional or metastatic extension, or other metastatic syndroms were not different in both groups. In the majority of cases (Ewert 1963; Jemenez et al. 1979; Marshall, Walsh 1977; Tveter 1973), patients with fever would also present other symptoms such an anorexia, asthenia, weight loss and anaemia. In these forms the diagnosis was delayed and could be missed, since the time between the first sign and the excretory urography was often over six months (an average of seven to ten months) in most of the publications (Cherukuri et al. 1977; Ewert 1963).

General fatigue was accompanied by a biochemical inflammatory syndrome. An elevated erythrocyte sedimentation rate (often more than 100 mm in the first hour), a refractory anaemia, alpha-2 globulin spike, and sometimes medullary plasmocytosis was noted. These biological signs gradually normalize after nephrectomy and may recur with the formation of metastases (Bowman, Martinez 1968; McPhadran et al. 1972; Marsh 1974). In some cases of the hyperpyretic form with severe inflammatory syndromes, hepatomegaly and hepatic dysfunction without evidence of hepatic metastases have been observed (Tartaglia 1970). Reduced liver function, evidenced by increased bromsulfthalein retention time, increased alkaline phosphatase, hypoalbuminemia, hyperglobulinaemia and abnormal prothrombin values were a prominent feature. In very rare instances an elevated alpha-foetoprotein could be observed (Piard et al. 1973). All of these signs decreased after

the removal of the tumor. In most of the febrile forms,
we noted the presence of clear cell type tumors (Battiger
et al. 1966; Bottiger, Ivemark 1959; Tveter 1973).

A certain number of facts in our study are different
from what has been previously stated. As far as we have
observed, a lumbar mass was seen more frequently and hematuria
was less frequently noted in febrile forms than in apyretic
ones.

The prognosis of the pyretic forms did not appear different from that of the apyretic one. This was in keeping
with Bottiger's observations (Bottiger 1958), but in contradiction with most of the other authors (Jimenez et al.
1979; Weinstein et al. 1961). The significance of fever
was not equivocal. The presence of fever was independent
of the pathological and anatomical conditions such as tumor
size and tumor invasiness. Necrosis and haemorrhage were
not likely to cause elevated temperature or the presence
of metastases.

Sometimes fever could be regarded as a result of an inter-
current complication as was stated in some clinical or
necropsy records. The infection was related or not to the
presence of the tumor or one of its metastases, throm-
bophlebitis and/or pulmonary embolism. In other cases,
fever was very likely neoplastic when it subsided completely
in less than 48 hours after the removal of the tumor or
when after subsiding, it flared up again simultaneously
with the appearance of a metastasis. The persistence of
fever after nephrectomy when it cannot be explained by
metastases or non-radical surgery suggests a probable
infection, or thromboembolic complication. We have
postulated two pathogenic hypothesis.

1) An immune mechanism where a tumor antigen induces
a delayed hypersensitivity reaction.

2) A secretion of endogenous pyrogens by the tumor
cells. These substances have been isolated in tumoral
extracts from pyretic patients operated on for a renal
cancer. The attempts to remove circulating endogenous
pyrogens in those patients have failed so far (Cranston et
al. 1973; Rawlins et al. 1971; Rawlins et al. 1970).
Roughly speaking the physiology of fever can be summed up
as follows. A exogenous pyrogen induces the formation

through phagocytes, of proteidic endogenous pyrogen that appear to cause fever by altering the activity of temperature sensitive neurons on the anterior hypothalamus that presumably determine the "set point" for normal body temperature. Endogenous pyrogens, however, may not act directly on these neurons but may work through other intermediates such as monoamines, prostaglandins, other metabolites of arachidonic acid, and cyclic adenosine monophosphate. These mediators can be inhibited by acetylsalicylic acid, indomethacine, alpha blockers and are potentiated by theophilline.

To conclude we would like to suggest some practical implications. It may appear advisable to suppress fever, when the tumor cannot be eradicated, for better comfort of the patient, though fever might stimulate the self defense mechanisms of the body. This point, however, is still being disputed (Ashman et al. 1976). The classical antipyretic non-specific-remedies can be proposed. Steroids, in spite of the risk of dependence (Gibbons et al. 1976), and non-steroid antiinflammatory agents (aspirin, indomethacin) can be used. Other substances thought of after understanding the physio-pathology of the fever (alpha-blockers, nicotinic acid) have not been tested under controlled conditions thus far.

Ashman RG, Gomez-Barrieto JW, Nahamias AJ (1976). The effects of temperature on the vitro transformation of human peripheral blood lymphocytes. Fed Proc 35:821.
Berger L, Sinkoff MW (1957). Systemic manifestations of hypernephroma: a review of 273 cases. Am J Med 22:791.
Bernheim HA, Block LH, Atkins E (1979). Fever: pathogenesis, pathophysiology and purpose. Ann Int Med 91:261.
Bottiger LE (1958). Fever in carcinoma of the kidney. Acta Med Scand 156:477.
Bottiger LE, Blanck C, Vonschrieb T (1966). Renal carcinoma: an attempt to correlate symptoms and findings with the histopathologic picture. Act Med Scand 180:329.
Bottiger LE, Ivemark BI (1959). The structure of renal carcinoma correlated to its clinical behaviour. J Urol 81:512.
Bowman HS, Martinez EJ (1968). Fever, anemia and hyperhaptoglobinemia. An extra renal tind of hypernephroma. Ann Int Med 68:613.
Cherukuri SV, Johenning PW, Ram MD (1977). Systemic effects of hypernephroma. Urol 10:93.

Chisholm GD, Roy RR (1971). The systemic effects of malignant renal tumors. Br J Urol 43:687.

Cranston WI, Luff RH, Owen D, Rawlins MD (1973). Studies on the pathogenesis of fever in renal carcinoma. Clin SC Mol Med 45:459.

Ewert EE, Conception RL, Pires EM (1963). Hypernephroma, The great imitator. Med Clin N Amer 47:431.

Gibbons RP, Montie JE, Correa RJ, Tate Masson J (1976). Manifestations of renal cell carcinoma. Urol 8:201.

Godeau P, Ghozlan R (1972). Syndromes paranéoplasiques et cancer du rein. R P XXII 1:43.

Grubb W, Drylie DM, Lade R, Fuller TJ (1977). Reversible systemic abnormalities associated with renal cell carcinoma. Urol 9:269.

Israel J (1896). Aus dem judischen krankenhaus in Berlin; ueher einige neue Erfahrungen auf dem gebiete der neurochi rurgie. Deutsh Med Wehnschr 22:345.

Jimenez Cruz JF, Rioja Sanz C, Garcia Lopez F, Sole-Bacelles F (1979). Les syndromes paranéoplasiques du cancer du rein. Sem Hop Paris 55:74.

Lange D (1972). Formes cliniques des tumeurs du rein de l'adulte. R P XXII 1:21.

McPhedran P, Finch SC, Nemerson YR, Barnes MG (1972). Alpha$_2$ globulin spike in renal carcinoma. Ann Int Med 76:439.

Marsh JC (1974). Renal carcinoma: fever, anaemia and hyperhaptoglobinemia. Ann Int Med 81:707.

Marshall FF, Walsh PC (1977). Extrarenal manifestations of renal cell carcinoma. J Urol 117:439.

Melicow MM, Uson AC (1960). Non urologic symptoms in patients with renal cancer. J A M A 192:146.

Piard A, Mabille JP, Putelat R, Mihiels R, Riflec, Justra bo E, Bourgeaux C, Juglaret M (1973). Syndrome paranéo plasique à manifestations multiples révélateur d'un hyper néphrome avec présence d'alpha foeto protéine. Sem Hop Paris 49:341.

Rawlins MD. Cranston WI, Luff RH (1971). Transferable pyrogen in human experimental fever. Clin Sc 40:193.

Rawlins MD, Luff RH, Cranston WI (1970). Pyrexia in renal carcinoma. Lancet 1:1371.

Tartaglia AP, Wolfe S, Propp S (1970). Hepatic dysfunction and fever associated with hypernephroma. N Y State J Med 1:2231.

Tveter KJ (1973). Unusual manifestations of renal carcinoma. Acta Chir Scand 401.

Warren M, Kelalis P, Utz D (1970). Changing concept of
  hypernephroma. J Urol 104:376.
Weinstein EC, Geraci, JE, Greene LF (1961). Staff meetings
  of the Mayo Clinic. 36:12.

Renal Tumors: Proceedings of the First International Symposium on Kidney Tumors, pages 293–300
© **1982 Alan R. Liss, Inc., 150 Fifth Avenue, New York, NY 10011**

HYPERCALCAEMIA

Geoffrey D. Chisholm, Ch.M. F.R.C.S.

University Department of Surgery/Urology
Western General Hospital
Edinburgh, Scotland, U.K.

Malignant disease is the commonest (55%) cause of hypercalcaemia in a hospital population although hyperparathyroidism is commoner in the general community. Less common causes of hypercalcaemia, in order of decreasing incidence, are vitamin D intoxication, sarcoidosis, thyrotoxicosis, immobilisation and milk-alkali syndrome and these account for 5% of patients with hypercalcaemia.

Of the cancers that metastasise to bone and cause hypercalcaemia, the commonest are carcinoma of the bronchus and breast. However, hypercalcaemia occurs in only about 5% of these cases whereas one third of the patients with multiple myeloma develop hypercalcaemia at some stage of their disease.

Hypercalcaemia in patients who have no evidence of bony metastases (also called humoral hypercalcaemia, tumour endocrinopathy or ectopic parathormone secretion) occurs mainly with squamous cell carcinoma of the lung and renal carcinoma.

Hypercalcaemia has been reported in about 10% of patients with renal carcinoma (Chisholm 1974; Sufrin, Murphy 1977). These skeletal metastases are typically osteolytic: bone destruction and resorption release large amounts of calcium which exceeds the capacity of renal and gastro-intestinal regulatory systems and result in hypercalcaemia. There is now evidence that some renal tumours secrete one or more humoral substances that cause hypercalcaemia (Powell, Singer, Murray, Minkin, Potts 1973).

AETIOLOGY

Parathormone (PTH)

The syndrome of pseudo-hyperparathyroidism i.e.
hypercalcaemia in the absence of bone metastases, hypo-
phosphataemia and normal parathyroid glands, was first
reported by Gutman, Tyson, Gutman (1936). Later, Albright
and Reifenstein (1948) suggested that a PTH-like substance
might account for at least some of the hypercalcaemia
associated with renal carcinoma. In 1964, Goldberg,
Tashjian, Order and Dammin demonstrated a PTH-like
substance both in a renal carcinoma and in its metastases.
The patient was known to have a renal tumour but because of
the symptoms attributed to primary hyperparathyroidism, the
neck was explored first; the parathyroid glands were
normal, no abnormality was found in the mediastinum but
pulmonary and pleural nodules showed metastatic renal
carcinoma. Tissue assay confirmed the presence of an
antigen indistinguishable from parathyroid hormone.

Further reports have confirmed the hypersecretion of a
PTH-like substance by some renal tumours by showing an A-V
gradient across the tumour (Buckle, McMillan, Mallinson
1970). There have also been reports of a co-existing
parathyroid adenoma with hypercalcaemia and renal carcinoma;
in one example, hypercalcaemia persisted after the
nephrectomy but responded promptly to a parathyroidectomy
(Herr, Martin 1973).

Thus, pseudo-hyperparathyroidism is a well recognised
phenomenon associated with some renal tumours and, based on
earlier reports, is cited as an example of ectopic production
of a PTH-like polypeptide. However, in some instances of
hypercalcaemia, there was no immunoreactive PTH either in
the tumour or in the circulation.

Prostaglandins

The possibility that prostaglandins might be important
arose from 2 observations: one, that the Prostaglandin E
series are potent stimulators of bone resorption in vitro
(Klein, Raisz 1970) and second, Prostaglandin E_2 appeared
to be the agent responsible for the hypercalcaemia seen with

mice fibrosarcomas (Tashjian, Voelkel, Levine, Goldhaber 1972). Subsequently, prostaglandins were shown to be the mediators of hypercalcaemia in several solid tumours, mainly carcinoma of lung and pancreas (Seyberth, Segre, Morgan, Sweetman, Potts, Oates 1975).

Clinical evidence for the role of prostaglandins in hypercalcaemia with renal carcinoma was reported by Brereton, Halushka, Alexander, Mason, Keiser, DeVita (1974). The patient had had a renal carcinoma removed but liver metastases were noted at operation. A persistent hypercalcaemia with a slightly depressed serum phosphate was noted 3 months later. There was no evidence for bone metastases and ectopic PTH secretion was postulated but no PTH was detected in the serum. Attempts to treat the hypercalcaemia failed but after giving indomethacin 25mg bd, the serum calcium promptly fell to normal. The patient died one year after nephrectomy and at autopsy there were no bony metastases and the parathyroid glands were normal. Liver and lung metastases were analysed for prostaglandins and showed markedly raised levels of PGE and PGF-like material in the liver metastases but not in the lung metastases.

Since then, a patient with hypercalcaemia and renal carcinoma was shown to have marked elevation of PGA, PGE and PGF in peripheral plasma and in all tumour samples assayed. At autopsy, 10 months after nephrectomy, there were no bony metastases and the parathyroid glands were normal (Robertson, Baylink, Marini, Adkinson 1975). Further evidence for the production of immunoreactive prostaglandins A and E has been provided from tissue culture and tumour tissue analyses (Cummings, Robertson 1977) and from in vitro studies culturing renal carcinoma tissue with mouse calvaria (Atkins, Ibbotson, Hillier, Hunt, Hammonds, Martin 1977). However, neither of these latter studies provides a complete explanation for hypercalcaemia with renal carcinoma. The fact that prostaglandins are produced by these tumours does not exclude the existence of other factors such as changes in cyclic AMP metabolism (Powell, McPartlin, Skrabanek 1978). The rapid metabolism of PGE has suggested to Atkins et al (1977) that PGE as a cause of hypercalcaemia occurs only when the tumour has massive non-bony deposits; this hypothesis is supported by the fact that the cases reported by Brereton et al (1974) and Robertson et al (1975) had large liver metastases.

Clinical Features

Hypercalcaemia can cause malaise, nausea, vomiting, constipation, thirst, polyuria, mental disturbance and loss of consciousness with death. If these features lead to the detection of hypercalcaemia in a patient with a known malignancy, then approximately $\frac{3}{4}$ of these patients will be found to have bone metastases. Xrays and/or bone scan will confirm the diagnosis. Thus, hypercalcaemia is usually a feature of advanced malignancy. Hypercalcaemia with non-metastatic renal carcinoma is often associated with a low serum phosphate and a mild hypokalaemic alkalosis.

If, by contrast, hypercalcaemia has been the presenting feature then the history, examination and investigation are directed to the main causes such as malignancy, thyro-toxicosis and vitamin D toxicity. If these are negative, hyperparathyroidism may be presumed and the diagnosis confirmed by means of serum PTH. (An elevated PTH confirms the diagnosis but these results may vary according to methodology and the interpretation of a PTH result should be checked with the laboratory). If the diagnosis is not confirmed, then the less common causes of hypercalcaemia must be considered.

The clinician must be alert to the possibility of primary hyperparathyroidism and renal carcinoma. The distinction between these two causes of hypercalcaemia may be difficult. The duration of hypercalcaemia in patients with renal carcinoma tends to be shorter and the symptoms more marked than with primary hyperparathyroidism. The occurrence of renal stones in patients with renal tumours and hypercalcaemia is rare, presumably because of the shorter history. PTH levels are generally higher in pseudo-hyperparathyroidism than in primary hyperparathyroidism (Riggs, Arnaud, Reynolds, Smith 1971). However the particular value of PTH levels lies in localising the site of abnormality by carrying out PTH assays on multiple samples obtained by neck vein catheterisation. In general, patients with parathyroid hypercalcaemia excrete more cyclic AMP than patients with non-parathyroid hypercalcaemia although an increase in cyclic AMP excretion has been noted with humoral hypercalcaemia. Discrimination between these groups can be achieved by expressing urinary cyclic AMP in relation to the volume of glomerular filtrate.

Management

The hypercalcaemia of primary hyperparathyroidism is treated either by removal of the tumour or by excision of $3\frac{1}{2}$ of the 4 hyperplastic glands.

Mild hypercalcaemia from other causes must be considered as potentially dangerous due to the risk of renal damage or soft tissue calcification. In patients with malignancy, the management of hypercalcaemia must be considered in relation to the overall management of the patient.

More severe hypercalcaemia may become an emergency and the general principles are to replace fluid loss from the body, to correct electrolyte abnormalities and to stop further input of calcium into the extracellular fluid by corticosteroids or mithramycin (Buescu, Dimich, Myers 1975).

The methods by which these aims are achieved depend upon the severity of the hypercalcaemia and the symptoms produced. In malignant diseases, even if the patient has only a short time to live, hypercalcaemia causing symptoms should be treated.

A high fluid intake should be encouraged as this maintains optimum renal calcium excretion. Intravenous saline may be given and this usually results in a rapid clinical improvement. Few patients can maintain an increased oral intake to 2-3 litres for a long period. The use of a diuretic to increase calcium excretion is acceptable only if close monitoring of fluid and electrolytes can be maintained.

In addition several other medications must be considered:

- Oral phosphate (Phosphate-Sandoz) 500mg qds effectively lowers the calcium, but one-third develop gastrointestinal side effects such as nausea and diarrhoea.

- Corticosteroids are effective (though unpredictable) in lowering calcium and relieve symptoms in about half the patients (Fulmer, Dimich, Rothschild, Myers 1972). Either hydrocortisone or prednisolone (30mg/day) is given in high doses; the dose is adjusted to maintain a normal serum calcium.

- A prostaglandin synthetase inhibitor, such as
indomethacin, will lower the serum calcium in few of these
patients. Unfortunately the response is rare so that the
clinical application is limited (Seyberth, Segre, Hamet,
Sweetman, Potts, Oates 1976). Several diphosphonates are
being assessed for their control of hypercalcaemia in
malignancy but further evaluation is required.

- Calcitonin has obvious attractions but its effect
is disappointing (Wisneski, Croom, Silva, Becker 1978).

- Mithramycin. If the above measures are ineffective,
then parenteral mithramycin can be used with good effect.
After a single injection of 25μg/kg there is a progressive
fall in serum calcium that is maintained for several days
(Slayton, Shnider, Elias, Horton, Perlia 1971). However,
there may be the serious side effects of bleeding or impaired
renal function.

It is important to emphasise that in the face of
terminal malignancy these measures are recommended only
to alleviate distressing symptoms and not in the expectation
of remission of the disease.

Albright F, Reifenstein EC (1948). Clinical hyperpara-
    thyroidism:metastatic malignancy. In "Parathyroid glands
    and Metabolic Bone Disease", Chapter 3, Baltimore, Md:
    Williams & Wilkins.
Atkins D, Ibbotson KJ, Hillier K, Hunt NH, Hammonds JC,
    Martin TJ (1977). Secretion by prostaglandins as bone-
    resorbing agents by renal cortical carcinoma in culture.
    Brit J Cancer 36:601.
Brereton HD, Halushka PV, Alexander RW, Mason DM, Keiser HR,
    DeVita VT Jr (1974). Indomethacin-responsive hypercalcemia
    in a patient with renal-cell adenocarcinoma. New Engl J
    Med 291:83.
Buckle RM, McMillan M, Mallinson C (1970). Ectopic secretion
    of parathyroid hormone by a renal adenocarcinoma in a
    patient with hypercalcaemia. Brit Med J 4:724.
Buescu A, Dimich AB, Myers WPL (1975). Cancer hypercalcemia -
    a pragmatic approach. Clin Bull Memorial Sloan-Kettering
    Cancer Center 5:91.
Chisholm GD (1974). Nephrogenic ridge tumors and their
    syndromes. Ann NY Acad Sci 230:403.
Cummings KB, Robertson RP (1977). Prostaglandin: Increased
    production by renal cell carcinoma. J Urol 118:720.

Fulmer DH, Dimich AB, Rothschild EO, Myers WPL (1972).
    Treatment of hypercalcemia. Comparison of intravenously
    administered phosphate, sulfate, and hydrocortisone. Arch
    Int Med 129:923.
Goldberg MF, Tashjian AH, Order SE, Dammin GJ (1964). Renal
    adenocarcinoma containing parathyroid hormone-like
    substance and associated with marked hypercalcemia. Amer
    J Med 36:805.
Gutman AB, Tyson TL, Gutman EB (1936). Serum calcium,
    inorganic phosphorous and phosphatase activity in
    hyperparathyroidism, Pagets' disease, multiple myeloma and
    neoplastic disease of the bones. Arch Intern Med 57:379.
Herr HW, Martin DC (1973). Primary or pseudohyperpara-
    thyroidism? Urology 2:62.
Klein DC, Raisz LG (1970). Prostaglandins: stimulating of
    bone resorption in tissue culture. Endocrinology 86:1436.
Powell D, McPartlin J, Skrabanek P (1978). Humoral
    hypercalcaemia in a patient with renal-cell carcinoma.
    Europ J Clin Invest 8:425.
Powell D, Singer FR, Murray TM, Minkin C, Potts JT Jr
    (1973). Nonparathyroid humoral hypercalcemia in patients
    with neoplastic diseases. New Engl J Med 289:176.
Riggs BL, Arnaud CD, Reynolds JC, Smith LH (1971).
    Immunologic differentiation of primary hyperparathyroidism
    due to nonparathyroid cancer. J Clin Invest 50:2079.
Robertson RP, Baylink DJ, Marini JJ, Adkinson HW (1975).
    Elevated prostaglandins and suppressed parathyroid hormone
    associated with hypercalcemia and renal cell carcinoma.
    J Clin Endocrinol Metab 41:164.
Seyberth HW, Segre GV, Morgan JL, Sweetman BJ, Potts JT Jr.,
    Oates JA (1975). Prostaglandins as mediators of
    hypercalcemia associated with certain types of cancer.
    New Engl J Med 293:1278.
Seyberth HW, Segre GV, Hamet P, Sweetman BJ, Potts JT,
    Oates JA (1976). Characterization of the group of patients
    with the hypercalcemia of cancer who respond to treatment
    with prostaglandin synthesis inhibitors. Trans Assoc
    Am Physicians 89:92.
Slayton RE, Shnider BI, Elias E, Horton J, Perlia CP (1975)
    New approach to the treatment of hypercalcaemia. The
    effect of short-term treatment with mithramycin.
    Pharmacol Ther 12:833.
Sufrin G, Murphy GP (1977). Humoral syndromes of renal
    adenocarcinoma in man. Rev Surg 149.
Tashjian AH Jr, Voelkel EF, Levine L, Goldhaber P (1972).
    Evidence that the bone resorption-stimulating factors

produced by mouse fibrosarcoma cells in prostaglandins E_2: a new model for the hypercalcaemia of cancer. J Exp Med 136:1329.

Wisneski LA, Croom WP, Silva OL, Becker KL (1978). Salmon calcitonin in hypercalcemia. Clin Pharmacol Ther 24:219.

Renal Tumors: Proceedings of the First International Symposium on Kidney Tumors, pages 301–316
© **1982 Alan R. Liss, Inc., 150 Fifth Avenue, New York, NY 10011**

THE NONMETASTATIC HEPATIC DYSFUNCTION SYNDROME ASSOCIATED
WITH RENAL CELL CARCINOMA (HYPERNEPHROMA):
STAUFFER'S SYNDROME

Kamal A. Hanash, MD, MS (Urology), FACS

Chief of Urology; Vice Chairman, Dept of Surgery
King Faisal Specialist Hospital & Research Centre
Riyadh, Kingdom of Saudi Arabia

Stauffer first reported the association of reversible
hepatic dysfunction with renal cell carcinoma (hypernephroma) at the Mayo Clinic in 1961 (Stauffer 1961). Since
then, several other reports have stressed this association
(Lemmon 1965, Mohamed 1965, Stewart 1967, Summerskill 1967,
Walsh 1968, Warren 1970, Utz 1971, Ramos 1972, Pirson 1973,
Jacobi 1975, Strickland 1977, Boxer 1978, Delpre 1979,
Robinson 1980). Initially, the syndrome was characterized
by abnormal sulfobromophthalein retention, increased serum
alkaline phosphatase, hypoprothrombinemia, and elevated α_2
globulin fraction of the protein electrophoresis in the
absence of hepatic metastases (Stauffer 1961). Subsequently,
several other clinical, biochemical, and histological
changes were associated with this syndrome (Utz 1970,
Boxer 1978). In an attempt to further characterize the
different clinical and biomedical aspects of this syndrome,
a prospective study including all cases of nonmetastatic
renal cell carcinoma seen at the King Faisal Specialist
Hospital and Research Centre from 1975 to 1980 was undertaken. (Table 1)

TABLE 1
NONMETASTATIC HEPATIC DYSFUNCTION SYNDROME ASSOCIATED
WITH RENAL CELL CARCINOMA
(STAUFFER'S SYNDROME)

- Hepatosplenomegaly
- Increased serum alkaline phosphatase
- Hypoalbuminemia
- Hypoprothrombinemia
- Prolonged prothrombin time

- Increased α_2 globulins (increased haptoglobulins)
- Increased serum bilirubin (indirect)
- Increased BSP retention
- Increased thymol turbidity
- Hypocholesterolemia
- Hypergammaglobulin (increase in IgM)
- Alkaline phosphatase isoenzyme
- Absence of hepatic metastases
- Nonspecific histologic hepatic changes
- Absence of osseous metastases
- Normal portal pressure
- Mainly clear cell type

MATERIALS AND MANAGEMENT

Thirty patients with hypernephroma and one patient with histologically proven renal leiomyosarcoma were included. A review of the clinical, laboratory, and histological findings revealed 11 patients with three or more characteristic parameters of the reversible hepatic dysfunction syndrome in the absence of liver diseases, hepatic, or osseous metastases. These 11 patients form the basis of our present study. Complete work-ups were carried out on all patients as delineated in Table 2.

TABLE 2

WORK-UP OF 31 PATIENTS WITH RENAL CELL CARCINOMA (HYPERNEPHROMA) WITHOUT DISTANT METASTASES

- Hemograms and platelet count
- Sedimentation rate
- PT, PTT, bleeding time
- SMAC 20™
- Serum protein electrophoresis
- Serum alkaline isoenzyme
- Urinalysis
- Urine culture and sensitivity
- Urine for schistosomiasis
- Urine cytology/antigen
- Chest x-ray
- Pulmonary tomography or scan (when indicated)
- Intravenous pyelography
- Retrograde pyelography (when indicated)
- Renal ultrasound/(scan)
- Flush aortogram and celiac arteriography
- Renal selective arteriography
- Liver scan

- Bone scan
- Tumor bone survey

Most of the laboratory tests were repeated several times pre- and postoperatively. In case of elevation of the serum alkaline phosphatase, isoenzyme determination was performed using the Titan® III cellulose acetate electrophoresis (The Helena Method*). Determination of the alkaline phosphatase was performed on a tumor extract from a patient with a serum alkaline isoenzyme and it was negative.

All patients underwent exploratory surgery and radical nephrectomies without lymphadenectomy were performed on all five patients with stage A, B, and C tumors (according to Robson, tumor staging) including one case of leiomyosarcoma (Robson 1968). Five patients with unresectable locally advanced tumors (Stage D) underwent tumor biopsy which confirmed the diagnosis. One patient with the characteristic findings of renal cell carcinoma on the IVP, ultrasound, renal scan and renal arteriography, refused surgery. Careful exploration for hepatic or other intraperitoneal metastases was carefully carried out. Four patients underwent wedge liver biopsies at the time of the nephrectomy or exploration. A periodic follow-up of the patients on a three-month basis during the first postoperative year and then every six months or until their deaths, was instituted with the repetition of most of the laboratory and radiologic studies including liver and bone scans. No autopsies were performed on any of the patients.

RESULTS

The sex distribution (seven men and four women) and the age group (81 percent in the fifth and sixth decades) were consistent with most of the reported series (Utz 1970). The most common clinical features were weight loss, fatigue, lassitude, fever, and weakness. Only two patients gave histories of gross hematuria. However, contrary to other series (Utz 1970, Boxer 1978) 70 percent of our patients complained of abdominal or flank pain.

On physical examination, eight patients had palpable abdominal masses. Hepatomegaly was present in six patients and splenomegaly, in two.

*Helena Laboratories, Beaumont, Texas 77704

On histologic examination, tumors in ten patients were of the clear cell type and one patient, a 45-year-old male, had a renal leiomyosarcoma of the right kidney. Sixty-five percent of the tumors were undifferentiated and 48 percent had invaded adjacent structures (Stage D) but spared the liver parenchyma. The histological hepatic changes are illustrated in Figures 1A and B.

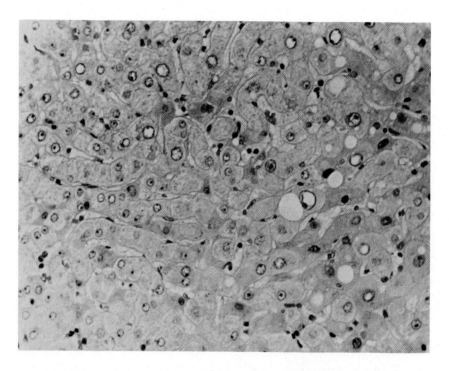

Figure 1A: Hepatic changes showing prominence of Kupffer cells, mild fatty change, variation in nuclear size and focal cellular degeneration. Magnified X120.

Figure 1B: Hepatic changes showing mild degenerative changes of hepatocytes and scattered lymphocytes indicating a mild nonspecific hepatitis. Magnified X 120

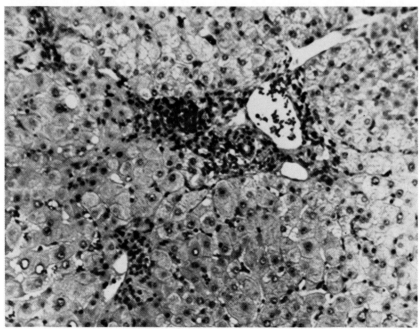

The most common biochemical abnormalities are shown in Table 3 with all the patients manifesting increases in serum alkaline phosphatase. The Regan and liver alkaline phosphatase

TABLE 3
ABNORMAL BIOCHEMICAL TESTS IN 11 PATIENTS WITH THE
HEPATIC DYSFUNCTION SYNDROME ASSOCIATED WITH
RENAL CELL CARCINOMA

Increased alkaline phosphatase	11
Prolonged prothrombin time	7
Increased α_2 globulin	7
Hypoalbuminemia	7
Hypergammaglobulins	6
Increased serum bilirubin	3
Increased gamma glutamyl transpeptidase	2
Liver isoenzyme	4
Renal cancer isoenzyme (Regan)	1

isoenzymes were demonstrated in one patient while in four others only the liver band was identified. (Figure 2)

Figure 2. Persistence of liver isoenzyme (alkaline phosphatase) following nephrectomy.

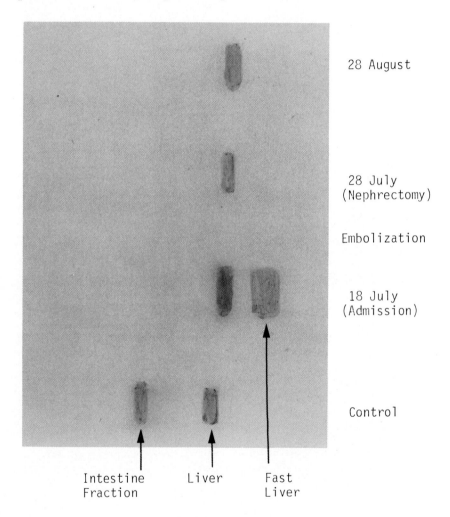

28 August

28 July
(Nephrectomy)

Embolization

18 July
(Admission)

Control

Intestine   Liver   Fast
Fraction   Liver

(Due to technical difficulties, this
 photo has been retouched.)

In one of the four, the liver isoenzyme disappeared following nephrectomy. Hypercalcemia (serum calcium of more than 10.5 mg/dl) was demonstrated in four patients having normal serum parathormone with reversal of the serum calcium to normal in two patients after nephrectomy. Eight patients with the non-reversibility of the hepatic dysfunction, including the five cases with the unresectable tumor died of metastases (pulmonary, brain, and liver) while one patient was lost to follow-up and presumed dead. Death occurred within two years from the time of surgery. Two patients with Stage A disease and normal liver function tests postoperatively are alive three and five years postnephrectomy without evidence of metastases. The stage and grade of the tumor had close correlation with the reversibility of the hepatic dysfunction in this series. The higher the grade and stage, the higher the incidence of nonreversibility of the hepatic dysfunction resulting in poor prognosis. The delay in diagnosis and treatment of the tumor was because of vague and nonclassical clinical symptoms. This was the major factor for the delay of several months on the part of the patient to seek medical advice and to a low rate of suspicion and correct diagnosis by the primary treating physician. This accounted for the high incidence of advanced stages encountered in this series with resulting poor survival as compared to other, large series (Warren 1970, Utz 1970).

DISCUSSION

Renal cell carcinoma may mimic, in its clinical presentation, a large number of medical conditions. Its multiple associations with unconventional signs, symptoms, and other diseases have become apparent over the years with an incidence of 20 to 40 percent (Warren 1970, Chisholm 1971, Boxer 1978, Regnier 1980). The classic triad of hematuria, flank pain, and abdominal mass, although present individually in 30 to 80 percent of the cases, is rare (five to ten percent) and it usually heralds a poor prognosis (Warren 1970, Skinner 1971, Regnier 1980). Among the nonurologic clinical symptoms, fever, weight loss, lassitude, weakness, cachexia, and neuromyopathy are the most common (Warren 1970, Chisholm 1971, Tveter 1973, Regnier 1980).

Several paraneoplastic signs and syndromes have been associated with renal cell carcinoma. These include raised sedimentation rate (5 to 80 percent), anemia (16 to 88 percent), hypertension (22 to 40 percent), hypercalcemia (4 to

12 percent), raised plasma alkaline phosphatase (9 to 24 percent), polycythemia (2 to 5 percent), amyloidosis (1 to 3
percent), and the reversible hepatic dysfunction (0 to 40
percent) (Utz 1970, Chisholm 1971, Ramos 1973, Pirson 1973,
Delpre 1979, Regnier 1980). Our incidence of 36% of reversible hepatic dysfunction associated with renal tumors cor-
roborates the Mayo Clinic series (Utz 1970). More recently
other syndromes have been described in association with
renal cell carcinoma. Increased blood levels of parathyroid
hormone, erythropoeitin, prostaglandins, renins, prolactin,
and calcitonin in some patients with renal cell carcinoma
were associated with the pathogenesis of the hypercalcemia,
polycythemia, and hypertension syndromes (Sufrin 1977,
Semaan 1979, Droller 1981). Awareness and early recognition of these different paraneoplastic syndromes in the
absence of specific tumor "markers" for renal cell carcinoma,
in contrast to testicular tumors, may lead to the proper
diagnosis in about one-third of the patients, namely, those
with nonurologic clinical and laboratory manifestations.
This may lead to a prompt surgical extirpation of the tumor
at its early stage with improvement of the prognosis. This
is also supported by the fact that up to 57 percent of
patients with hypernephroma present, initially, with metastatic disease which is usually refractory to radio therapeutic, chemotherapeutic, and immunotherapeutic treatments
(Lokich 1975).

Among all of these paraneoplastic syndromes, the
reversible hepatic dysfunction of Stauffer's syndrome which
has been more commonly identified when carefully looked for,
is manifested by several particular clinical and biochemical
features. It may be considered as a possible "tumor marker"
for some cases of renal cell carcinoma. Although nonspecific, its presence in the absence of liver diseases or
osseous and hepatic metastases may be the first indicator
of the presence of an unsuspected hypernephroma (Utz 1970).
It may rarely occur with renal infections (Vermillion 1970,
Robinson 1979) and has been associated with two renal sarcomas, including one in our series (Summerskill 1967). The
most common presenting clinical manifestations of fever,
fatigue lassitude, weight loss, and anemia (Utz 1970,
Boxer 1978, Robinson 1980) corroborate our findings although
the presence of a higher incidence of abdominal or flank
pain in our series may be related to the more locally
advanced tumors encountered in our patients. The presence
of hepatomegaly in 66 percent and splenomegaly in 33 percent

as reviewed by Delpre (Delpre 1979) adds another clinical
feature to this syndrome and is confirmed by our own findings. Its almost universal association with the clear cell
type of renal cell carcinoma is in accord with our own
findings except for one case of renal leiomyosarcoma in our
series (Utz 1970, Boxer 1978). The most consistent common
histologic hepatic findings include proliferation of the
Kupffer cells associated with dilated sinusoids, degenerative
changes of the hepatocytes, focal lymphocytic infiltration,
moderate steatosis and focal necrosis (Stauffer 1961,
Summerskill 1967, Utz 1970, Jacobi 1975, Boxer 1978, Delpre
1979). These changes, although encountered in several other
situations such as bacteremia, surgery, anesthesia, shock
and nonrenal malignancies (Utz 1970) and described as "non-
specific reactive hepatitis," are consistent findings, as
found in our own cases, and seem to confirm the reversible
hepatic dysfunction syndrome as a separate medical entity
produced by the renal cell carcinoma.

The common biochemical abnormalities found in our
patients with the hepatic dysfunction syndrome shown in
Table 3 compare with those reported in the literature
(Utz 1970, Delpre 1979). Their reversals to normal following nephrectomy, except in cases of persistent or late
metastases, are considered as important tumor markers and
prognostic signs as illustrated in several series, including
ours (Utz 1970, Boxer 1978, Delpre 1979). Their identification should not be considered as a sign for nonoperability
or cure.

These findings are certainly nonspecific to this
syndrome and may be associated with intestinal tumors (Abels
1942, Nieburgs 1965) and many other medical conditions (Utz
1970). The identification of the Regan alkaline phosphatase
isoenzyme in two cases including our own and the liver pattern in four cases, as in four of ours, (Lemmon 1965,
Girmann 1975, Strickland 1977, Stewart 1967, Delpre 1979)
points more towards the hepatic origin of the raised serum
alkaline phosphatase in patients with the reversible hepatic
syndrome associated with hypernephroma. This seems to be in
contradiction to other reports by Durocher, et al. and
Nathanson, et al. (Durocher 1969, Nathanson, et al. 1971)
who associate the elevation of the serum alkaline phosphatase and its isoenzyme to tumor secretion, as in the case
of breast and colon cancer, myeloma and reticulum cell
sarcoma (Stolbach 1969). However, the negative finding of

a tumor extract isoenzyme in one of our cases with elevated
serum alkaline phosphatase isoenzyme gives more support to
the hepatic origin of the isoenzyme. In spite of several
theories, the etiology and pathogenesis of the reversible
hepatic dysfunction syndrome are still obscure (Bottiger
1960, Chalmers 1960, Schersten 1969, Cachin 1970, Delpre
1979).

In recent years, the secretion of "ectopic" hormones
by tumors arising from different tissues with no endocrino-
logic function has been more frequently recognized and
reported. These hormones, including parathyroid, adreno-
corticotropic, melanocyte stimulating, antidiuretic,
gastric-like, thyrotropin-like, erythropoeitic, gonadotropic,
have been identified in various tumors (Tashjian 1964,
Goldberg 1964, Liddle 1968, Semaan 1979, Droller 1981).

A toxic substance secreted by the renal tumor cells
has been held responsible as the etiologic factor of the
reversible hepatic dysfunction. Our experimental attempts
to identify such a hepatotoxic substance that could be
responsible for the insult to the liver cells were unsuccessful (Hanash 1971). In addition, the injection of saline
and acetone extracts of hypernephroma removed from patients
with and without the hepatic dysfunction syndrome into mice
failed to produce any biochemical or histological hepatic
dysfunction (Hanash 1971). This failure to identify such a
hepatotoxic substance does not exclude the existence of such
an implicating factor. New radioimmunologic and enzymatic
techniques may be helpful in this respect. Our observation
of a quantitative, morphologic change in the thymuses of
patients with renal cell carcinoma as compared to controls
matched for age and sex (Hanash 1971b) raised the possibility of an immunologic factor responsible for the reversible
hepatic dysfunction syndrome. This possibility was further
strengthened by finding a specific immunocellular response
in cases of hypernephroma (Stjernsward 1970).

Recently, much emphasis has been placed on the role of
the liver as an "immunoregulatory organ" and the effect of
liver disease on the T cell dysfunction (Eddleston 1980).
The immunopathogenic mechanism advanced by Eddleston
(Eddleston 1980) relating to the hepatocellular damage seen
in different types of hepatitis seems to be an attractive
theory to explain the pathogenesis of the reversible hepatic
dysfunction associated with hypernephroma. This hypothesis

adapted with minor modifications is illustrated in Table 4.

TABLE 4

HYPOTHETIC IMMUNOPATHOGENESIS
OF THE NONMETASTATIC REVERSIBLE HEPATIC DYSFUNCTION
ASSOCIATED WITH RENAL CELL CARCINOMA

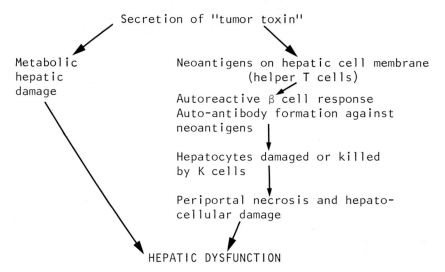

Defective renal cell cancer specific immunity?

Development and growth of renal cell cancer

Secretion of "tumor toxin"

Metabolic
hepatic
damage

Neoantigens on hepatic cell membrane
(helper T cells)

Autoreactive β cell response
Auto-antibody formation against
neoantigens

Hepatocytes damaged or killed
by K cells

Periportal necrosis and hepatocellular damage

HEPATIC DYSFUNCTION

Adapted with modifications from: A.L.W.F. Eddleston (1980):
Immunology and the Liver. In: Parker C. W. (Ed.):
Clinical Immunology. Philadelphia, Saunders p. 1009

The possible secretion of an hepatotoxic substance by the
tumor cells may cause liver damage by either direct metabolic
derangement or by the stimulation of an autoimmune reaction.
The latter, based on the recruitment of helper T cells,
stimulates an autoreactive β cell response and autoantibody
formation against the neoantigens formed on the cell membrane
of the hepatocytes. The hepatic dysfunction thus produced
may, on the other hand, decrease the number of T cells and
affect the immunologic response against the tumor.

A successful nephrectomy, on the one hand, by eliminating the secretion of the hepatotoxic substance by the tumor cells may lead to the reversal of the hepatic dysfunction, which presages a good prognosis. (Table 5).

TABLE 5
HYPOTHETIC EFFECT OF NEPHRECTOMY
ON THE IMMUNOPATHOGENESIS
OF THE REVERSIBLE HEPATIC DYSFUNCTION ASSOCIATED
WITH RENAL CELL CARCINOMA

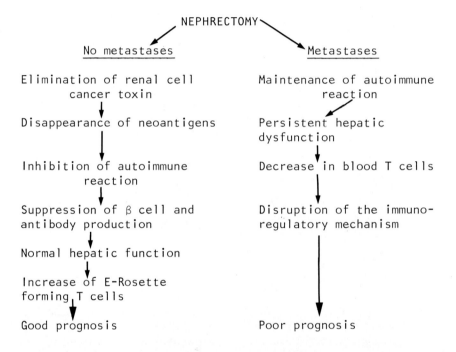

Persistence of the renal cancer or subsequent development of metastases, on the other hand, results in the persistence of the insult and damage of the liver cells and may be considered as an ominous sign for poor survival.

REFERENCES

Abels JC, Rekers PE, Binkley GE *et al.* (1942). Metabolic studies in patients with cancer of the gastrointestinal tract II. Hepatic dysfunction. Ann Intern Med 16:221.

Bottiger LE (1960a). Studies in renal carcinoma II. Biochemical investigations. Acta Med Scand 166:455.

Boxer RJ, Waisman J, Lieber MM, Mamfraso FM, Skinner DG (1978). Nonmetastatic hepatic dysfunction associated with renal cell carcinoma. J Urol 119:468.

Cachin M, Lévy CL, Monnier JP (1970). Perturbations réversibles des fonctions hépatiques au cours d'un cancer du rein. Sem Hop Paris 46:814

Chalmers TC (1960). Pathogenesis and treatment of hepatic failure. N Eng J Med 263:213.

Chisholm GD, Roy RR (1971). The systemic effects of malignant renal tumors. Br J Urol 43:687.

Delpre G, Ilie B, Papo J, Streifler C, Gefel A (1979). Hypernephroma with nonmetastatic liver dysfunction (Stauffer's syndrome) and hypercalcemia. Amer Col Gastroenterology 72:239.

Droller MJ (1981). Prostaglandins and neoplasia. J Urol 125:757.

Durocher J (1969). Alkaline phosphatase and hypernephroma. N Eng J Med 281:1369.

Eddleston ALWF (1980). Immunology and the liver. In: Parker CW (ed), *Clinical Immunology*. Philadelphia, Saunders, p 1009.

Girmann G, Gratzel M, Pees H, *et al.* (1975). Contribution to the aetiology of reversible hepatic dysfunction (Stauffer's syndrome) associated with renal tumors. Dtsch Med Wochenschr 100:480.

Goldberg MF, Tashjian AH, Order SE, Damiu GJ (1964). Renal adenocarcinoma containing a parathyroid hormone-like substance and associated with marked hypercalcemia.

Am J Med 36:805

Hanash KA, Utz DC, Ludwig J, Wakim KG, Ellefson RD, Kelalis
   PP (1971a). Syndrome of reversible hepatic dysfunction
   associated with hypernephroma: an experimental study.
   Investigative Urol 8:399.

Hanash KA, Souadjian TV, Utz DC, Kelalis PP, Titus JL
   (1971b). Quantitative morphologic studies of the thymus
   in hypernephroma. J Urol 105:488.

Jacobi GH, Philipp TH (1975). Stauffer's syndrome: diagnostic help in hypernephroma. Clinical Nephrology 4:113.

Lemmon WT Jt, Holland PV, Holland JM (1965). The hepatopathy
   of hypernephroma. Am J Surg 110:487.

Liddle GW (1968). Preliminary characterization of some
   ectopic hormones. Vitamins Hormones (NT) 26:293.

Lokich JJ, Harrison JH (1975). Renal cell carcinoma:
   natural history and chemotherapeutic experience. J Urol
   114:371.

Mohamed SD (1965). Reversible nonmetastatic liver-cell
   dysfunction and thrombocytosis from a hypernephroma.
   Lancet 2:621.

Nathanson L, Fishman WH (1971). New observations on the
   Regan isoenzyme of alkaline phosphatase in cancer patients.
   Cancer 27:1388.

Nieburgs HE, Parets AD, Parez V, et al. (1965). Cellular
   changes in liver tissue adjacent and distant to malignant
   tumors. Arch Path (Chicago) 80:262.

Pirson Y, Descos L, Mestrallet G, et al. (1973). L'hepato-
   pathie non metastatique des hypernephromes. A propos de
   deux nouvelles observations. Ann Gastroenterol Hepatol
   Paris 49:341.

Ramos CV, Taylor HB (1972). Hepatic dysfunction associated
   with renal carcinoma. Cancer 29:1287.

Regnier J (1980). Retrospective study of the clinical manifestations of 50 adenocarcinomas of the kidney in adults.
Rev Med Suisse Romande 100:909.

Robinson TJ, Graham WJN, Mulligan TO (1979). The nephrogenic hepatic dysfunction syndrome associated with renal
sepsis. Br J Clin Practice 33:329.

Robinson TJ (1980). Hepatic dysfunction associated with
hypernephroma. Irish Med J 73:277.

Robson CJ, Churchill BM, Anderson W (1968). The results of
radical nephrectomy for renal cell carcinoma. Trans Am
Assoc Genitourin Surg 60:122.

Schersten T, Wahlquist L, Johannson LG (1969). Lysosomal
activity in liver tissue from patients with renal carcinoma. Cancer 23:608.

Semaan NA (1979). Paraneoplastic syndromes associated with
renal carcinoma. In: Johnson DE, Samuels ML (eds).
Cancer of the Genito-Urinary Tract. New York, Raven
Press, p 73.

Skinner DG, Colvin RB, Vermillion CD, Pfister RC, Leadbetter WF (1971). Diagnosis and management of renal cell
carcinoma. Cancer 28:1165.

Stauffer MH (1961). Nephrogenic hepatosplenomegaly (abstract).
Gastroenterology 40:694.

Stewart AG, Spront JG (1967). Epilepsy and liver dysfunction
in association with hypernephroma. Br Med J 4:660.

Stjernsward J, Almgard LE, Franzen S (1970). Tumor-
distinctive cellular immunity to renal carcinoma. Clin
Exp Immunol 9:963.

Stolbach L, Sprunt JG, Fishman WH (1969). Ectopic production
of an alkaline phosphatase isoenzyme in patient with
cancer. N Eng J Med 281:757.

Strickland RC, Schenker S (1977). The nephrogenic hepatic
dysfunction syndrome: a review. Am J Dig Dis 22:49.

Sufrin GEA, Mirand CS, Moore RH, Chu TM, Murphy GP (1977). Hormones in renal cell cancer. J Urol 117:433.

Summerskill WHJ, Shorter RG (1967). Progressive hepatic failure: its association with undifferentiated renal tumor. Arch Intern Med 120:81.

Tashjian AH Jr, Levine L, Munson PH (1964). Immunochemical identification of parathyroid hormone in non-parathyroid neoplasms associated with hypercalcemia. J Exp Med 119:467.

Tveter KJ (1973). Unusual manifestations of renal cell carcinoma. Acta Ch Scand 139:401.

Utz DC, Warren MM, Gregg JA, Ludwig J, Kelalis PP (1970). Reversible hepatic dysfunctiion associated with hypernephroma. Mayo Clinic Proc 45:161.

Vermillion SE, Morlock CG, Bartholomew LG, et al. (1970). Nephrogenic hepatic dysfunction secondary to tumefactive xanthogranulomatous pyelonephritis. Ann Surg 171:130.

Walsh PH, Kissane JM (1968). Nonmetastatic hypernephroma with reversible hepatic dysfunction. Arch Intern Med 122:214.

Warren MM, Kelalis PP, Utz DC (1970). The changing concept of hypernephroma. J Urol 104:376.

**Renal Tumors: Proceedings of the First International Symposium on
Kidney Tumors, pages 317–336**
© **1982 Alan R. Liss, Inc., 150 Fifth Avenue, New York, NY 10011**

METASTATIC RENAL CELL ADENOCARCINOMA

Wafic S. Tabbara, Amira M. Mehio and George P.
Aftimos
Pathology Department, St. Joseph University
Medical School, Hotel Dieu de France and Barbir
Medical Center, Beirut

INTRODUCTION

This study will be limited to renal cell carcinoma, the
so-called hypernephroma, because of its peculiar metastatic
patterns. This tumor is described as having metastasized to
every site and organ in the body, including such uncommon
locations as the eye, the parotid region or the gingiva.
The tumor has provided some of the most bizarre growth
behavior in the realm of neoplasia (Grabstad 1964). Sudden
explosive growth with widespread metastases is matched by
slow silent asymptomatic growth for years (Mostofi 1967).
In a number of cases the occurence of a solitary metastasis
leaves a chance for cure after removal of the metastatic
growth. On the other hand metastases may appear in patients
who have had nephrectomy for renal carcinoma 1031 years
prior to discovery of the metastatic focus (Kradjian, Bennington 1965). In other instances, renal tumor was not
detectable clinically or radiographically at the time the
metastasis was discovered and became obvious only months or
years later. Another interesting feature of this tumor is
its occasional regression without treatment (Everson 1964;
Everson, Cole 1966). We are more concerned in this study by
the possible regression of metastatic tumor particularly
from the lung after nephrectomy for renal carcinoma (Rafla
1970, Garfield, Kennedy 1972). Renal cell carcinoma also
remains the most common malignancy for the curious phenomenon
of metastasis of a cancer into another cancer (Campbell et
al 1968).

MATERIALS AND METHODS

We reviewed the pathological material from Hotel-Dieu de France (HDF) and Barbir Medical Center (BMC) in Beirut for the period from 1979 thru September 15, 1981. We selected 38 renal cell adenocarcinomas in a total of 152 renal specimens including biopsies and nephrectomies and 12 biopsies from metastatic foci. We discarded all the other renal malignancies: Wilms' tumor, transitional cell carcinoma, primary sarcomas and metastatic tumors to the kidney. Some of the latter tumors were associated with renal cell carcinoma in the same metastatic focus in our material and deserve special attention. We will discuss the specific features of metastatic renal cell carcinoma in light of the data from our material (Tables 1, 2 and 3) compared to information from the medical literature.

TABLE 1

PATHOLOGICAL MATERIAL - H.D.F. AND B.M.C.

1979	14 cases
1980	9 cases
1981	15 cases
Total	38 cases

TABLE 2

ANATOMICAL AND TOPOGRAPHICAL DISTRIBUTION OF THIS SERIES

Nephrectomies	26 cases
Liver biopsies	2 cases
Bone biopsies	3 cases
Bronchial biopsies and lobectomies	3 cases
Lymph node (supra-clavicular)	1 case
Retroperitoneum	2 cases
Parotid area	1 case
Total	38 cases

In two instances renal cell carcinoma was suspected cytologically in our laboratory on smears from fresh urine. We discarded these cases because of poor follow-up.

TABLE 3

AGE INCIDENCE OF RENAL CELL ADENOCARCINOMA IN MATERIAL FROM H.D.F. AND B.M.C.

Minimum	5	years
Maximum	77	years
Mean age	55.2	years

This tumor occurs almost exclusively in adults and exhibits a rapidly increasing incidence with advancing age in both sexes (Bennington 1973). Thru 1973, less than 60 cases were reported in children (Dehner et al, 1970, Pratt-Thomas et al, 1973). Our unique patient in this group is a 5-year old girl who presented a deep midline abdominal tumor with striking calcifications on frozen-section. Routine sections revealed a characteristic clear cell adenocarcinoma of the kidney. Figure 1 shows the characteristic histological features.

Renal cell adenocarcinoma is usually reported as occurring twice as frequently in males as in females. Our figures are slightly low; they may be corrected if they are compared to the total number of men and women in the population (Table 4). In the State of California, this correction was

TABLE 4

SEX DISTRIBUTION IN PATHOLOGICAL MATERIAL FROM H.D.F. AND B.M.C.

Males	25	65.7%
Females	13	34.3%

was carried on at the California Tumor Registry and resulted
in an incidence ratio in excess of 3:1.

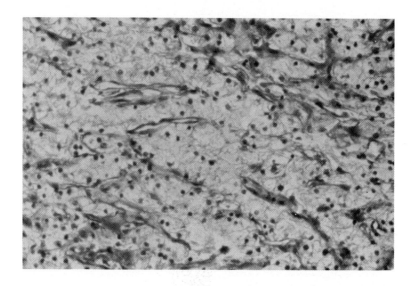

Fig. 1. Characteristic pattern of clear cell carcinoma of
kidney H.E. x 10.

Renal cell carcinoma is reputed for its high metastatic
potential. Ninety-five percent of all renal carcinomas
produce metastatic inclusions at autopsy (Creevy 1935;
Soloway 1938 and Kozoll, Kirshbaum 1940). The following
figures from Bennington (1973) are highly demonstrative.

1)   Sites where metastases are common include lungs,
      lymph nodes, liver, bone, adrenal, opposite
      kidney, brain, skin etc... with an incidence
      ranging from 55.0% (lung) to 3-2% (skin).

2)   Sites where metastases are less common include
      pancreas, thyroid, ureter, epididymis, muscle
      and gall bladder with an incidence <2%.

3)   Sites where metastases are uncommon include
     mesentery, corpus. cavernosum, bladder, dura,
     ovary with an incidence <1%.

The sites of highest metastatic incidence (lungs, bones,
liver and lymph nodes) are presented in our purely surgical
material (Table 5). Our material also includes brain, skin,
thyroid and bladder metastases of renal cell adenocarcinoma,
observed prior to 1979. The parotid gland metastasis is a
very rare site; the patient was a 65-year old male who underwent nephrectomy for renal cell adenocarcinoma 8 months earlier.

TABLE 5

SITES OF METASTASES IN PATHOLOGICAL MATERIAL FROM
H.D.F. AND B.M.C.

Broncho-pulmonary	3
Bone	3
Liver	2
Lymph nodes	4
Retroperitoneum	2
Parotid gland	1
Total	15

The clinical staging of renal cell carcinoma prior to
surgery is of utmost importance. The possible regression of
metastases postoperatively is rather remote. New techniques
have been introduced for the detection of metastatic sites
adapted to different types of cancer. The detection of
metastases from renal cell carcinoma can be achieved by the
radionuclide imaging of metastases by I^{131} labelled antitumor antibody (Belistsky et al, 1979).

The percentage of metastases contributed by this tumor
at sites in which metastases are common and at sites in
which metastases are less common is greater than would be
expected from the frequency of this carcinoma among all
malignant neoplasms. In our material, renal cell carcinoma

represents 1.06% of all malignancies, compared to 1-1.2% in the literature. Several hypothesis are raised to explain this high metastatic potential of renal cell adenocarcinoma (Bennington 1973). These are:

1) Survival time of patients with renal carcinoma is long enough to provide greater opportunity for metastases to develop.

2) The routes of dissemination available for metastases from this tumor are particularly varied.

3) Cells from renal cell carcinoma are better able to reach some sites or to survive there, than cells from other carcinoma, most probably because of peculiar immunologic properties. Some combination of these different mechanisms seems most likely (Table 6, Figure 2).

TABLE 6

GROSS CHARACTERISTICS OF RENAL CELL ADENOCARCINOMAS IN PATHOLOGICAL MATERIAL FROM H.D.F. AND B.M.C.

Size of Tumors	Minimum	3	cm
	Maximum	20	cm
	Mean size	7.9	cm
Encapsulated tumors		12	
Multifocal tumors		3	
Extension to pelvic cavities		3	
Extension to fat		5	
Lymph node metastases		3	
Vascular permeation		8	

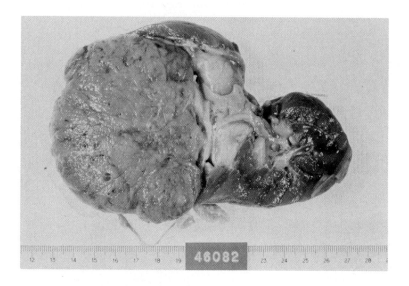

Fig. 2. Renal cell carcinoma, massive polar, encapsulated.

It is generally accepted that larger tumors give a
poorer prognosis. Among 45 patients with tumors less than
3cm in diameter, only one had metastases (Bell 1938). Many
authors designate tumors that are less than 3cm to the
category of renal adenomas. But it is now known that renal
tumors less than 2 cm had metastasized and a large percentage
of tumors larger than 10 cm in greatest diameter had not
(Hicks 1954; Long et al, 1966; Xipell 1971). Some authors
draw a comparison between renal adenocarcinoma and prostatic
adenocarcinoma (Bennington 1973). They see no conceptual
distinction between occult carcinoma of the prostate and
renal tumors under 3cm which have metastasized, or between
latent carcinoma of the prostate and renal tumors under 3 cm
which have not metastasized.

It is not yet resolved whether renal cell carcinoma
arises de novo from the renal tubule cell or by evolution
through adenomatous hyperplasia and renal cortical adenoma
(Holland 1973). Adenomatous hyperplasia or adenoma have been
found in 14% of patients with renal carcinoma (Whisenand et
al, 1962). This may serve to explain the multicentric

occurrence of renal carcinoma and its bilateral incidence.
Three of our 26 renal tumors were multifocal. Mostofi (1967)
found that the 5- and 10-year survival rates for patients
with single tumors were 54% and 40% respectively; these values
are in contrast to 40% and 20%, respectively, for those with
multiple tumors (Figure 3). Similar figures are presented
by Petkovic (1959).

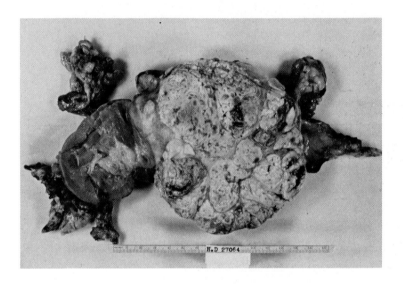

Fig. 3. Gross pattern of a multifocal renal carcinoma.

None of our renal carcinomas involved the adrenal. On
the other hand none of the metastatic tumors in our material
was found in that site. The problem of vascular permeation
and lymph node metastases is related to the routes of
metastasis of renal carcinoma. It will be reconsidered in
the general discussion.

Most metastases from renal cell carcinomas in our
material were of the clear cell type. This was also the
dominant histological type in our renal tumors (Table 7).

TABLE 7

HISTOLOGICAL CLASSIFICATION OF RENAL CELL ADENOCARCINOMAS
IN MATERIAL FROM H.D.F. AND B.M.C.

Clear cell adenocarcinoma	28
Glandular cell adenocarcinoma	4
Renal adenoma cortical with schisto-somiasis of urinary tract	1
Transitional cell carcinoma with cortical adenoma	1
Renal cell carcinoma + angiomyolipoma (Riopelle's tumor)	1
Sarcomatoid hypernephromas	3

These figures are correlated with those in the literature
(Cabanne, Bonenfant 1980). The clear cell pattern had
become almost synomymous of renal cell carcinoma. These
considerations are important for the differential diagnosis
of renal cell carcinoma in particular sites of metastasis
and will be further discussed.

DISCUSSION

We will limit this discussion to three major aspects of
metastatic renal cell adenocarcinoma. (1) The routes of
metastasis are mainly responsible for the widespread distribution of metastases and the high incidence of metastases in
peculiar sites. (2) The peculiar patterns of metastatic
renal cell carcinoma outside the kidney and the problems of
histological differential diagnosis which they induce and
(3) the spontaneous regression of metastases after nephrectomy
are also clearly important to the understanding of this
disease.

Renal cell carcinoma spreads by direct extension or
invasion of intrarenal veins and lymphatics. Approximately
one-third of the patients already have metastases when the
diagnosis of the primary is made (Middleton 1967).

Local extension is manifest in involvement of the pelvis of the ureter, the perinephric tissue, the adrenal gland or the liver. Direct extension to the adrenal occurs within Gerota's fascia in 6-10% of operated patients (Robson et al, 1969).

Lymphatic spread results in involvement of the lumbar lymphatics. Lymphatic plexuses of the renal parenchyma and perinephric fat communicate freely with each other before draining into the lateral aortic nodes. Most efferents from these nodes drain into the cysterna chyli though some may join the thoracic duct directly (Gray 1966). Occasionally, the thoracic duct will divide into two branches; the right one then empties into the right subclavian vein (Holland 1973). Thus both supraclavicular areas must be examined for suspicious nodes in preoperative staging.

Lymphogenous spread affects chiefly the regional lymph nodes. The most proximal are first involved. Other retroperitoneal, abdominal and mediastinal nodes are less frequently involved. Rarely tumor deposits are located in supraclavicular, cervical, axillary and inguinal lymph nodes.

A lymphohematogenous spread needs to be individualized. It is due to the proximity of the lateral aortic nodes to the cysterna chyli. Malignant cells carried by lymphatics gain access to the thoracic duct and are carried to superior vena cava, right heart and lungs.

The thoracic duct was one route of spread for 67% of the primary extraperitoneal abdominal carcinomas. Thus this lymphohematogenous route provides a mean for metastases to bypass the liver via the thoracic duct and to reach the lungs and the pulmonary artery (Schwedenberg 1905; Pick et al, 1944).

Hematogenous spread is probably more important in renal adenocarcinoma than fro most cancers. Venous invasion and growth of tumor thrombus into the intrarenal veins is seen in about 30% of operative specimens (Angervall et al, 1969; Robson et al, 1969). An unbroken tumor thrombus may extend to the vena cava and even to the right atrium. Blood borne metastasis is frequently a feature of the disease, but its occurrence is unpredictable. The venous drainage of the kidney through the caval system and its tributaries helps to explain the frequency and wide distribution of metastases

from renal adenocarcinoma (Mostofi 1967). Embolic tumor
cells in the renal vein may spread by retrograde to pelvic
structures via left spermatic or ovarian vein. This results
in embolisation of the pampiniform or the ovarian plexus and
the consequent development of metastatic deposits in the
spermatic cord, epididymis, testicle, broad ligament, ovary,
vagina or vulva. Abeshouse in 1956 documented 50 cases of
metastases of renal adenocarcinoma to genitourinary organs.
He discounted lymphatic and arterial spread as well as intra-
ureteral implantation as most unlikely. Although Abeshouse's
arguments against implantation metastases are most convincing,
there are occasional reports of this unlikely phenomenon
occurring in the bladder and the ureter (Heslin et al, 1955;
Howell 1944; Sargent 1960). Reports of extension of renal
adenocarcinoma in the ureteric vein in conjunction with
ureteral metastases seem to indicate that this is the actual
route of so-called implantation metastases (Batson 1942;
Mitchell 1958).

    Embolic tumor cells in the renal vein may also spread
to the exial skeleton via paravertebral veins. The latter
form an extensive plexus from pelvis to skull, which
anastomoses freely with the canal system at each segmented
level. Cancer cells entering the canal system can be shunted
in the paravertebral veins, presumably during periods of
increased intra-abdominal pressure. This route not only
explain the frequent bone metastases, but may also account
for the relatively high frequency of involvement of the
thyroid gland which is in close proximity to the paravertebral
veins. Twenty-five percent of metastases to the thyroid are
from renal carcinoma (Tuaillon et al, 1959). Tumor cells can
also ascend in the vena cava. The latter provides the channel
for the great majority of metastases, especially those
ultimately reaching the lung. Another metastatic route
involves migration through pulmonary circulation to arterial
circulation. Zeidman and Buss (1963) have shown that
malignant cells reaching the lung are not necessarily arrested
there. They may pass via the pulmonary capillary as single
cells or small emboli into the arterial circulation to
produce widespread metastases. It is important to remember
that metastases from this tumor to any organ may reach that
site by more than one route.

    Metastatic deposits from renal adenocarcinoma are
recognized rather easily when composed of large clear cells.
But not all metastatic deposits from renal cell carcinoma

are of the clear cell type and they may often be considerably
less well differentiated than the primary cancer. On the
other hand, not all clear cell carcinomas should be considered
from renal origin. There are several microscopic features
that suggest primary renal tumor including:

1)   The large clear cells. They contain intra-
     cytoplasmic glycogen demonstrated with the
     periodic acid Schiff (P.A.S.) reaction, neutral
     lipid stainable with oil red O, Sudan IV or
     perchloric acid-naphtaquinone on frozen sections
     and phospholipids stainable with Sudan black
     on routine sections (Figure 4).

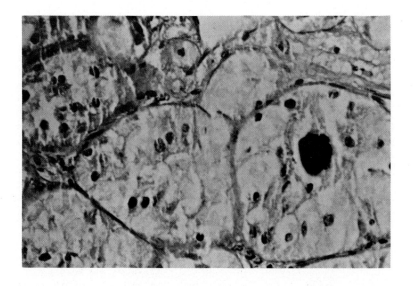

Fig. 4. Papillary pattern of renal cell adenocarcinoma with
calcification. H.E. x 10.

     Glycogen and lipids are also present in the glandular
cells, in a small amount (Figure 5).

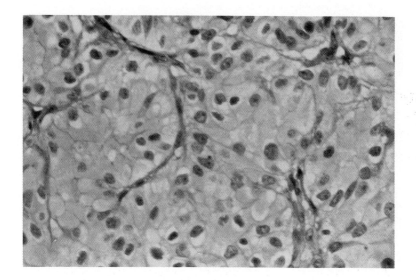

Fig. 5. Glandular cell pattern, renal cell adenocarcinoma
of kidney. H.E. x 10.

2)   The characteristic architectural patterns including
       endocrinoid arrangement of cells in highly vascular
       stroma, tubular, papillary, solid or cystic configu-
       rations. Intratumoral calcification is also a
       suggestive feature.

3)   The sarcomatoid type of renal cell carcinoma
       mimics fibrosarcoma, rhabdomyosarcoma or lipo-
       sarcoma. As seen in Figure 6, its constituent
       cells retain electron microscopic features similar
       to the large clear cell or the glandular cell,
       thus allowing a differential diagnosis (Farrow
       et al, 1968).

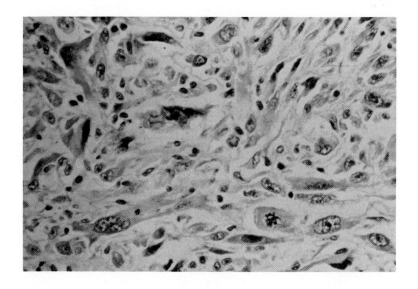

Fig. 6. Sarcomatoid pattern of renal cell carcinoma. Transi-
tion with differentiated carcinoma of kidney. H.E. x 25.

    Adrenal cortical carcinomas are most frequently confused
with renal adenocarcinomas. These tumors are usually more
bizarre, with pleomorphism, giant cells, and nuclear hyper-
chromasia. The differential diagnosis with sarcomatoid
renal carcinoma is only possible by electron microscopy
(Tannenbaum 1971).

    Two conditions in the lung derserve discussion. The
first is the benign clear cell tumor of Libow and Castleman
(1963). Constituent cells contain diastase resistant PAS +
material and scanty lipids. These cells are characterized
by the presence of neurosecretory granules in the cytoplasm
(Becker et al, 1971). The second is bronchiolo-alveolar
carcinoma of the lung, which may also be confused with renal
cell carcinoma. Mucin stain is a good clue for this diagnosis.

    In the parotid area, muco-epidermoid carcinoma and

some variants of acinic cell carcinoma may raise diagnostic problems. Demonstartion of mucin characterizes the first tumor. The cells of acinic cell carcinoma of salivary glands contain PAS + diastase resistant material which is absent in renal cell adenocarcinoma (Figure 7).

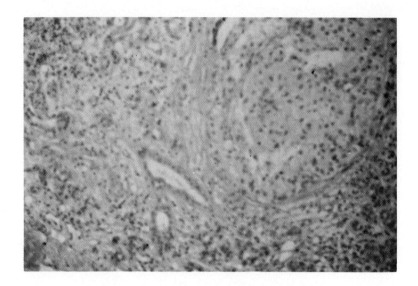

Fig. 7. Metastatic clear cell adenocarcinoma in the parotid gland. P.A.S. x 10.

Bone deposits raise diagnostic problems with prostatic primary or osteogenic sarcomas as well as the rare clear cell adenocarcinoma of the thyroid or any clear cell sarcoma of soft tissues involving bones. Electromicroscopy may be of help.

Primary hemangioblastomas of the central nervous system may be confused with a metastatic renal adenocarcinoma to the brain. The presence of a prominant capillary network and the absence of tubular, papillary or trabecular patterns

are good indications for hemangioblastoma. One should
remember the well-known association of this condition with
renal cell tumors in the Von-Hippel-Lindau syndrome.

Lipoid cell tumors and clear cell (mesonephric)
carcinoma of the ovary may be confused with renal cell
primary. This is also true of clear cell carcinomas of
uterus and vagina. The differential diagnosis may be
impossible by optic microscopy alone (Scully 1970).

Sebaceous cell carcinoma and clear cell nodular
hidradenoma of the skin raise difficult problems with primary
renal cell adenocarcinoma (Rulon, Helwig 1974). Lobulation,
resemblance to sebaceous cells, foci or keratinization and
nuclear pleomorphism characterize subaceous carcinoma. In
favor of nodular hidradenoma we should consider the multi-
lobular pattern, the lack of papillary configurations and
intracellular lipids. Occasionally, ballon cell melanoma
may mimic renal cell adenocarcinoma. In one of our observations to skin was very much similar to renal cell carcinoma.
The absence of lipids and the positive reaction with Fontana
stain characterize ballon cell melanoma (Figure 8).

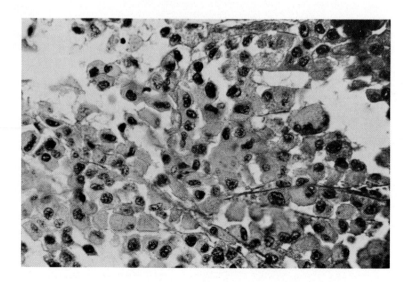

Fig. 8. Balloon cell melanoma of skin, metastatic Fontana x
25.

Spontaneous regressions have prompted controversy over whether the primary tumor should be removed if multiple metastases are already present. This fact of the natural history of the disease is important to ascribe fairly the benefit of various treatments and to understand immunologic factors useful in diagnosis and treatment.

Acceptable regression of metastatic lesions of renal cell carcinoma have now been reported in more than 40 cases. Regressive metastases are in the main pulmonary, but only a few were confirmed histologically. Because many other pulmonary conditions such as sarcoidosis, collagen and fungal diseases may regress too, and can mimic metastatic lesions, spontaneous regression of metastatic renal carcinoma appears more scarce than thought. It is statistically predominant in lung lesions and in an elderly masculine population.

Multiple causes may be responsible for spontaneous regression of metastasis predominantly in elderly males. Fever and infection have also been associated with regression. However the intervention of a host immune response seems to be the most likely explanation.

In conclusion, we would like to stress the absolutely ubiquetous nature of the dissemination of metastatic renal cell carcinoma. They are the manifestations of a rich network of routes of spread available for this tumor on one hand, and are responsible for major problems of differential diagnosis on the other. The spontaneous regression of these metastases is possible but scarce and does not indeed reverse the dictum "Those having hypernephroma, if they live long, will eventually succumb to the disease".

REFERENCES

Abeshouse BS (1956). Metastases to ureters and urinary bladder from renal carcinoma. Report of 2 cases. J Int Coll Surg 25:117.

Angervall L, Carlstrom E, Wahlqvist L, Ahren Ch (1969). Effects of clinical and morphological variants on spread of renal carcinoma in an operative series. Scand J Urol Nephrol 3:134.

Arner O, Blanck C, Von Shreeb T (1965). Renal adeno-carcinoma: morphology, grading of malignancy, prognosis study of 19 cases. Acta Chir Scand (Suppl) 346:11.

Batson OV (1942). The role of the vertebral veins in metastatic processes. Ann Intern Med 16:38.

Becker NH, Soifer (1971). Benign clear cell tumor "sugar tumor" of the lung. Cancer 27:712.

Bell ET (1938). Classification of renal tumors. J Urol 39:238.

Bell ET (1950). Renal diseases. Philadelphia: Lea and Febiger, p 428.

Bennington JL (1973). Cancer of the kidney - etiology, epidemiology and pathology. Cancer p 1017.

Bennington JL, Kradjian RM (1967). Distribution of metastases from renal cell carcinoma. In "Renal Carcinoma", Philadelphia: W.B. Saunders Co., p 156.

Cabanne F, Bonenfant JL (1980). Principes de pathologie générale et spéciale. In Maloine SA (ed): "Anatomie Pathologique" , Paris: Les Presses de˙ l'Université Laval, Québec, p 997.

Campbell LV Jr., Gilbert E, Chamberlain CR Jr., Watne AL (1968). Metastases of cancer to cancer. Cancer 22:635.

Creevy CD (1935). Confusing clinical manifestations of malignant renal neoplasms. Arch Intern Med 55:895.

Dehner LP, Leestma JE, Price EB Jr. (1970). Renal cell carcinoma in children; a clinicopathologic study of 15 cases and review of the literature. J Pediatr 76:358.

Everson TC, Cole WH (1966). Spontaneous regression of adenocarcinoma of the kidney (hypernephroma). In "Spontaneous Regression of Cancer", Philadephia: W.B. Saunders, Co., p 11.

Everson TC (1964). Spontaneous regression of cancer. Ann NY Acad Sci 114:721.

Farrow GM, Harrison EG Jr., Utz DC (1968). Sarcomas and sarcomatoid and mixed malignant tumors of the kidney in adults - Part III. Cancer 22:556.

Garfield DH, Kennedy BJ (1972). Regression of metastatic renal cell carcinoma following nephrectomy. Cancer 30:190.

Grafstad W (1964). Renal cell carcinoma: I - incidence, etiology, natural history. NY State J Med 64:2539.

Grafstad W (1964). Renal cell carcinoma: II - diagnostic findings. NY State J Med 64:2658.

Grafstad W (1964). Renal cell carcinoma: III - types of treatment. NY State J Med 64:2771.

Gray H (1966). The lymphatic system. In Goss CM (ed): "Anatomy of the Human Body", Philadelphia: Lea and Febiger, p 735.

Heslin JE, Milner WA, Garlick WB (1955). Lower urinary
tract implants or metastases from clear cell carcinoma of
the kidney. J Urol 73:39.

Hicks WK (1954). Benign tubular adenoma with malignant
transformation. J Urol 71:162.

Holland JM (1973). Cancer of the kidney - natural history
and staging. Cancer p 1030.

Howell RD (1944). Ureteral implantation of renal adenocarcinoma. J Urol 66:561.

Kay S (1968). Renal carcinoma; a 10-year study. Am J Clin
Pathol 50:428.

Kozoll DD, Kirshbaum JD (1940). Relationship of benign and
malignant hypernephoid tumors of kideny. Clinical and
pathological study of 77 cases in 12,885 necropsies.
J Urol 44:435.

Kradjian RM, Bennington JL (1965). Renal carcinoma recurrent
31 years after nephrectomy. Arch Surg 90:192.

Liebow AA, Castleman B (1963). Benign clear cell tumor of
the lung. Am J Pathol (Abstract) 43:13a.

Long RJ, Utz DC, Dockerty MB (1966): Malignant transformation
of a renal adenoma. Report of a case. Cancer J Surg
9:266.

Mitchell JE (1958). Ureteric secondaries from a hypernephroma.
Brit J Surg 45:192.

Middleton RG (1967). Surgery for metastatic renal cell
carcinoma. J Urol 97:973.

Mostofi FK (1967). Pathology and spread of renal cell
carcinoma. In King JS Jr. (ed): "Renal Neoplasia",
Boston: Little, Brown and Co., Inc., p 41.

Oberling C, Riviere M, Haguenau F (1960). Ultrastructure
of the clear cells in renal carcinoma and its important
for the demonstration of their renal origin. Nature
186:402.

Petkovic SD (1959). An anatomical classification of renal
tumors in the adult as a basis for prognosis. J Urol
81:618.

Pick JW, Anson BJ, Burnett HW (1944). Communication between
Lymphatic and venous system at renal level in man.
Q Bull Northwestern Univ Med Sch 18:307.

Pratt-Thomas HR, Spicer SS, Upshur JK, Greene WB (1973).
Carcinoma of the kidney in a 15 year old boy - unusual
histologic features with formation of microvilli. Cancer
31:719.

Rafla S (1970). Renal cell carcinoma - natural history and
results of treatment. Cancer 23:26.

Robson CJ, Churchill BM, Anderson W (1969). The results of

radical nephrectomy for renal cell carcinoma. J Urol
101:297.

Rulon DB, Helwig EB (1974). Cutaneous subaceous neoplasus.
Cancer 33:83.

Sargent JW (1960). Ureteral metastases from renal adenocarcinoma presenting a bizarre urogram. J Urol 83:97.

Schivedenberg TJ (1905). Uber die carcinose des ductus
thoracicus. Virchow Arch (Pathol Anat) 181:295.

Scully RE (1970). Recent progress in ovarian cancer. Hum
Pathol 1:73.

Skinner DC, Colvin RB, Vermillion CD, Pfister LC, Leadbetter
WF (1971). Diagnosis and management of renal cell
carcinoma, a clinical and pathologic study of 309 cases.
Cancer 28:1165.

Soloway HM (1938). Renal tumors. A review of one hundred
thirty cases. J Urol 40:477.

Tannenbaum M (1971). Ultrastructural pathology of human
renal cell tumors. Pathol Ann 6:249.

Tuaillon MM, Colson P, Planchu M (1959). Les métastases
intrathyroidiennes des tumeurs à cellules claires du rein.
Lyon Med 91:939.

Utz DC, Warren MM, Gregg JA, Ludwig JA, Kalalis PP (1970).
Reversible hepatic dysfunction associated with hypernephroma. Mayo CLinic Proc. 45:161.

Whisenand JM, Kostas D, Sommer SC (1962). Some host factors
in the development of renal cell carcinoma. West J
Surg 70:284.

Xipell JM (1971). The incidence of benign renal nodules - a
clinicopathologic study. J Urol 106:503.

Zeidman I, Buss JM (1962). Transpulmonary passage of tumor
cell emboli. Cancer 12:731.

Renal Tumors: Proceedings of the First International Symposium on Kidney Tumors, pages 337–340
© 1982 Alan R. Liss, Inc., 150 Fifth Avenue, New York, NY 10011

CLINICAL SIGNS IN RENAL NEOPLASIA. A COMPARISON OF TWO
SERIES OF THREE HUNDRED CASES

A. Haertig, R. Küss

Clinique Urologique - Hôpital Pitié

Paris, France

Among the clinical signs which are indicative of renal
neoplasia, some are characteristically urological, for
example the triad of haematuria, pain, growth of the lesion.
Others are less characteristic, and may be non-urological in
origin. These may be misleading, but can lead to the discovery of metastases. A third group can lead to the
discovery of latent pathology quite fortuitously (Table 1).

TABLE 1

PREOPERATIVE CLINICAL PRESENTATION IN A SERIES OF
309 RENAL TUMORS*

Clinical Symptom	Number of Cases
Haematuria	183 (59%)
Pain	127 (41%)
Palpable Neoplasm	139 (45%)
Fever	21 (7%)
Weight Loss	85 (28%)
Varicocoele	7 (2%)
Preoperative Secondary Disease	31 (10%)
Chance Discovery	20 (7%)

*(Skinner, DG)

Urological Signs

The principal warning sign is haematuria, since this was found in 50% of the studies. It is almost always a macroscopic haematuria and it should always give rise to investigations for renal neoplasia, irrespective of the age of the patient. In the study carried out at la Pitié we noted one such case in a man less than 20 years of age.

The haematuria is complete, spontaneous, and unpredictable. It may occur once or be repeated, and it occurs quite independently of other difficulties with micturition or infection. In our series, it was the diagnostic indicator in 36% of all positive cases of renal neoplasia.

About one-third of the cases in our series presented with atypical thoracic pain, lumbar pain, renal colic or cruralgia. It was difficult to assess the diagnostic significance of these signs. They were rarely isolated and are frequently misleading so that, in general, it was another symptom which helped to finalize the diagnosis (Table 2).

TABLE 2

CLINICAL SIGNS IN 311 CASES OF RENAL NEOPLASM FROM 1965-1980*

Clinical Symptoms	Number of Cases	Number of Cases Where Symptom was Revealing
Haematuria	143 (46.0%)	114 (36.6%)
Pain	74 (23.8%)	
Palpable Tumor	94 (30.0%)	16 (5.0%)
Para-Neoplasia	57 (18.3%)	
Fever	51 (16.4%)	32 (10.0%)
Neurological Symptoms	1	
Phlebitis	5	
Weight Loss	83 (26.7%)	53 (17.0%)
Varicocele	8 (2.5%)	2
Preoperative Metastases	114 (36.6%)	60 (20.0%)
Chance Discovery	26 (8.3%)	26 (8.3%)

*Urology Clinic, Pitié Hospital - Professor René Küss.

Only rarely was a tumor directly palpable from the beginning (16 cases, i.e. 5% in our series). Conversely, full
clinical examination revealed a palpable tumor in 30-45% of
cases, depending on the study. Varicocele was found in less
than 2% of cases.

Non-Urological Signs

These can be more interesting, and they represented
about 10-20% of diagnostic indicators in cases where no
urological sign existed.

Among these signs are weight loss, para-neoplasia
syndromes, and finally, the preoperative discovery of
metastases.

The weight loss could be as much as 6 kg per month, and
it was found in over 25% of cases in all the series. Isolated
weight loss was the sympton of renal tumor in 53 of 311
patients in our series, i.e. 17%. It was found in association
with other clinical signs in 28% of cases (Table 2).

Among the para-neoplastic syndromes, fever was the most
frequently encountered sign, occurring at a rate of between
7% and 16%, depending on the series. The rate was 10% in our
series.

Neurological syndromes unrelated to metastases were
found much less frequently (2% of cases).

It is, however, imperative that an investigation for
signs of metastasis should be initiated with the first
clinical examination. The percentage of positive findings
varies according to the author Skinner (Table 1), for example,
having found 10% and we, in our series, 20%. In our series,
114 cases of visceral metastases were found in 60 of the 311
patients. Such a figure is exceptional when compared with
other series, and it is probably related to the unusual
environment of the Urology Service at la Pitié, which accepts
patients from neurology, neurosurgery, rheumatology and
respiratory medicine. Among the 20% of our patients who had
metastases, 27% had neurological lesions and 42% bony lesions.

All the different studies agreed on the percentage of
cases where renal neoplasia was discovered by chance (7-8%

of cases). The neoplastic lesion in these cases was found during investigation of arterial hypertension, proteinuria, preoperative work-up, radiological studies (barium series, echotomography) or during investigation of renal stones or hydronephrosis.

If these cases which are diagnosed by chance have a greater chance of five-year survival, they should not allow one to forget that, in the majority of cases, the diagnosis of renal neoplasm is based on clinical signs of established disease (haematuria, palpable tumor, para-neoplastic syndrome or metastases).

Renal Tumors: Proceedings of the First International Symposium on Kidney Tumors, pages 341–344
© 1982 Alan R. Liss, Inc., 150 Fifth Avenue, New York, NY 10011

POSITIVE AND DIFFERENTIAL DIAGNOSIS, AND DIAGNOSTIC
PITFALLS OF MALIGNANT TUMORS: I.V.P.

J. Grellet, M.D.

Department of Radiology, Hopital LA PITIE
83 Bld de l'Hopital, 75013 Paris

Since its introduction in 1929, I.V.P. has undergone
considerable change. At first, renal cancer research
was limited, for all intent and purposes, to detection
of a distorsion in the collecting system. Then, the use
of non-toxic contrast media in nephrotomography permitted
more precise analysis of the renal outline, and even
though less precise, that of the kidney area. Efficiency
of intravenous angiography is increased using digital
video subtraction (A.D.V.S), a method which has given
I.V.P. almost the same diagnostic power as non-selective
arteriography.

The positive diagnosis of renal cancer

Only malignant epithelial tumors are considered in
this paper. Traditionally, positive diagnosis is
established in two stages related to finding 1) a
tumoral syndrome and 2) signs of malignancy.

Discovery of a renal tumoral syndrome must include a
search for the following signs:
  a)   displacement and rotation of kidney
  b)   distortion of the collecting system
  c)   change in renal outline
  d)   nephrographic anomalies

False negatives are uncommon when these rules are
observed. I.V.P., as part of the initial screening
examination, is not always repeated when it is of poor

quality. As a matter of fact, practically one out of ten
cancer cases can be over looked with the first urography.
The reasons for this are rarely the fault of the physician
reading the X-ray, but are due to poor technical quality
of the I.V.P. examination.

Once a tumoral syndrome has been discovered, signs
of malignancy must be determined which include:
  a) renal calcification
  b) invasion of calyces or renal pelvis. Filling
      defects from masses of tumor projecting into the
      pelvis or calyces may be distinguished from
      primary epithelial tumors of the renal pelvis
      or from blood clots.
  c) nephrotomographic anomalies. This phase is often
      neglected, but A.D.V.S. enhances the diagnostic
      power of this technique. However, numerous false
      positives and negatives have limited the interest,
      trust in the accuracy of this procedure. Ac-
      cording to data in the literature (Curet et al.
      1981; Depner et al. 1976; Felson, Moskowitz 1969;
      Folin 1967), one can hypothesize that the precision
      of urography (benign versus malignant) is about
      65 to 75% and that use of A.D.V.S. can increase
      its accuracy from 5 to 10%.

Differential diagnosis of renal cancer

Over the last 10 to 15 years a certain number of
false positives of renal tumours have been described.
Differential diagnosis requires recognition of numerous
constitutional or acquired conditions of the kidney or
nearby organs. These include the following:
  a) Morphological anomalies of the left kidney may
      be caused by variations of the spleen.
  b) Cortical nodules.

Thornbury et al. recently classified the fusion
anomalies of individual renal lobules which normally form
the kidney. The nodules which represent an excess of
cortex tissue, are hypervascularized and can, depending
on their situation and size, deform the renal outline and
stretch the collecting system. Subcapsular nodules,
prominence of hilar lip, prominent column of Bertin, and
foetal lobulation fall into the category of cortical nodules.

c) The kidney can be rotated either entirely or partially. Kyaw and Newman (1971) illustrated a particular case of partial rotation which concerned the inferior pole.

d) Regeneration of a pathologic kidney is often focal and causes a regenerating nodule. Such nodules are secondary to acquired conditions such as lonephritis (Felson, Moskowitz 1969), glomeru-lonephritis (Depner et al. 1976), trauma, infarction and obstruction. Under X-ray, these conditions behave as any renal mass which could protude from the renal outline or compress the calyces and the pelvis.

e) Renal sinus lipomatosis, extrarenal tumors, including nearby organs, subcapsular and perirenal hematomas and non visualizing kidney are additional conditions that relate to different diagnosis of renal cancer. 10 to 25% of cancers show up as a non visualizing kidney, and the importance of this high percentage should be emphasized.

Conclusion

After 50 years, I.V.P. is still used in screening examination for kidney tumors. Its utility has improved as a result of discoveries in arteriography. Consequently an entire range of diagnostic pitfalls can be eliminated. However, two limitations of I.V.P. are the near impossibility of diagnosing cancer without supplementary examination, and the limited accuracy in defining local invasion of a renal tumor.

Curet PH, Fransioli C, Richard F, Grellet, J (1981). Fiabilité de l'artériographie rénale. Séminaires d'uro-néphrologie. Masson p. 21.

Depner TA, Ryan KG, Yamaucho H (1976). Pseudo tumor of the kidney: a sequel to regional glomerulonephritis. Am J Roentegnol 126:1197.

Felson B, Moskowitz M (1969). Renal psuedotumors: the regenerated nodule and other lumps, bumps, and dromedary humps. Am J Roent 107:720.

Folin J (1967). Angiography in renal tumors: its value in diagnosis and differential diagnosis as a complement to conventional methods. Acta Radiol Suppl. STOCK p. 267.

Kyaw M, Newman M (1971). Renal pseudotumors due to ectopic accessory renal arteries. The angiographic diagnosis. Am J Roent 113:443.

Thornbury JR, McCormick TL, Silver TM (1980). Anatomic radiologic classification of renal cortical nodules. Am J Roent 134:1

Renal Tumors: Proceedings of the First International Symposium on
Kidney Tumors, pages 345–347
© 1982 Alan R. Liss, Inc., 150 Fifth Avenue, New York, NY 10011

NEPHROTOMOGRAPHY IN PATIENTS WITH RENAL CARCINOMA

Karen Damgaard, M.D. and Flemming Lund, M.D.

University of Copenhagen Medical School

The role of nephrotomography in the assessment of renal
masses and particularly in the discrimination between
solid tumours and cystic formations deserves thorough
attention. Nevertheless the number of publications discussing this subject is rather limited.

In 1955 Evans reported a diagnostic accuracy of 96%,
examining one hundred cases of suspected renal mass
lesions (Evans et al. 1955). Two years later, his analysis of a larger series of 252 patients revealed an accuracy
of 95% (Evans 1957). In a similar series of 274
thoroughly analysed patients with proven diagnosis, Lang
reported a diagnostic accuracy of only 44% (Lang 1971).

The last decade has not essentially resolved this issue, and we therefore believe it is important to attempt
to answer the question of whether nephrotomography can
establish a definitive diagnosis in renal masses with an
acceptable high level of confidence. If not, the question
remains whether nephrotomography still represents a
valuable supplement to intravenous urography.

Nephrotomography possesses the advantages of a non-
invasive modality, which at a low risk improves the evaluation of the renal morphology, and increases the discrimination of the renal pathology. The criteria for discrimination between cyst and solid lesion have to be strict. A
cyst must exhibit a well defined, thin wall with distinct,
sharp lines, radiolucent throughout and with a homogenous
density. In contrast a neoplasm exhibits a thick, ir-

regular wall with poorly defined margins, with irregular opacifications and highly to slightly decreased density.

Our technique has been to inject a bolus of 1.5 ml Urografin (60%) in less than 15 seconds. The first exposure follows after 15 seconds showing the angiographic phase. After five minutes the ensuing exposure shows the pyelogram, following which tomography is carried out within five to ten minutes, with eventually additional tomographies.

Materials and Results

Our series is comprised of 53 patients with proven renal carcinoma (1976-1980). In 43 cases the clinical symptoms prompted intravenous urograms, which confirmed the suspicion. In six cases the lesions were incidental findings, as urography was carried out for reasons other than tumor suspicion. Another four cases were incidental findings where abdominal angiography or CT-scanning unexpectedly exhibited tumours in the kidneys. Thus about 20% of the tumour cases were incidentally detected. The median age of the patients was 62 years (range 29 - 80 years), and male to female sex ratio was 3/2. In 25 patients it was found necessary to supplement urography (IVU) with an immediate nephrotomography. The results thus obtained were studied and evaluated blindly by one of us (K.D.), revealing the following (Table 1).

Table 1

A comparison of IVU and Nephrotomography

IVU normal - nephrotomography diagnostic	0
IVU inconclusive-tomography indicat. of the abnormal	2
IVU and tomography equally informative	14
IVU abnormal, informative value improved by tomography	9
Total	25

Thus, in two cases the urograms were inconclusive, but the nephrotomograms were indicative, and in another nine cases the urograms were abnormal and the nephrograms improved the diagnosis, revealing a diagnostic accuracy of 11 out of 25 cases (44%).

Discussion

Nephrotomography as a supplement to urography undoubtedly has valuable significance in clinical routine. It clarifies the existence of the contralateral kidney, it describes the size of the suspect kidney and it draws attention to a possible pathologic, space occupying mass. In patients of advanced age it may incidentally contribute to the finding of an unsuspected tumour. It is, however, less reliable in discriminating between benign and malignant processes in the kidney.

Conclusions

Nephrotomography per se is not capable of establishing a definite diagnosis with acceptable confidence. It serves as a first generation diagnostic modality for use in search of the final diagnosis.

Evans JA, Monteith JC, Dubilier W (1955). Radiology 64:655.
Evans JA (1957). Radiology 69:684.
Lang EK (1971). Radiology 98:119.

Renal Tumors: Proceedings of the First International Symposium on Kidney Tumors, pages 349-368
© **1982 Alan R. Liss, Inc., 150 Fifth Avenue, New York, NY 10011**

ARTERIOGRAPHY AND CANCER OF THE KIDNEY

C Bollack and J.J. Wenger

Department of Urological Surgery (Prof. Bollack)
Department of Radiology (Prof. Warter)
C.H.U. Strasbourg

Renal arteriography has been used in the pathology of renal tumors for several years in the positive diagnosis of a tumor, in pretherapeutic assessment, and, occasionally, as additional or isolated therapy in the form of embolisation.

DIAGNOSIS

Renal adenocarcinoma can be diagnosed by arteriography in approximately 95% of cases. Selective opacification can be obtained with midstream aortogram.

A. The following represents an analysis of arteriographical signs. As signs appear at different times of the arteriograph it is possible to distinguish both chronological and morphological anomalies.

a) at the arterial phase:
an increase in the caliber of the renal artery: This is judged on the midstream aortogram but it is not always clear if the kidney has several arteries; global opacification can also make it possible to detect contralateral arterial stenosis (Fig. 1). Abnormal tumoral vessels and similar modifications are more often than not evident, i.e., dilated, twisted and irregular neovessles (Fig. 2). Occasionally the modifications are more discreet and are hidden by normal vessels; behavioural modifiers, especially vasoconstrictors would reveal them to be neovessels which are irregular in their caliber, their course and their

division.

The displacement of arterial branches is very often
visible and it demonstrates a space occupying
lesion (a cyst or a tumor). A second oblique
incidence (true profile of the kidney) can serve
to make them more precise. These displacements
are less marked in solid tumors than in cysts.
They are often limited in tumors by vascular invasion.

The enlargement of the capsular vessels is seen
often as hypertrophied in hypervascularized tumors
which derive a part of their vascularisation from
perirenal vessels. This demonstrates the invasion
of the perirenal space.

b)   at the parenchymatous phase:
     Tumorography (tumoral parenchymography) is only
     manifest in hypervascularized tumors, or following
     vasoconstriction of normal vessels (pharmacoangio-
     graphy) where the normal parenchyma disappears.
     Different forms are noted:
     1)   homogeneous tumor strictly limited to the
          contiguous tissue
     2)   heterogeneous tumor, more often with vascu-
          lar lacunae, signifying intratumoral necro-
          sis
     The limits of these occasionally are very distinct
     (20%) but hardly ever when the very extensive
     tumor derives its vascularisation from the
     neighboring organs. This participation is not
     synonymous with inextirpability.

c)   at the venous phase:
     Advanced venous opacification may be evident,
     explosive, signifying a true arterio-venous fistula,
     classical but are very rare. More usually the
     opaficiation is only a little advanced, but it is
     particularly more intense. Elective opacification
     of a venous branch is more often than not consistent
     with an intravenous hypervascularized tumor
     thrombus. The absence of the renal vein (40% of
     the cases) can be observed despite a sufficient
     filling of the tumor at a late seriography. It
     is consistent with either a propagation of the
     tumor or with a compression of the vein by the
     tumor or, more frequently, by hilar lymph nodes.

A collateral venous circulation often exists. The preoperative assessment should include a study of the renal vein on the arteriogram or else a cavography. A selective renal phlebography may be necessary, especially for the left renal vein.

Venous collaterals are identified in 34% of the cases, whether capsular, ureteral or gonadic veins, they correspond to the drainage of the neighboring organs, or to an actual circulation where there is an obstruction of the renal vein; there is usually a delay in their opacification which makes it difficult to determine the type of drainage.

B. Practical circumstances of diagnosis:

The diagnosis is evident and in more than 80% of the cases, the association of symptoms confirms the diagnosis. The diagnosis is difficult when there are limitations of arteriography. For example, in hypervascularized tumor the tumor is small (under 2 cms) and the urographic modifications are discreet. It is in this clinical condition or the assessment of metastases which leads to the arteriography and even echography is not helpful. The diagnostic arguments are that the vascular anarchy is rarely distinct and the vasoactive drugs risk causing a vasoconstruction of the afferent vessels. A small adenocarcinoma is often very limited and separated from the adjacent parenchyma; moreover, it is rarely heterogeneous and the site of necrosis. Thus, a heterogeneous tumor with hypervascularized zones could be of another etiology (angiomyolipoma, metastasis). In certain angiomyolipomas the tumor may be hypervascularised with vascular anomalies (dolicho-arteries, aneurysms) that can give some indication but the diagnosis is often impossible since these abnormal vessels also do not react with vasoconstrictors. These tumors are frequently associated with a tuberous sclerosis and are sometimes bilateral. On occasion a surgical biopsy, with its associated risks of haemorrhage can provide confirmation. In the slightly vascularised tumor, the diagnosis can be missed through insufficient study either by single frontal incidence, or a single midstream aortogram or the lack of

arterial modifiers. This is why, even if the urography is conclusive in showing another cause of
haematuria (bladder, prostate) if the echograph is
positive (solid formation or hypoechogenesis) all
the technical refinements should be used. The
diagnosis can also be imprecise between a metastasis
and a hypervascularised tumor. A kidney which has
been modified by an anterior pathology (pyelonephritis or tuberculosis) can pose problems which
can be difficult to resolve. Slight arterial ir-
iregularities could be the sole arguments in favour
of surgical exploration.

CONCLUSION

The role of arteriography in the positive diagnosis of
cancers of the kidney is decreasing in importance in
comparison with non-invasive methods (urography, echography,
CT scan). Pretherapeutic assessment can benefit from an
angiographic study: arteriography and eventually phlebography to decide the surgical technique. Finally, in
certain cases, embolisation, preoperative or palliative is
valuable for stopping haematuria or relieving pain. These
3 different approaches can be executed simultaneously.

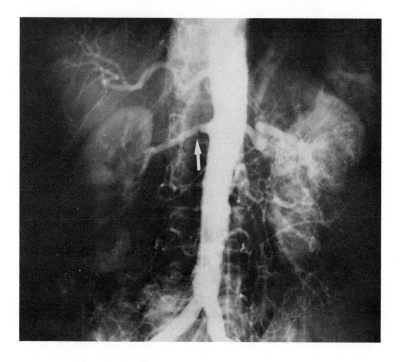

Figure 1 : Midstream aortogram
Hypervascularized tumor of the left kidney, and
stenosis of the right renal artery (_____)

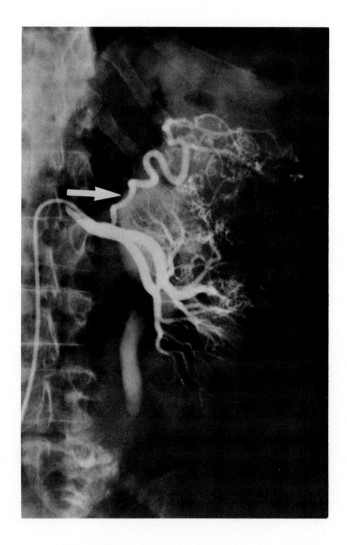

Figure 2a : Arterial phase :
Hypertrophy of a capsular branch vascularising
the tumor (⎯⎯→) on the external edge of the
upper pole.

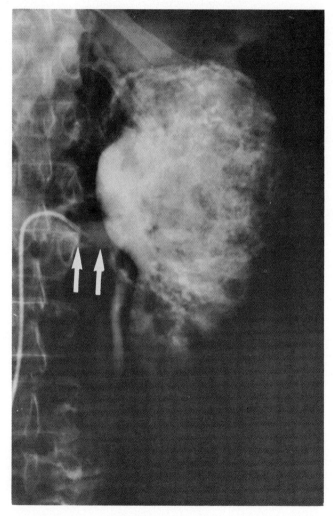

<u>Figure 2b</u> : Venous phase :
The tumor is well limited : the renal vein is
opacified (⟹)

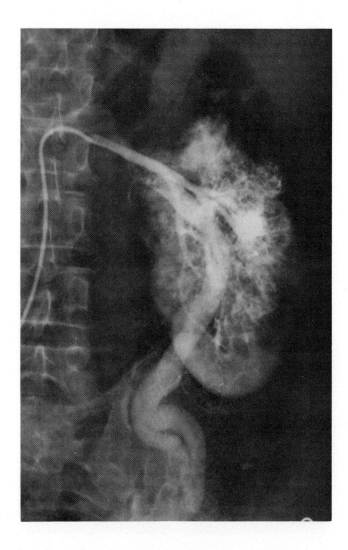

Figure 3 : Very large tumor with polycyclic hilar masses ;
venous drainage is effected through the dilated
vein of the left ovary ; the renal vein is
compressed by lymph nodes.

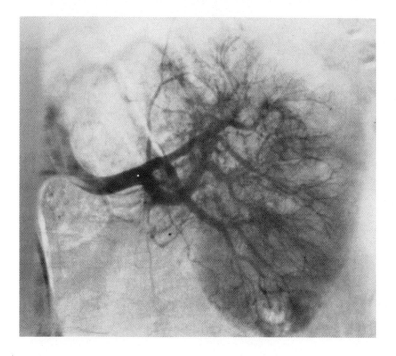

<u>Figure 4</u> : Tumor of the upper pole : the linear opacities
under the renal artery correspond to the vascularisation of the intravenous neoplastic thrombus.

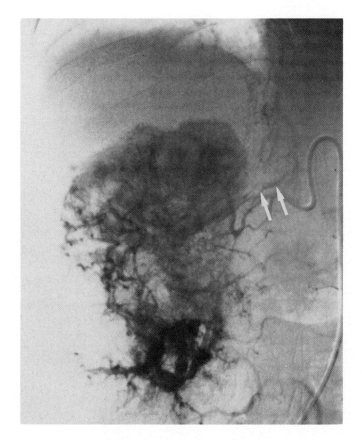

<u>Figure 5a</u> : Very extensive hypervascularized tumor ; linear
hilar and right paravertebral opacities (vascularisation of the intravenous tumor thrombus).

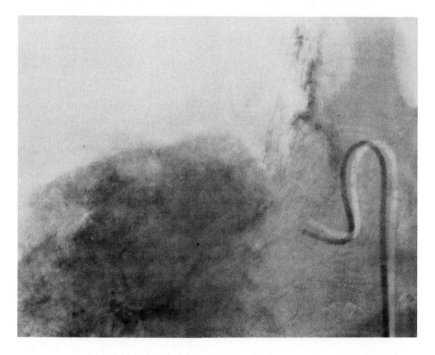

Figure 5b : Later phase and at increased magnification : intra-caval extensions are clearly visible.

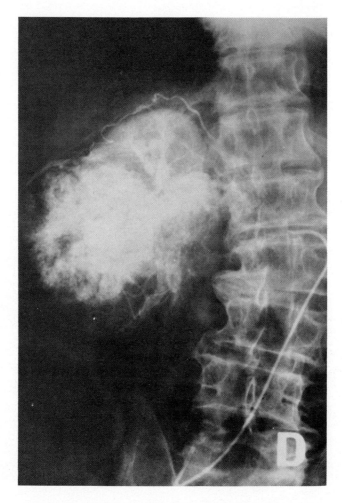

Figure 6 : Peripheral renal tumor and paravertebral tumoral
bud : indication of a cavography to distinguish
a lymph node of the intravenous thrombus.

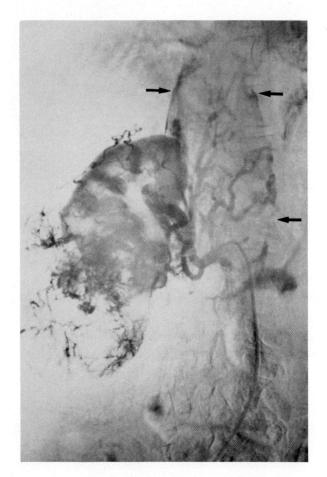

Figure 7 : Very extensive intravenous thrombus of the vena cava : cardiac opacification detected an extension in the right atrium.

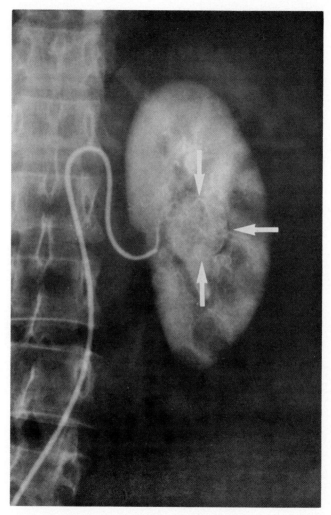

Figure 8 : Small centrohilar tumor : the I.V.P. was performed for signs of urinary infection.

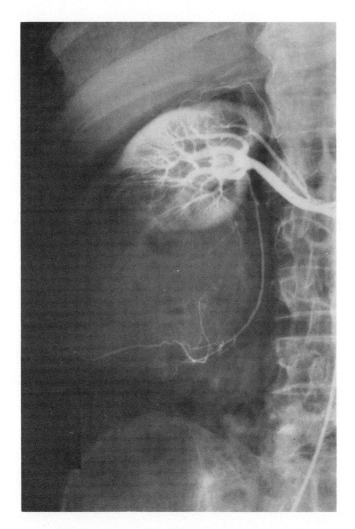

Figure 9 : Extensive hypervascularized tumor with apparently malignant neovessels ; this was not
determined by echography (very significant tumoral necrosis).

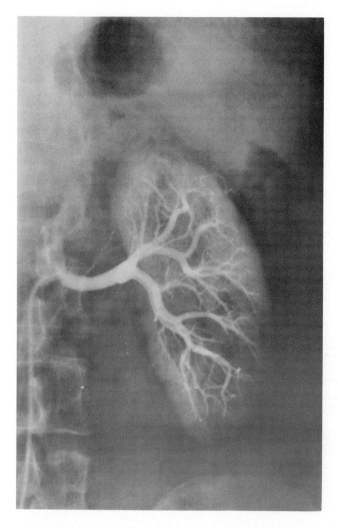

Figure 10a: Limits of arteriography : in straight Frontal projection
1976 : minimal displacement of a retropyelic branch

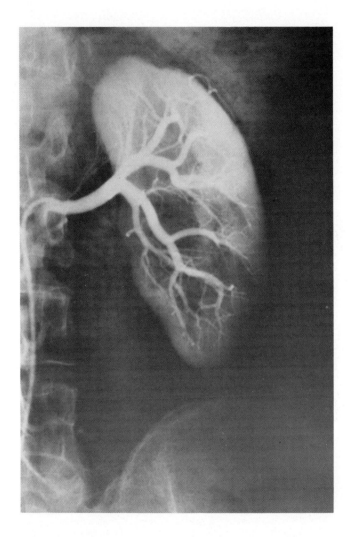

Figure 10b : Limits of arteriography : in straight Frontal
              projection
              1979 : more marked displacement : the vascular
                     irregularity is marked

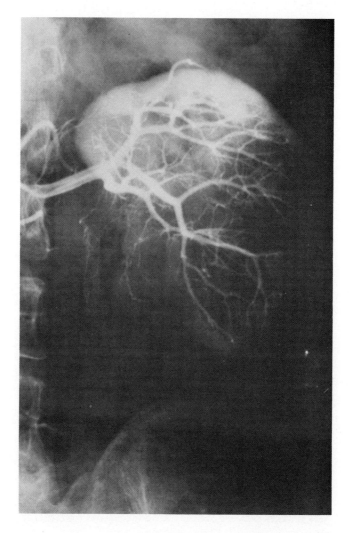

Figure 10c : Limits of arteriography : in straight Frontal projection
1980 : obvious malignant tumor
An incomplete arteriographical examination of the patient suggested the diagnosis of a cyst (1976 end 1979) which could have been at variance with an oblique projection and behavioural modifiers.

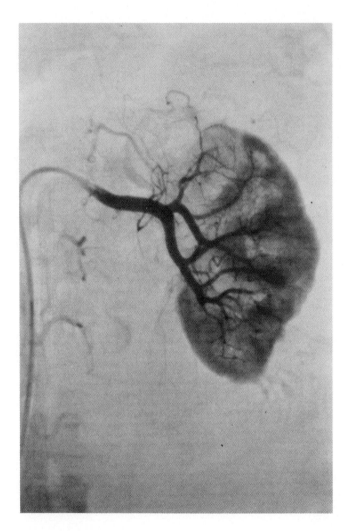

<u>Figure 11a</u> : arterial phase

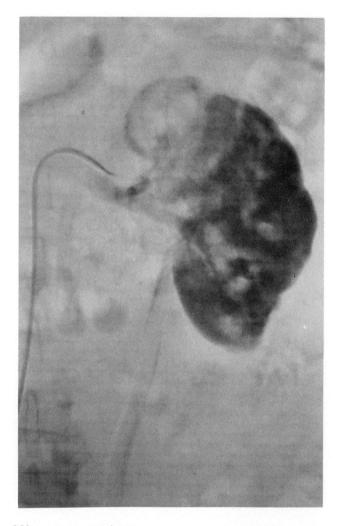

Figure 11b : venous phase
hematuria in a patient with chronic pyelonephritis. The minimal arterial disorders suggest an invasion, and justify the decision to
operate.
The pathological examination reveals the co-
existence of an adenocarcinoma and an excreto-
urinary epithelioma (transitional cell carcinoma)

Renal Tumors: Proceedings of the First International Symposium on Kidney Tumors, pages 369–375
© **1982 Alan R. Liss, Inc., 150 Fifth Avenue, New York, NY 10011**

HOW DOES ULTRASOUND SHOW RENAL CANCER, DIAGNOSTIC
DIFFICULTIES AND RELIABILITY

M. CH PLAINFOSSE, M D., S. MERRAN, M.D.
Central Radiology
Hôpital Broussais 96, rue Didot
Paris 75 674

In the ultrasound features of renal cancer, typical
renal cancer is made of an echogenic mass, the structure of
which is not the same as renal parenchyma. The contours
are regular in small and encapsulated cancers and irregular
in the other cases. These contours are always clear. The
mass distorts the normal renal shape. If it grows near
the sinus, the latter can be obliterated, thinner or displaced.

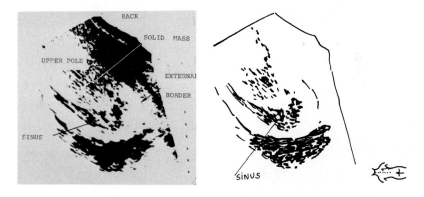

Fig. 1. The tumor area is surrounded by sinus echoes. The
tumor breaks the contours of the posterior face of the
kidney and makes the upper part of the sinus thinner.

If the tumor grows near the capsule, the external
renal border is displaced (Fig. 2). If it is near the
pyelo-ureteral junction, it can induce an hydronephrosis.
The ultrasound scans have to be numerous and in various
planes in order to give information about the tumoral
volume. Ultrasound is better than IVP to see an anterior
or posterior extent of the tumor. Tumoral spread is a very
important problem but a very difficult one. With ultrasound
alone it is often possible to see an intracaval thrombosis,
as seen in Fig. 3.

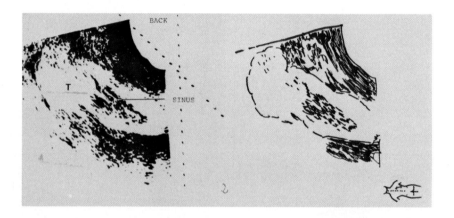

Fig. 2. The borders of the kidney are discontinuous and
pelvicaliceal echoes are displaced.

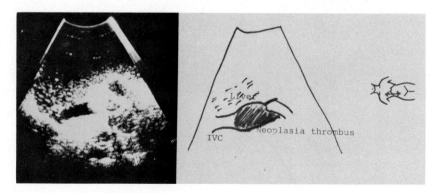

Fig. 3. Extension of a renal cell-carcinoma in the IVC.
Echogenic pattern corresponding to a neoplastic thrombosis.

One may also suspect this condition if the caval vessel is wider than normal or unmoved while breathing. When this thrombosis grows in a renal vein, and especially in the left renal vein, it is unlikely to be seen. The spread must be looked for in the other kidney, adrenals and liver. Ultrasound is the best method to see metastasis. However, there is a problem with adenopathy because it is difficult to recognize an edematous increase or normal size lymph node from a pathologic lymph node. Yet it is the same with all the techniques. Of course the patient must be fasting for this medial retroperitoneal exploration.

With ultrasound some cancers are less typical. For example, tumors are hardly echogenic in cases when the vascularity is poor (for example sarcoma) and when it comes from the excretory tract. In the latter case the tumor is always continuous to the sinus. Renal cancers can also be necrotic and become liquid. The ultrasound structure of this is made by a few echoes. This picture looks like cysts. But there is no acoustic enhancement and the borders are well drawn. The necrotic process cannot occur in small masses.

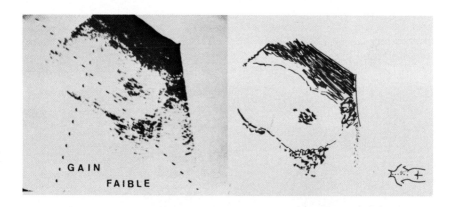

Fig. 4. Cystic like tumor of the upper pole of the kidney. The lateral borders of the "cyst" are too clear and there is no acoustic enhancement behind the lesion.

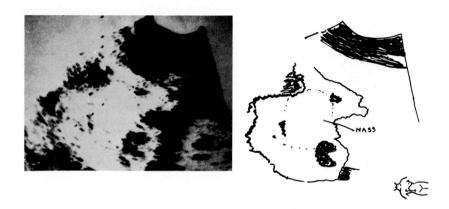

Fig. 5. This cystic-like tumor was a renal cell carcinoma of the anterior face of the kidney. The normal anterior outlines of the kidney and the pelvic are erased. Note the visible lateral borders of the tumor, and the absence of posterior acoustic enhancement.

With ultrasound some cancers appear like septated cysts but a lot of diseases can give such an impression. Calcifications also create difficulty in recognizing the structure of a mass because of the acoustic shadows. In such cases ultrasonography is not the best method for diagnosis. When the mass is less than 2 cm in diameter it is impossible to recognize it by ultrasound because image definition is poor.

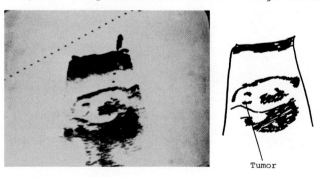

Tumor

Fig. 6. The smallest renal carcinoma we have diagnosed by ultrasound.

When a mass originates from renal borders, it is impossible to know if it is a renal mass or an extra renal on which pervades the kidney (Fig. 7).

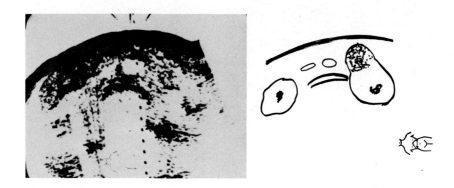

Fig. 7. Retroperitoneal, extra-renal malignant tumor infiltrating the kidney. Ultrasonography cannot distinguish such a tumor from a renal cell carcinoma.

Every renal structure we have described in renal cancer can be found in other masses. If the renal mass is of the same echogenicity as the renal parenchyma, we can easily recognize renal pseudo tumor (a huge Bertin column or a regenerative nodosity). Sinus lipomatosis also always enlarges the sinus. Its structure is very echogenic. Lipomatosis tumors have a very echogenic structure with very strong echoes. The most frequent in the kidney is angiomyolypoma (Fig. 8). It can be suspected if the X-ray film shows a radiolucency in the lipomatosis area. If the mass is almost sonolucent, we have to suspect cancer with hydatic cyst and abscess, but in all of these diseases the clinical symptoms are very different. Moreover, we should not forget cysts with parasitic echoes, (electronic noise, reverberation echoes, delayed echoes or penumbra echoes). The quality of the echographist may frequently determine an accurate diagnosis. In the case of a septated mass we have to consider not only hydatic cyst and abscess but also the multilocular (Fig. 9).

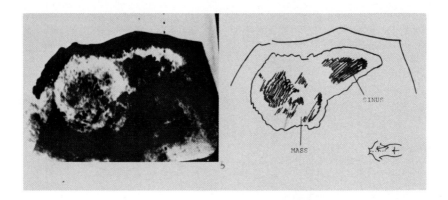

Fig 8. Echogenic tumor of the kidney with well drawn borders.
The kidney is deformed and the pelvic echoes are obliterated
by a huge and very echogenic mass. This tumor was an angiomyolipoma. Can ultrasound alone make the differential diagnosis? This is the problem.

     In each doubtful diagnosis another method must be used:
puncture, arteriography or CT scan. a) If the puncture
shows blood or colored liquid or nothing we have to suspect
a tumor. Arteriography can show the small masses and calcified tumors but in the case of necrotic tumors arteriography
can fail. CT scan is a very good means of diagnosis in
both situations. Focal renal tumor spread can be approached
with the best accuracy by CT scan. For bone metastasis
we used scintigraphy and for lung metastasis X-ray and CT
scan.

     Accuracy in our experience based on 165 cases of renal
cancers studied during the last six years was 94% of true
positive cases and 6% of false negatives cases. Out of
those 6%, 1.5% were small sized cancers and could not be
studied because of technical difficulties in seeing the
upper pole of the left kidney and 3% were calcified tumors.
Apart from these 165 cases, in another study, we found 3.5%
false positive diagnosis. These errors occur in some parasitic echoes, in abnormal thickening of renal parenchyma
without any tumors, and in incomplete exams. On the other
hand the true negative cases with ultrasound are important
and cannot be questioned.

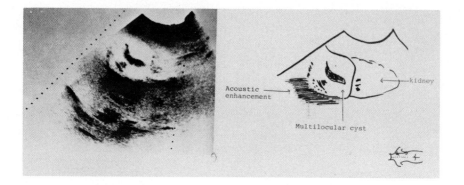

Fig. 9. A multilocular cyst.

In fact ultrasound allows us to differentiate solid
masses from liquid masses. In doubtful cases or in solid
masses, CT scan is the best way to clarify the diagnosis
and to know the spread. But, in our opinion, ultrasound
is also the cheapest way to achieve the best accuracy.

Renal Tumors: Proceedings of the First International Symposium on Kidney Tumors, pages 377–397

COMPUTED TOMOGRAPHY IN THE DIAGNOSIS AND EVALUATION OF RENAL
CELL CARCINOMA

Francois Richard, Saad Khoury, René Küss

Clinique Urologique, Hôpital de la Pitié

Paris, France

INTRODUCTION

    Computed tomography (CT) scan gives without any
contrast media an excellent display of cross sectional renal
anatomy. The kidneys are outlined clearly by the surrounding perinephric fat. CT scans can also reveal tissue densities.
Alteration of densities by I.V. injection of a contrast media
gives valuable information allowing one to distinguish between a benign renal cyst and a solid renal neoplasm. Computed
tomography is an extremely accurate method of obtaining more
definitive diagnostic information about a renal mass and the
evaluation of its extension.

MATERIALS AND METHODS

    This study includes 79 patients with a final diagnosis
of renal cell carcinoma, all of whom had CT scan examination.
Of these, 78 were studied with a third generation CT scan,
and in one case a prototype scanner was used, the results of
which were regarded as invalid. In most cases, density
studies were carried out before and after the administration
of soluble iodinated contrast medium. In ten cases, the
disease was so extensive that removal was deemed impossible;
the diagnoses were confirmed radiologically and clinically.
In the remaining 69 cases, surgery was possible, and an
anatomoclinical staging was made using the following
criteria (Weyman et al, 1980).

1)   The degree of accuracy, i.e. the rate of the sum

of true positive and true negative cases over the
total number of cases.

2) The degree of sensitivity, ie., the probability of
having a true positive answer.

3) The degree of specificity, i.e., the probability
of having an extension of the disease actually,
along with a positive CT scan.

4) Negative predictive value, i.e., the probability
that there is no extension in the presence of
a negative CT scan (Table 1).

RESULTS

A correct prospective diagnosis of renal malignancy by
CT scan was made in 77 out of 79 cases, i.e., 97.5%. In
one case, a small neoplasm of the upper pole was missed.
This was because the scan was done without injection of
contrast medium, and because only one slice was made in the
upper pole. A second CT scan, carried out one month later,
established the true diagnosis. In the remaining case, it
was uncertain whether the increased attenuation noted
represented a renal cell neoplasm or a tumor of the pelvis.
Because this study was carried out using prototype equipment, its technical validity is doubtful.

During this period, four false positives were recorded.
These were two tumors of the pelvis, invading the parenchyma,
one oncocytoma and one strumum. In four cases where the
lesions were calcified, the diagnosis remained uncertain
(three multicompartmental cysts and one calcified tuberculoma).

Staging

The CT scan is a valuable diagnostic aid in the study
of perinephric extension of a growth, in the study of lymph
node involvement, and in renal vein involvement. Perinephric
extension was evaluated and the results are given in
Table 2. There were five false positive diagnoses, which
were due to adherence to the psoas muscle (2), parietal
adherence (1), liver metastases (1) and adrenal extension (1).
Tables 3 and 4 list the results of renal vein and vena cava
involvement, and Table 5 gives the data on lymph node involvement. One CT scan was considered ambiguous, as it was uncertain
whether the patient had a biliary cyst or hepatic metastases.

TABLE 1

STAGING CRITERIA

C.T. \ Pathology	Cancer	Normal
Cancer	a	b
Normal	c	d

ACCURACY $\dfrac{a+d}{a+b+c+d}$

SENSITIVITY $\dfrac{a}{a+c}$

SPECIFICITY $\dfrac{d}{b+d}$

PREDICTIVE VALUE POSITIVE $\dfrac{a}{a+b}$

PREDICTIVE VALUE NEGATIVE $\dfrac{d}{c+d}$

TABLE 2

LOCAL-REGIONAL INVOLVEMENT

True Positive	7	Accuracy	91%
True Negative	56	Sensitivity	100%
False Positive	5	Specificity	90%
False Negative	0	Predictive Value Positive	58%
Indeterminate	1	Predictive Value Negative	100%
Total	69		

TABLE 3

RENAL VEIN INVOLVEMENT

True Positive	16	Accuracy	86%
True Negative	44	Sensitivity	76%
False Positive	1	Specificity	91%
False Negative	0	Predictive Value	94%
Indeterminate	8	Predictive Value	100%
Total	69		

TABLE 4

VENA CAVA INVOLVEMENT

True Positive	5	Accuracy	97%
True Negative	62	Sensitivity	100%
False Positive	2	Specificity	96%
False Negative	0	Predictive Value Positive	71%
Indeterminate	0	Predictive Value Negative	100%
Total	69		

TABLE 5

LYMPH NODE INVOLVEMENT

True Positive	7	Accuracy	94%
True Negative	58	Sensitivity	88%
False Positive	2	Specificity	95%
False Negative	0	Predictive Value Positive	78%
Indeterminate	2	Predictive Value Negative	100%
Total	69		

DISCUSSION

Evaluation of a renal mass can be identified by CT scanning because they differ in density from normal parenchyma or because they project beyond the normal kidney margin (Caron Poitreau et al, 1979; Lecudonnec et al, 1981; Love et al, 1979; Rampal et al, 1980; Richard et al, 1980; Sagel et al, 1977; Struyven et al, 1979). The investigation of CT scanning has proved extremely valuable in accurately distinguishing a benign renal cyst from a renal neoplasm (Figures 1 and 2). If an intravenous contrast medium is used, the accuracy in this respect is even greater (Figure 3) (Caron Poitreau et al, 1979; Lamarque et al, 1980; Magilner, Obtrum 1978). Table 6 shows the CT characteristics of renal cysts and solid masses.

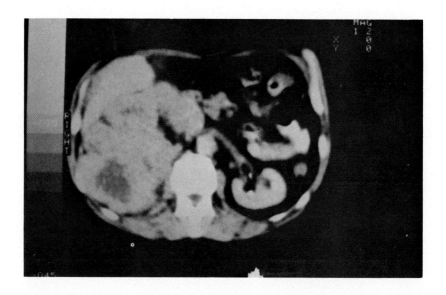

Fig. 1.   Large renal cell carcinoma of the right kidney with central necrosis.

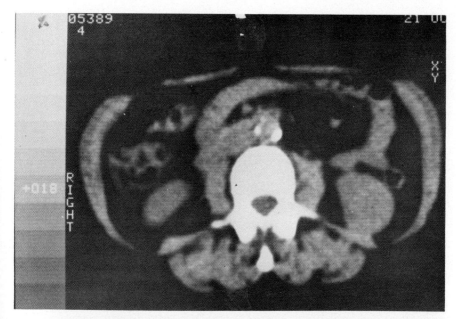

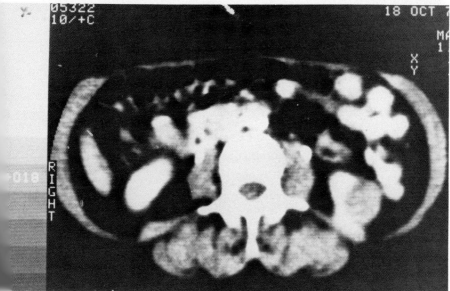

Fig. 2. Small renal cell carcinoma of the left kidney. The study of densities before and after contrast medium injection allows diagnosis.

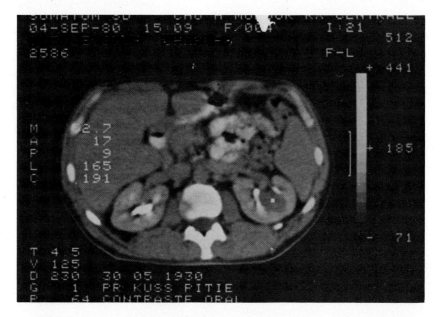

Fig. 3. Small intrarenal tumor undetected by other means of diagnosis.

TABLE 6

COMPUTED TOMOGRAPHY CHARACTERISTICS OF SOLID MASSES (CANCER) AND RENAL CYSTIS

Features	Cancer	Cyst
Margins	Irregular	Smooth
Wall thickness	Thick	Thin
Parenchymal interface	Indistinct	Distinct
GT densities without injection	Heterogenous approximate renal tissue 30-50 UH	Homogenous approximate water 0-10 UH
Contrast enhancement	Yes 40-80 UH	No 0-10 UH

Sources of Error

1) Artifacts produced by partial volume averaging may
    give misleading information in tumors less than 2
    cm in diameter (Hounsfield 1973; Love et al, 1979;
    Richard et al, 1980; Sagel et al, 1977). The
    densities recorded in a reconstructed slice
    represent the attenuation of x-rays by all tissues
    within the volume of that slice. Thus, if a slice
    includes a portion of normal parenchyma as well as
    a cyst, the attenuation volume will be greater
    than if only the cyst were included. Conversely,
    small solid masses projecting beyond the renal
    contour may be averaged in with the adjacent
    perinephric fat, and thus seem lower in density.
    Fortunately, the infusion of contrast media and
    the use of collimators thinner than 1 cm provide
    an alternative solution to the problem of partial
    volume averaging (Weymon et al, 1980).

2) Very large tumors distorting and pressing on
    adjacent organs may be difficult to differentiate
    from tumors of the adrenal or from retroperitoneal
    tumors if there are no slices which show their
    actual attachment to the kidney (Elie et al, 1980).

3) A CT scan can easily distinguish a tumor from
    foetal lobulation hypertrophy, a culum of Bertin,
    or a sinusal lipomatosis (Hadar, Levine 1980;
    Richard et al, 1980).

4) Angiomyolipomata (Figure 4) is relatively easy
    to diagnose when negative density areas (fat)
    are represented in the tumor (Bush et al, 1979;
    Frija et al, 1980; Hansen et al, 1978; Jardin
    et al, 1980; Rao et al, 1981; Shawker et al,
    1979; Totty et al, 1981).

5) A tumor of the renal pelvis can be identified
    (Figure 5) when it protrudes into the lumen of the
    excretory system. However, an accurate diagnosis
    might be difficult when it represents a parenchymal
    infiltration mass (Richard et al, 1980, 1981).

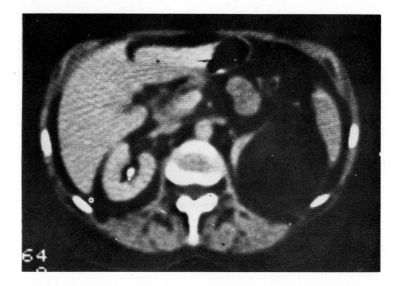

Fig. 4. Angiomyolipoma with negative densities.

6) A CT scan cannot distinguish between histofocal varieties of tumors with positive densities. However, renal cell carcinoma remains the most likely diagnosis (Wojtowicz et al, 1979).

7) A renal abscess may be indistinguishable from a febrile necrotic tumor despite the fact that in the case of an abscess the wall of the tumor is smooth. Central densities on two consecutive scans may differ because of changes in volume of the lesion (Mendez et al, 1979).

8) A calcified tumor can be difficult to assess by CT scanning (Richard et al). The other available diagnostic aids share this same problem. However, the diagnosis of a calcified growth can be made when the calcification is within a high density tumor. Also, the attenuation index of the tumor increases when contrast medium if injected. If this density remains unchanged after the injection of contrast medium, then the diagnosis becomes more difficult. In cases of low positive density (15-25 UH), tumor necrosis may be

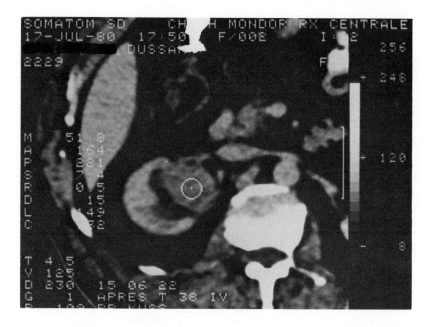

Fig. 5.   Tumor of the renal pelvis.

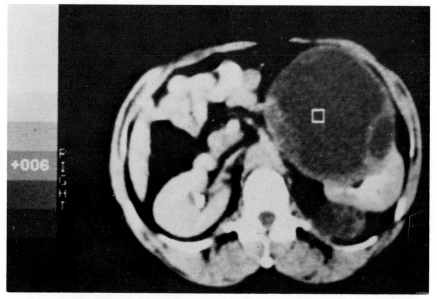

Fig. 6.   Hydatid cyst of left kidney.

difficult to differentiate from renal abscess or
tuberculoma. In cases where the attenuation value
is approximately that of water, the most probable
diagnosis is that of a calcified cyst or a
hydatid cyst compartmentalized within the lesion
(Figure 6). In general the presence of calcification
can lead to a false negative diagnosis of renal
neoplasm or it can present an accurate diagnosis
being made.

Evaluation of Extension

The CT scan allows one to identify, with good accuracy,
the presence or absence of extrarenal extension. It can
provide valuable information about operability, the usefulness of embolisation, or the correct surgical approach
(Lamarque et al, 1981; Levine et al, 1979).

1)   Perinephric extension, that is the invasion of
      a tumor of the perinephric space (Parienty et al,
      1981; Weymon et al, 1980), can be identified on a
      CT scan by the presence of an indistinct tumor
      margin with strands of soft tissue density extending
      into or obliterating completely the preinephric
      fat (Figures 7 and 8). However, such irregular

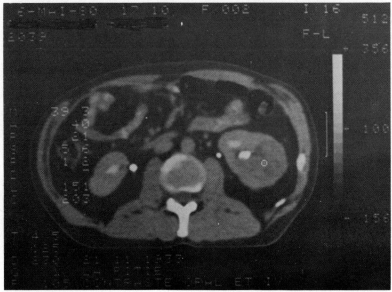

Fig. 7. Renal cell carcinoma Stage 1 Gerota's facia is well
outlined.

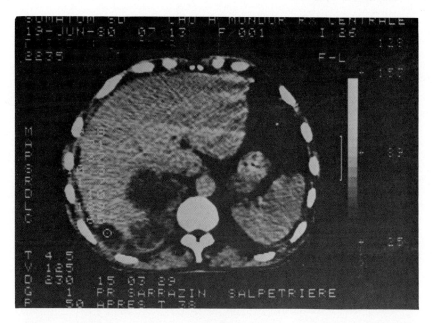

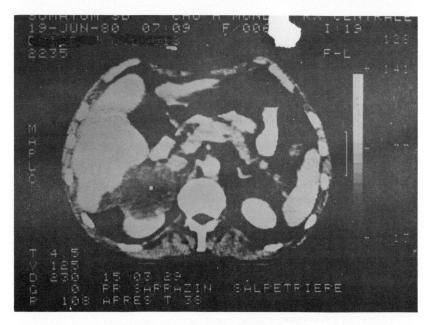

Fig. 8. Renal cell carcinoma of right kidney with hepatic extension.

densities in this perinephric space can also be
seen with intracapsular tumors. This is presumably
due to the presence of collateral vessels and/or
connective tissue septa. Small neoplastic extensions
into the perinephric fat without actually involving
Gerota's fascia or without obliterating the perinephric fat are difficult to assess using CT scanning.
Most of the incorrect or indecisive scans are of this
nature, but because radical nephrectomy is now the
standard operation (en bloc resection of the kidney
and perinephric fat), such minor perinephric
extension does not alter the surgical approach. It
is, however, critically important to identify
extension beyond perinephric fat.

Thickening of Gerota's fascia does not in itself
indicate neoplastic involvement, but any loss of
fat planes between the tumor and the adjacent
structure should be considered very carefully.
The presence of any tissue of non-uniform density
invading the surrounding organs indicates neoplastic
extension.

2) Renal vein involvement (Figure 9) can be seen as
enlargement of the main renal vein, often accompanied
by lower density defects within the vein, and this may
accurately indicate renal vein invasion (Ferris et
al, 1979; Marks et al, 1978; Smith, Levine 1980;
Steele et al, 1978; Zerkouni et al, 1980). Sometimes, renal vein involvement should be suspected
from enlargement of the renal vein by itself
(>1.5 cm in diameter). This diagnosis is
sometimes made difficult because of obliquity and
shortness of the right renal vein, cases of
duplicity, and in cases where the main renal
vein is enlarged by lymph nodes. In some cases
one can detect findings indirectly on the angio-
scans, for example intraparenchymal stasis with
collateral shunts, or an asymetrically specified
vena cava. The diagnosis of tumor trombus in the
vena cava can be directly identified on the CT Scan
as a lower density tumour present beforehand, after
the injection of the contrast media. In some cases,
this lower density zone can be surrounded by a high
density zone after the contrast media has been injected.
This may be caused by blood influx, in the case of

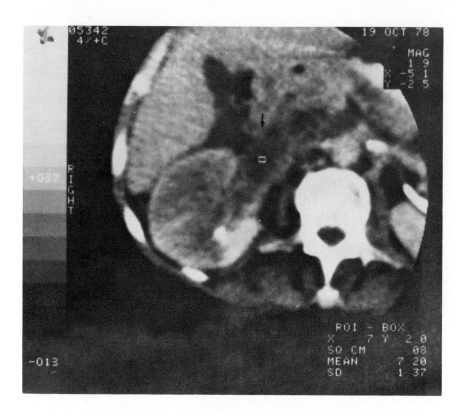

Fig. 9a. Renal vein involvement.

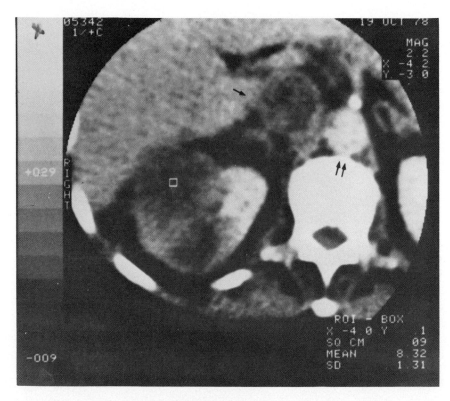

Fig. 9b. Vena cava thrombosis.

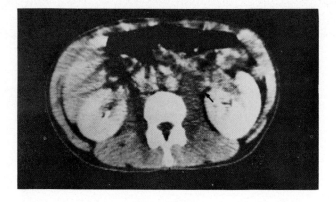

Fig. 10. Lymph nodes involvement.

partial thrombosis, or to soaking of the thick, inflammed wall of the vena cava by dye.

The vena cava can often be very enlarged (>3 cm in diameter) when there is enlargement of the renal veins, and with a normal caliber vena cava below that level, this can imply the presence of thrombus. Vein contrast infusion as part of the CT study may help identify intraluminal tumor thrombus, and especially its cephalad extension. In addition, it can distinguish external compression of the vena cava by nodes or tumor from an intraluminal tumor thrombus. High slides must be taken in order to explore properly the upper limit of a neoplastic thrombus. Tables 4 and 5 give the data on our analysis of renal vein and vena cava involvement.

3) Lymph node involvement can be detected by CT scan (Figure 10) only when the lymph nodes are enlarged (Weyman et al, 1980). However, this type of study cannot distinguish between hyperplastic enlargement and tumor metastases.

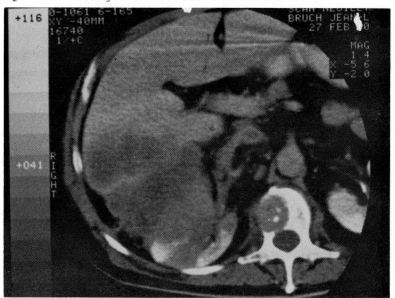

Fig. 11. Metastasis to liver and vertebra.

Microscopic enlargement is similarly undetectable. However, the value of the CT scan over lymphangio-

graphy or angiography is that it can direct the
surgeon to suspicious areas. Microscopic lymph
node metastasis cannot be detected by any means
at present. In some cases, hilar extension of a
renal tumor can be mistaken for lymph node enlargement and this should be regarded as a possible
source of error.

4)   Tomodensitometry can detect intra-abdominal
      metastases (Figure 11) from a renal primary
      (Richard et al; Weyman et al, 1980). This is
      easily done in the liver and suprarenal because
      the metastases is contralateral to the tumor.
      Conversely, it is more difficult when the invasion
      or metastasis is local since the affected organs
      are ipsilateral. In addition one can detect with
      this method a contralateral neoplasm, a second
      neoplasm, or a metastasis.

In conclusion, tomodensitometry is a means whereby one
can diagnose renal carcinoma in about 98% of cases, and
which can identify precisely any extension of a malignant
tumor in about 85% of cases. It has, accordingly, a routine
role in the examination and diagnosis of renal carcinoma
and consequently has reduced the indications for arteriography. New technical improvements (Bolus injection and
faster scanning time) may further improve our results.

REFERENCES

Bush W, Freeney P, Orme B (1979). Angiomyolipoma: charac-
  teristic images by ultrasound and computed tomography.
  Urology 14:531.
Caron Poitreau C, Soret J, Lavenet F, Rieux D, Viallem et
  Rognon L (1979). L'apport de la tomodensitométrie au
  diagnostic des masses rénales. Chirurgie 105:481.
Elie G, Dilhudy M, Ksas D, Le Treut A, Lagarde C (1980).
  Masses rénales et surrénaliennes en tomodensitométrie.
  J Radiol 61:89.
Engelstad BL, MacClennan BL, Levitt RG, Stanley RV, Sagel SS
  (1980). The role of precontrast images in computed tomo-
  graphy of the kidney. Radiology 136:153.
Ferris RA, Kirschner LP, Mero JH, McCabe DJ, Moss ML (1979).
  Computed tomography in the evaluation of inferior vena
  caval obstruction. Radiology 130:710.

Frija J, Larde D, Belloir C, Botto H, Martin M, Vasile N
(1980). Computed tomography diagnosis of renal angiomyolipoma. J Comput Assist Tomogr 4-6:843.
Hadar H, Meiraz D (1980). Renal sinus lipomatosis: differentiation from space occupying lesion with aid of computed
tomography. Urology 15:86.
Hansen G, Hoffman R, Sample W, Becker R (1978). Computed
tomography diagnosis of renal angiomyolipoma. Radiology
128:789.
Hounsfield GN (1973). Computerized transverse axial scanning
(tomography). Br J Radiol 46:1016.
Jardin A, Richard F, Leduc A, Chatelain C, Leguillou M,
Fourcade R, Camey M, Kuss R (1980). Diagnosis and treatment
of renal angiomyolipoma (based on 15 cases). Europ Urol
6:69.
Lamarque JL, Rouanet JP, Bruel JM, Tavera G (1981). Place
de la scannographie dans le bilan d'extension du cancer du
rein. Communication au 83è Congrés Francais de Chirurgie
Actualités chirurgicales Masson ed Paris A paraître.
Lamarque J, Bruel J, Rouanet J, Lopez P et Call (1980). La
tomodensitométrie rénale. Rev Prat 30:1667.
Lecudonnec B, Botto H, Duval F, Auvert J, Ferrane J (1981).
Scannographie et urologie. Concurs Med 103:3683.
Levine E, Lee KR, Weigel J (1979). Preoperative determination
of abdominal extenst of renal cell carcinoma by computed
tomography. Radiology 132:395.
Levine E, Maklad NF, Rosenthal SJ, Lee KR, Weigel J (1980).
Comparison of CT and ultrasound in abdominal staging of
renal cancer. Urology 16:317.
Love L, Churchill R, Reynes C, et al (1979). Computed tomo-
graphy staying of renal carcinoma. Urol Radiol 1:3.
Magilner AD, Obtrum BJ (1978). Computed tomography in the
diagnosis of renal masses. Radiology 126:715.
Marks WM, Korobkin M, Callen PW, Kaiser JA (1978). CT
d diagnosis of tumor thrombosis of the renal vein and inferior
vena cava. Ann J Roentgenol 131:843.
Martin N, Botto H, Vasile N. (1981). Incidence of tomodensito-
métre sur le coût diagnostique des syndromes tumoraux
renaux. Nouv Press Med 10:2081.
Mendez G, Isikoff MB, Morillo G (1979). The role of CT in
the diagnostic of renal and perineal abcess. J Urol 122:
582.
McClennan BL, Stanley RJ, Melson GL, Levitt RG, Sagel SS
(1979). CT of renal cyst: is cyst aspiration necessary?
AJR 133:671.
Meaney FF, Vacka LJ, Gallagher JH (1980). Contribution of

CT of relative costs in the operative management of parents with renal cell carcinoma. CT 4:185.

Parienty RA, Pradel J, Picard JD, Ducellier R, Lubrano JM, Smolarski N (1981). Visibility and thickening of the renal fascia ou computed tomograms. Radiology 139:119.

Rao PN, Obborn DE, Barnard RJ, Best JJM (1981). Symptomatic renal angiomyolipoma. Br J Urol 53:212.

Rampal M, Huguet JF, Pons G, Aumi JC, Tassy JP, Coulange C (1980). Valeur de la tomodensitometrie dans le diagnostic du tumeur du rein. Ann Urol 14:183.

Richard F, Khoury S, Parienty R, Ducellier R, Fourcade R, Kuss R (1980). Le rein en tomodensitométrie. J Urol 86:91.

Richard F, Lecudonnec B, Fourcade R, Jardin A, Chatelain C, Kuss R (1980). Apport de la tomodensitométrie dans le diagnostic et le bilan d'extension de tumeur de la voie excrétrice supérieure. Ann Urol 14:301.

Richard F, Vallancien G, Larde D, Parienty R, Kuss R (1981). Interet de la tomodensitométrie dans le diagnostic des lacunes de la voie excrétrice supérieure (23 cas). Société Francaise d'Urologie. Ann Urol A paraitre

Richard F, Chatelain C, Jardin A, Grellet JP, Curet Ph, Kuss R (1981). Résultats comparatifs de l'échotomographie de la tomodensitométrie et de l'artériographie dans l'exploration des masses rénales. Sem Urol Néphrol 7ème série 1-20, Paris, Masson ed.

Sagel SS, Stanley RJ, Levitt RG, Geisse G (1977). Computed tomography of the kidney. Radiology 124:359.

Shawker T, Horvath K, Dunnick N, Javadpour N (1979). Renal angiomyolipoma diagnosis by combined ultrasound and computerized tomography. J Urol 121:675.

Smith WP, Levine E (1980). Sagittal and coronal CT image reconstruction: application in assening the inferior vena cava in renal cancer. J Comput Assist Tomogr 4:531.

Steele JR, Sones PJ, Heffner LT (1978). The detection of inferior vena cava thrombosis with computed tomography. Radiology 128:385.

Stewart BH, Haaga JR, Alfidi RJ (1978). Urological applications of computed axial tomography: a preliminary report. J Urol 120:198.

Struyven J, Gregoir W, Schulman CC (1979). La tomographie axiale computerisee dans les affections urinares. Ann Urol 13:81.

Totty WG, McClennan BL, Melson GL, Pater (1981). Relative value of CT and ultra sacography in the assessment of renal angiomyolipoma. J Comput Assist Tomogr 5-2:173.

Weyman PJ, McClennan BL, Stanley RJ, Levitt RG, Sagel SS (1980). Comparison of computed tomography and angiography

in the evaluation of renal cell carcinoma. Radiology 137:
417.

Wojtowicz J, Karwowski A, Konkiewicz J, Lukaszewki B (1979).
Renal oncocytoma. J Comput Assist Tomgr 3:124.

Zeman RK, Cronan JJ, Visconi GN, Rosenfield AT (1981).
Coordinated imaging in the detection and characterization
of renal. CRC Crit Rev Diagn Imag 15:273.

Zerhouni EA, Barth KH, Siegelman SS (1980). Demonstration
of venous thrombosis by computed tomography. Ann J
Roentgenol 134:753.

Renal Tumors: Proceedings of the First International Symposium on Kidney Tumors, pages 399–408
© **1982 Alan R. Liss, Inc., 150 Fifth Avenue, New York, NY 10011**

COMPUTED TOMOGRAPHY DETECTION OF INFERIOR VENA CAVA
OBSTRUCTION IN RENAL CANCERS

L.M. Rognon and Ch. Caron-Poitreau

C.H.U. Angers

49040 Angers Cedex France

Inferior vena cava (IVC) invasion during the development of renal cancers has always been a serious factor.
Detection of such invasion and appreciation of its nature
and extent, factors that are essential to the management
of the disease, are usually obtained by caval venography
and sometimes by aretriography. Currently, the use of
computed tomography provides additional interesting information as ten of our cases show.

MATERIALS AND METHODS

Among the latest cases of renal cancer examined by
computed tomography, ten showed fairly extensive IVC
modifications indicating obstruction by tumoral invasion
or thrombosis. The patients were mostly male (seven out
of ten), relatively young (seven under 60 years and three
under 45 years) and suffered from large tumors mostly
situated on the right (seven on the right and three on
the left). In three cases the tumors were discovered in
patients with urological disorders while five cases
showed, in addition, severe inflammatory syndromes
(sedimentation rate greater than 100, fever etc.) together with a general run-down condition. In two cases
the patients were admitted for phlebitis of the limbs.

In each case the tumor syndrome was brought to light
by intravenous urography, nephrotomography and echography.
The diagnosis was then confirmed by computed tomography.
The apparatus used is a third generation type with a six-
second scan.

Each exploration consisted of:

1) guiding sections without opacification
2) serial sections after rapid injection of 60 ml of a 38% iodine compound
3) sections covering the entire height of the renal region during slow perfusion of the same solution
4) analyses of the pictures obtained by reconstruction in the orthogonal, sagittal and frontal planes.

Once the IVC anomaly was detected, its characteristics were determined by caval venography through the femoral vein or, when necessary, through the jugular vein. Except in one case, arteriography was not used.

Three of the patients were not operated on because of general weakness, the presence of metastases or because or computed tomography results concerning the tumor itself and the state of the IVC.

One patient underwent surgical exploration for an enormous inextirpable tumor invading the IVC up from the diaphragm. Histology showed the the neoplasm, considered renal, was more likely a malignant adrenal cortical carcinoma spreading to the wall of the IVC.

In the remaining six cases, extensive nephrectomy was associated with operations on the IVC ranging from extirpation of tumoral thrombosis (3 cases) to segmentary resection of the IVC (3 cases). In all of these cases, histological examination of the renal tumor led to the conclusion of adenocarcinomas (Grawitz tumors). The venous extension turned out to be malignant in four of the patients but in the other two it corresponded to infiltration of the veinous wall caused by a former thrombosis and showed no neoplastic lesions.

RESULTS

Case 1: Ma...Male aged 61. 1978: hematuria. 1980: subocclusive syndrome of undetermined origin. 1981: recrudescence of hematuria. Intravenous urography: tumor syndrome spreading to the upper pole of the right kidney; opacification at the lower pole. Computed tomography: voluminous tumor occupying two-thirds of the upper rear region of the right kidney; peripheral hypervascularisa-

tion; between sections at 45 mm and 90 mm, hypodensity of
the vena cava (27 EMI units) above the hilus surrounded
by a dense ring on the inside and outside faces; this
segment being thrust forward by dense prevertebral formations suggesting adenopathies; the right renal vein enlarged and irregular; the vena cava under the junction
of the left renal vein showing a normal aspect. Caval
Venography through the femoral vein: reduced diameter,
stagnation of the injected compound at the lower and
with considerable collateral circulation; the IVC pushed
forward as seen in profile. Operation (V-1981): tumoral
hardening of the right side of the IVC in the sub-hepatic
section going below the end of the right renal vein. After
clamping, extensive right nephrectomy with resection of
the infiltrated right wall of the IVC. Resolvent postoperative renal insufficiency. Postoperative phlebography
(+ 45 days): complete thrombosis of the vena cava with
derivation through azygous rachidial systems, permeability
of the left renal vein.

Histology: Nephroepithelimoa (Grawitz tumor). Tumoral
obliteration of the initial branches and the trunk of
the renal vein. Infiltration of the wall of the re-
sectioned vena cava by a fibro-hyaline callus, dense and
pigmented, identified as a former thrombosis and showing
no neoplastic extension.

Case 2: Ch...Female aged 58. Acute abdominal syndrome,
painful and feverish. Laparotomy revealed a large tumor
in the right kidney. Postoperative phlebitis on the
right side. Intravenous urography: no secretion of the
right kidney. Phlebography (right femoral and right
jugular veins): iliac thrombosis and extensive lacuna
of the IVC, considerable collateral circulation. Computed
tomograph : large tumor in the right kidney. Sub-
hepatic vena cava enlarge (3.74 cm), homogenous, hypodense (30 EMI units). (Fig. 1).

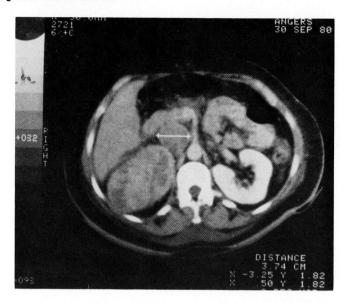

Fig. 1. Case 2. Grawitz tumor: fibrino cruoral
thrombosis invading the IVC. Post contrast C.T. Scan.
Sub-he atic V.C. enlarged (.74) cm) homogenous - hypodense
(30 EMI unit).

The right renal vein appeared enlarged and irregular;
the left renal vein distally obstructed; the subpedicular **vena** cava recovered normal diameter, hypodense
center (23 EMI units) with an opaque surrounding periphery continuing up to the iliac (Fig. 2). Reconstruction:
overall hypodensity of the vena cava with dilatation at
the upper end and well-defined limits at the lower end
(Fig. 3). Operation: extensive right nephrectomy with
segmental cavectomy removing the base of the thrombosed
left renal vein. Histology: Grawitz tumor; tumoral
invasion of the base of the right vein together with a
fibrino-cruoral thrombosis invading the vena cava and
in the process of organization. Absence of tumoral
elements in the vena cava.

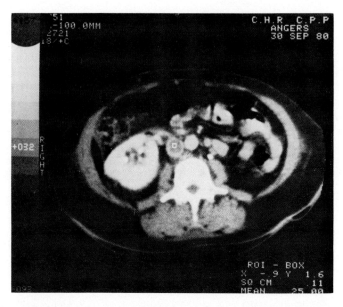

Fig. 2. Case 2. The subpedicular V.C. recovered normal diamater; hypodense center surrounded by an opaque fringe.

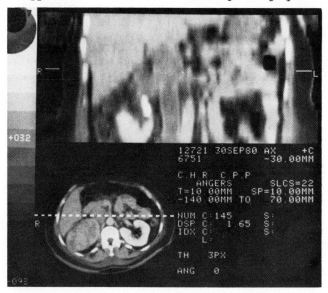

Fig. 3. Case 2. Coronal reconstruction of IVC: overall hypodensity with dilatation at the upper end and well defined limits at the lower end.

In two of our observations, the IVC was not sufficiently identifiable to judge its invasion. As shown by the operations, it was obstructed by a massive tumoral extension and additionally masked by the opacity of the renal tumor surrounding it closely with its prolongations and adenopathies. The identification was only possible on a section showing the end of the left renal vein draining the unaffected kidney.

In the eight other cases, the invasion of the IVC was demonstrated by computed tomography showing the decreased opacity of one of the segments associated with diverse other signs.

The hypodensity was especially evident after contrast and on reconstructed sections. It appeared as a fairly homogenous zone contrasting against the opacity of the blood circulating over or under the IVC and that in the aorta. Its density, sometimes slightly increased after iodine opacification, remained usually between 20 and 30 EMI units with some variation according to the plane examined.

In two of the observations, the clear segment of the IVC was short (3 cm and 4.5 cm). It began at the junction of the renal vein and developed upwards. In the first case, it corresponded to a tumoral bud (Grawitz tumor) covered by a few fibrino-cruoral clots; in the second, to a former thrombosis with no signs of a tumor (Case 1).

On the other hand, in six cases the hypodense zone covered the IVC almost entirely, sometimes continuing along the iliac axes. As confirmed surgically, this aspect corresponded usually to a tumoral invasion of the IVC together with an extensive thrombosis. However, in one of these cases, the thrombosis alone was found in the IVC (Case 2).

The hypodense aspect of the obstructed IVC was quite often surrounded by an irregular opaque fringe. (Figs. 4 5, and 6). The interpretation of this rosette figure is not simple (Van Breda et al. 1979). Zernouni has shown that in the case of hepatic cancer the rosette corresponds to hypervascularization of the wall of the IVC invaded by a tumoral extension as demonstrated by arteriography (Zernouni et al. 1978). It could also be attributed to parietal thickening due to the organization of a former throbmosis or to free blood circulating at the periphery of a thrombus. In two of the patients we observed that the rosette figure only appeared after very strong opacification by a massive dose of the contrasting compound. In one case, the rosette appeared to be in direct continuity with a dilated lumbar vein.

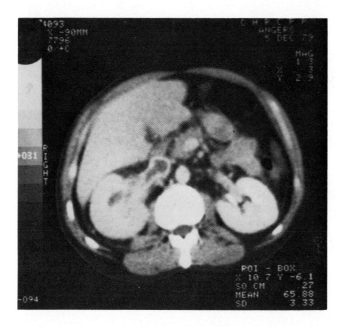

Fig. 4. Grawitz tumor. Tumoral invasion of the renal vein and of the IVC with extensive thrombosis; hypodense aspect surrounded by an irregular opaque fringe.

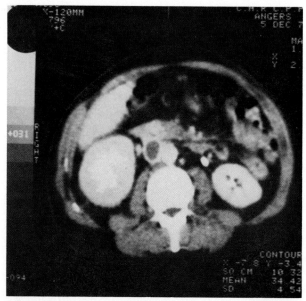

Fig. 5. Case of Fig. 4 - Section at a lower level "Rosette" figure.

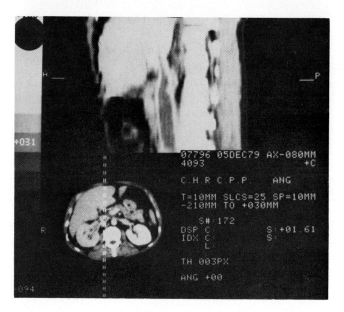

Fig. 6. Case of Fig. 4 - Coronal reconstruction.

The images of hypodense centers surrounded by an opaque fringe were, according to the cases observed, accompanied by:

1) a displacement of the IVC by tumoral prolongations or adenopathies; and

2) an irregular aspect of the sections of the invaded segment (Fig. 7);

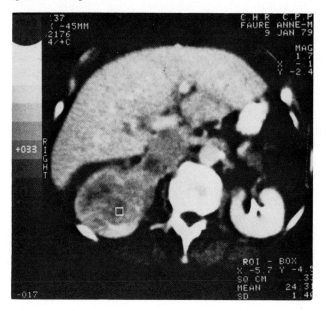

Fig. 7.   Irregular and hypodense enlargement of right renal vein and of IVC.

3) a segmentary dilation (Fig. 7). From 50 computed tomographies, Marks gives a mean value of 2.7 cm for the normal diameter of the IVC at the upper part of the abdomen, with extreme values of 1.5 cm and 3.7 cm (Marks et al. 1978). Thus, any enlargement exceeding the maximum value should be considered pathologic if accompanied by:

1) an increase in the diameter of the vein draining the renal tumor;

2) a normal diameter of the other renal vein, and

3) a sharp return to the normal diameter along the axis of the vena cava.

4) considerable collateral circulation especially in the perirenal cavity.

CONCLUSION

Computed tomography currently appears to be the most useful method for the detection of inferior vena cava invasion during the evolution of renal cancers. In most cases, it demonstrates the presence as well as the general extent of the obstruction but not, however, its nature. In the cases examined, it was not possible to distinguish between the contribution of thrombosis and that of tumoral invasion to the obstruction. Usually, the two processes are associated but, as we observed in two of our patients, vena cava lesions can correspond to the organization of simple thrombosis without any association of a malignant infiltration, a fact that should be borne in mind when making therapeutic decisions.

Fernis RA, Kirschner LP, Mero JH, McCabe DT, Moss ML (1979). Computed tomography in evaluation of the inferior vena canal obstruction. Radiology 130:710.
Marks WM, Korobkin M, Callen PWC, Kaiser JA (1978). CT diagnosis of tumor thrombosis of the renal vein and inferior vena cava. Am J Roentgenology 131:843.
Smith WP, Lepine E (1980). Sagittal and coronal CT image reconstruction. Application in assessing the inferior vena cava in renal cancer. J Comput Assist Tomogr 4:531.
Steele JR, Sones PJ, Heffner LT (1978). The detection of inferior vena cava thrombosis with computed tomography. Radiology 128:385.
Van Breda A, Rubin BE, Druy EM (1979). Detection of inferior vena cava abnormalities by computed tomography. J Computed Assist Tomogr 2:164.
Zernouni EA, Barth KH, Siegelman SS (1978). C.T. demonstration of inferior vena cava invasion in a case of hepatocellular carcinoma. J Computed Assist Tomogr 2:363.

Renal Tumors: Proceedings of the First International Symposium on Kidney Tumors, pages 409–415
© **1982 Alan R. Liss, Inc., 150 Fifth Avenue, New York, NY 10011**

LOCAL RECURRENCE AFTER NEPHRECTOMY FOR RENAL CANCER : CT
RECOGNITION

Roger A. Parienty, Janine Pradel, François Richard
and Saad Khoury
Scanner Hartmann Inter-Cliniques
I, rue des Dames Augustines
92200 - Neuilly sur Seine. France

This study is motived by the following considerations :
I - Up to present, there is a striking discrepancy between
the low-rated clinical estimation (I0-20%)of local recurrence
(LR) and the high frequency of such lesions at autopsy(4I%)(I)
It is likely that we miss their early recognition.
2 - LR are generally considered of a poor prognosis. However, when they are early diagnosed and treated, survival
may be slightly improved (2).
3 - Computed tomography (CT) has been proven the most
efficient means of evaluation of the retroperitoneum (3)
4 - To our knowledge two comprehensive studies only have
been published about CT in post-nephrectomy patients (4,5)
we lack large series of systematic CT follow-up after nephrectomy for renal cancer. Our own presentation also is
limited : it is proposed as a contributive preliminary communication of a work in process.

METHODS :

CT was performed with a third generation CT scanner
(General Electric 7800 then upgraded 8800) with a scan
time of II seconds. Scans were obtained with a I0mms col-
limation at a I0 to 20 mms interval. Patients lied supine.
Only one patient had a complementary study in lateral decubitus to make sure the identification of the shifted pancreas
after left nephrectomy. The alimentary tube was opacified by
ingestion of dilute gastrografin. Iodinated contrast medium
was injected in I.V. bolus. Plain CT scans were usually judged not necessary. In one case, the demonstration of a small
LR in an asymptomatic patient was ascertained by sequential

C.T. scans following a fast bolus of contrast : this "dynamic
CT study" doubled a usual one.

PATIENTS :

Our 25 cases were classified in 3 groups according to
the motives for the CT examination.

Group A : II asymptomatic patient, 30-70 year-old (mean = 58)
underwent a merely systematic CT examination I2 to 38 months
(mean = 20) after nephrectomy for renal adenocarcinoma, right
in 6 cases, left in 3, bilateral in one (complete left, partial right nephrectomy). The last case presented a bilateral
carcinoma and underwent a partial nephrectomy for transitional cell carcinoma at right and complete nephrectomy for
adenocarcinoma at left.

Group B : 8 patients presented a clinical suspicion of recurrence but no local symptom at the nephrectomy site : 4 had
pulmonary metastasis, 3 a worsening condition, and the last
one complained of controlateral back pains which were in
fact due to trauma. Their age ranged from 23 to 65 years
with a mean of 53 years. CT was performed between 8 and 58
months (mean = 20) after nephrectomy for renal cancer (5
right and 2 left adenocarcinoma, I left nephroblastoma
in the youngest patient).

Group C : 6 patients presented local symptoms at the nephrectomy site : a palpable mass in 2 and local pains in 4. Their
age ranged between 35 to 70 years (mean = 49). CT was carried
on between 6 and 48 months (mean = I9) after nephrectomy
for renal adenocarcinoma in 5 cases (2 right, 2 left and I
bilateral with complete left and partial right nephrectomy)
and for right squamous-cell cancer in the last case.

RESULTS :

Out of 25 patients, CT demonstrated 5 LR surgically
proven. We had no false positive and no false negative. In
3 cases, a first CT study was inconclusive, but subsequent
CT examinations allowed to rule out a cancer recurrence. The
main features of these LR are summarized in Table I.

Most often the local tumoral recurrence appeared on CT
(Fig. I) as a muscle-like mass with hypodense necrotic
areas, stuck to the posterior wall and/or close to the psoas
muscle and to the spine, blurring the great vessels. Its

contours were irregular but well outlined and smooth. In one case (Fig.2) necrosis in a parietal LR produced cystic cavities, mimicking an evisceration at palpation. It was easily diagnosed by CT.

CT was at first inconclusive in the following circumstances : in two patients a parietal thickening did not change on subsequent CT scans and was considered scartissue ; once, questional ileal loops shifted close to the spine and great vessels were identified by better oral opacification or repeated CT scans. Pitfalls due to shifted viscus are well-known (4,5) and usually are easily ruled out by CT while interposed intestinal gaz may impede ultrasonography. On the other hand, the possibility of a persistent sterilized fibrotic mass after radio or chemotherapy remains to be demonstrated.

DISCUSSION :

Our 5 LR were easily diagnosed by CT, but we deem that LR is unexpectedly voluminous and too late a discovery when CT is requested for local symptoms (Table 2). However, our asymtomatic LR measured only 3 cms in diameter (Fig.3) This case pleads for systematic C.T. follow-up. Alter et al (5) proposed to select high risk patients for such periodic CT scanning, since their 5 LR were found in 3 stage III and 2 stage IV renal cancers. In these patients they advise to get a baseline CT examination soon after surgery to document any change on further follow-up. Our results are concordant (Table 2 and 3), although our series is short : out of 5 LR, 2 followed incomplete nephrectomy (because of bilateral renal cancer), I followed nephrectomy for stage III adenocarcinoma, and the 2 last followed nephrectomy for stage II adenocarcinoma. Therefore, while we agree to give a priority to high risk patients, we still need a larger experience of systematic CT follow-up of asymptomatic patients :that is perhaps the price to pay for an earlier diagnostic of LR and an improved survival of these patients.

REFERENCES

I. Bennington JL, Kradjian RM (I967) Renal carcinoma. Philadelphia, Saunders : I58.
2. Mur-phy GP, Moore RH, Kenny GM (I970). Current results
from primary and secondary treatment of renal cell carcinoma. J. Urol. I04 : 523.
3. Stephens DH, Sheedy PFII, Hattery RR (I977). Diagnosis
and evaluation of retroperitoneal tumors by Computed Tomography. Am J Roentgenol I29 : 395.
4. Bernardino ME, De Santos LA, Johnson DE (I979).Computed
Tomography in the evaluation of post-nephrectomy patients.
Radiology I30 : I83.
5. Alter AJ, Uehling DT, Zwiebel WJ (I979). Computed Tomography of the retroperitoneum following nephrectomy.
Radiology I33 : 663.
6. Bernardino ME, Green B. Goldstein HM (I978). Ultrasonography in the evaluation of post-nephrectomy renal cancer
patients. Radiology I28 : 455.

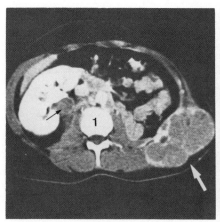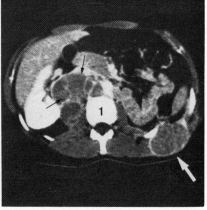

Fig. I : (case n°3 in Table I). 26 year-old woman, I4
months after left nephrectomy for stage III adenocancer.
CT requested for palpable mass + pulmonary metastases. Parietal recurrence at the nephrectomy site (white arrows),
and controlateral paraspinal mass (black arrows), are obvious.

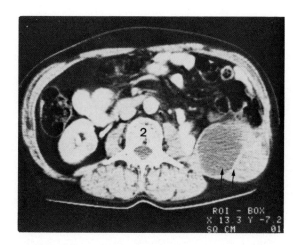

Fig. 2 : (Case n°2 in Table I). 70 year-old man, 48 months
after left nephrectomy for stage II adenocarcinoma. A questionable mass at palpation was considered as an evisceration by
the referent physician. The parietal tumoral mass (arrows)
appeared at surgery made of solid tissues + cystic pouches,
as suggested by the CT scans.

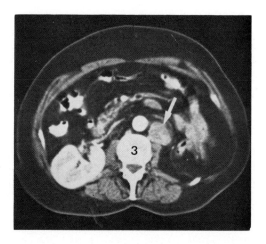

Fig. 3 : (case n°I in Table I). 70 year-old woman, 24
months after left nephrectomy for stage II adenocarcinoma
and partial right nephrectomy for transitional cell cancer.
This patient was absolutely asymptomatic and included in a
series of systematic CT follow-up. The tumoral mass (arrows)
measured 3x4 cms in diameter and was proven at surgery a
local recurrence of thetransitional cell cancer.

TABLE I : SUMMARIZED FEATURES IN 5 L.R. OUT OF 25 PATIENS

	I	2	3	4	5
SEX	F	M	F	M	M
AGE	70	70	26	35	70
PATHOLOGY	transitional cells (+ controlateral adenocarcinoma)	adenocarcinoma stage II	adenocarcinoma stage III	adenocarcinoma stage III (bilateral)	squamous cell carcinoma
TREATMENT	partial nephrectomy (+controlateral nephrectomy)	nephrectomy	nephrectomy (+ chimiotherapy for pulmonary metastases 6 months after surgery	partial nephrectomy (+ controlateral nephrectomy)	nephrectomy + radiotherapy
MOTIVES FOR C.T.	systematic C.T. follow-up	palpable mass	palpable mass	local pains + hematuria	local pains
N° OF MONTHS AFTER SURGERY	24	48	I4	6	28

TABLE 2 : FREQUENCE OF LOCAL RECURRENCE (L.R.) ACCORDING TO
CLINICAL PRESENTATION

Clinical presentation	Group	n° of cases	n° of L.R.	% of L.R.
asymptomatic	A	II	I	9
symptomatic but no local symptoms	B	8	O	O
local symptom	C	6	4	66;6
TOTAL		25 .	5	20

TABLE 3 : FREQUENCE OF LOCAL RECURRENCE (L.R.) ACCORDING TO STAGE
AT NEPHRECTOMY FOR RENAL ADENOCARCINOMA

Stage	n° of cases	n° of L.R.	% of L.R.
I	3	0	0
II	9	I	II,I
III	9	2	22,2
IV	2	0	0
TOTAL	23	3	I3

TABLE 4 : CUMULATIVE LIST (ALTER ET AL. I979, AND PARIENTY ET AL.I98I)
OF LOCAL RECURRENCE ACCORDING TO STAGE AT NEPHRECTOMY FOR
RENAL ADENOCARCINOMA.

Stage	n° of cases	n° of L.R.	% of L.R.
I	9	0	0
II	9	I	II,I
III	I9	5	26,3
IV	4	2	50
TOTAL	4I	8	I9,5

Renal Tumors: Proceedings of the First International Symposium on Kidney Tumors, pages 417–423
© **1982 Alan R. Liss, Inc., 150 Fifth Avenue, New York, NY 10011**

DOES PERCUTANEOUS PUNCTURE STILL HAVE A ROLE TO PLAY IN
THE DIAGNOSIS OF RENAL TUMORS

Professor Adolphe Steg

Chief of the Department of Urology
Hopital Cochin
75014 Paris, France

Does percutaneous puncture still have a role to play
in the diagnosis of renal tumors? Such a question, unthink-
able only four or five years ago, emphasizes the considerable progress brought to urological diagnosis by ultrasonography and computed tomography. This question is still
unanswered. It could be put in other equally provocative
terms: "can we do without percutaneous puncture in the
diagnosis of renal tumors today?", or, more precisely,
"in the diagnosis of renal cysts". Here we are asking a
question of crucial importance to urological practice.
Simple cysts represent, by far in fact, the most frequently
found renal masses. Everyone agrees that this lesion,
by itself, does not necessitate surgical treatment provided that, and this provision is imperative, the diagnosis
is affirmed with certainty. The practical problem thus
presents itself in these terms: is there today another
non-invasive method than cyst puncture which allows us
to affirm the diagnosis of cyst with as much certainty?

I) THE DIAGNOSIS VALUE OF PERCUTANEOUS PUNCTURE
The percutaneous puncture of a renal mass supposed
to be cystic generates, as shown in Table I, six pieces
of information. When these six criteria are examined
together we think that one can declare with certainty
that the lesion punctured is in fact a kidney cyst.

TABLE I
CRITERIA GENERATED BY CYST PUNCTURE AND ASPIRATION IN CASE
OF RENAL CYST

I) Liquid mass
2) Clear, straw colored aspirate
3) No cytologic abnormality
4) No histochemical abnormality
5) Cyst is regular and thin-walled on cystography
6) Perfect superimposition of the opacified cyst upon the
   negative defect seen on I.V.P.

In our study of I342 cases of renal cysts, analyzed
in the Report to the I975 Meeting of the French Urological
Association (Steg I975),we did not find a single case in
which all six of these criteria had been obtained and the
lesion turned out to be anything other than a renal cyst.

It should go without saying that the information
which percutaneous puncture brings concerns only the
lesion punctured and tells us nothing about the existence
in the same kidney of other lesions in contact with, or at
a distance from the cyst. The argument which was often put
forward not so long ago in favor of an aggressive attitude
towards cysts was that systematic surgery occasionally
permitted the discovery of an associated cancer in contact
with or near the cyst. We strongly believe that when a
totally asymptomatic cyst is discovered by an intravenous
urogram performed for an unrelated cause and when all six
of the criteria are observed, surgical intervention has no
more chance of finding an associated cancer than in a
urographically normal kidney.

II) COMPARISON OF THE INFORMATION OBTAINED BY PERCUTANEOUS
   PUNCTURE AND THAT OBTAINED BY THE MODERN INVESTIGATIVE
   METHODS : ULTRASONOGRAPHY AND COMPUTED TOMOGRAPHY

Besides the wealth of information that it brings, the
percutaneous puncture has the tremendous advantage of
being harmless. In 443 punctures (Steg I975) we observed
only I2 complications (2.7 %) :
- 2 cases of hematuria which resolved spontaneously
- 3 cases of intracystic hemorrhages   which only I
  necessitated draining
- 7 cases of infection which were treated in 4 cases by
  antibiotics, in I case by percutaneous draining, and
  in 2 cases by surgical draining

One can therefore legitimately conclude that local
regional complications are entirely exceptional and,

ordinarily, entirely lacking in gravity. However, as low
as this level of morbidity is, one can always wonder if it
could not be avoided altogether, and if the same diagnostic
results could not be obtained with exams totally innocuous,
i.e., ultrasonography and computed tomography.

Table 2 compares the information obtained by these
two methods with that of percutaneous puncture. It is
obvious that the latter furnishes the most numerous and
most precise data and, most importantly, that its specificity is total (Lang 1980).

TABLE 2
ULTRASONOGRAPHY, COMPUTED TOMOGRAPHY AND PERCUTANEOUS
PUNCTURE IN THE DIAGNOSIS OF RENAL CYSTS

	Ultrasonography	C.T.	Puncture
Liquid mass	+	+	+
Clear, straw colored aspirate	0	0	+
No cytologic abnormality	0	0	+
No histochemical abnormality	0	0	+
Cyst is regular and thin walled on cystography	+	+	+
Perfect superimposition of the opacified cyst upon the negative defect seen on IVP	±	±	+

But one may wonder if all these data which the puncture furnishes are really indispensable to the diagnosis.
Do not ultrasonography and computed tomography have sufficient accuracy to allow avoiding further investigations ?

The answer to that question cannot be positive without reserve, as the following three arguments will show :

A) First argument : most of the statistics give ultrasonography and computed tomography an accuracy of between
90 and 95 % of the cases (Sanders 1981); this therefore
leaves a percentage of error which, if not large, is not
negligible either.

In contrast, percutaneous puncture, under the condition that all the criteria for confirming a cyst are
insisted upon, has, in our view, an accuracy of 100 %, in
the sense that there are no false positives. The only
errors are false negatives and hence inconsequential
(Steg 1975).

In fact, whenever by percutaneous puncture we find a
murky or bloody aspirate or a fat content or an irregular
looking wall on cystography, we prefer for safety sake
to formally challenge the diagnosis of cyst. We do this

knowing that authentic cysts can hemorrhage and contain a
low dose of fat, and that a cyst wall deformed by clots is
irregular in cystography. We prefer, however, in these
cases to keep the patient from running the risk entailed
by a diagnosis error.

B) Second argument: ultrasonography and computed tomography in demonstrating a lesion free of internal echoes
and with liquid density can suggest the diagnosis of cyst
when in fact the lesion is one of the following:
- a renal abscess which sometimes presents a smooth, echo
  free image (Fallon, Gershon 1981; Goldman et al. 1977).
- localized hydronephrosis in a kidney with duplication of
  the ureter
- a necrotic tumor
- or, even, a tumor grown on the base of a cyst and too
  small to be seen by ultrasonography or computed tomography (Marshall 1980; Murphy, Marshall 1980).

In all these cases, however, percutaneous puncture
easily solves the diagnostic problem because:
- in the case of an abscess, it brings forth pus,
- in the case of localized hydronephrosis, it opacifies
  and often even shows the corresponding ureter
- in the case of a tumor, necrotic or associated with a
  cyst, it aspirates blood.

C) Third argument: ultrasonography and computer tomography can suggest the presence of a solid mass even though
the lesion turns out to be a cyst. The following cases
well illustrate this last argument.

Case n° 1: Advanced osteoporosis and a crush fracture
of the twelfth thoracic vertebra in a 69-year-old male
suggested the possibility of metastases. Accordingly, the
search for a primary tumor was carried out by barium meal,
barium enema and chest X-ray studies, and tracheal biopsies, all of which proved normal. Finally, an intravenous
urogram was performed; it revealed a mass at the upper pole
of the left kidney (Fig 1) evoking a simple cyst, but for
which two successive ultrasonograms demonstrated a lesion
with mixed contents, giving off more echoes in the periphery
than at the center (Fig 2). A computerized tomogram
confirmed these findings and led to the conclusion of a
necrotic tumor at the anterior-superior pole of the left
kidney (Fig 3). This patient was directed to our urology
department for nephrectomy. However, because of the
contract between the ultrasound and scanner findings, and
those of the intravenous urogram, a percutaneous puncture
was performed. It produced data typical for a renal

cyst (Fig 4). In order to rule out a tumor associated with this cyst, an arteriography was practiced and it revealed the avascular image of a cyst, and no other abnormality.

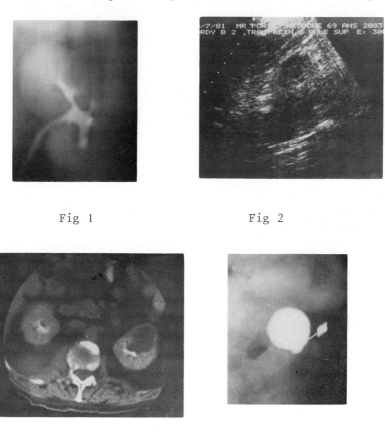

Fig 1   Fig 2

Fig 3   Fig 4

Case n° 2 : In a 58-year-old man with polycythemia, an IVP suggested a space occupying lesion between the upper and the middle calix of the left kidney (Fig 5). At ultrasono-graphy the lesion was partially echoic (Fig 6). Computed tomogram demonstrated a lesion with a densitometric value of 3I HE (Fig 7). Both examinations were performed a second time and confirmed the high suspicion of a solid mass. Per-cutaneous puncture produced data typical of a cyst (Fig 8)

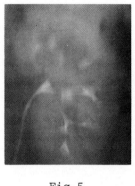

Fig 5

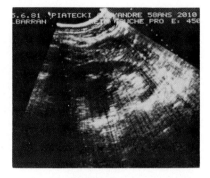
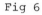

Fig 6

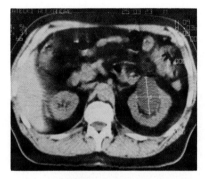

Fig 7

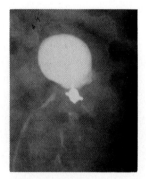

Fig 8

III) CONCLUSION

Percutaneous puncture of cysts still has, today, a non negligible role to play in the diagnosis of renal tumours. Its indication is a question of good sense and should depend essentially on the X-ray and clinical findings.

On the one hand, consider a totally asymptomatic lesion whose urogram strongly suggests a cyst and which fails to capture the contrast medium in the tomograms. If ultrasonography and computerized tomography demonstrate an undoubtable liquid lesion, the diagnosis of a cyst can be affirmed with sufficient probability to authorize the abstention from surgery. But whenever the ultrasound and

computerized tomography yield images which are not absolutely indisputable, especially whenever there is a discrepancy
between these exams and the X-ray and clinical findings,
the diagnosis of cyst cannot be affirmed without percutaneous puncture.

On the other hand, when the cystic mass is not totally
asymptomatic, the diagnosis of cyst should not be considered except with great care because a simple uncomplicated
renal cyst fails to cause renal colic, general deterioration, fever, an elevation of the erythrocyte sedimentation
rate, or, especially, hematuria.

Here, ultrasonography and computed tomography, even
when demonstrating a typical liquid mass, cannot by themselves permit the affirmation of the diagnosis of a cyst,
and percutaneous puncture is absolutely indispensable.
Either it reveals that the criteria of a cyst are not all
present and then one is led to seek surgical verification
of the mass. Or it produces all the signs of a cyst and
then the puncture permits the affirmation that it is not
that mass which is the cause of the troubles because an
authentic cyst is asymptomatic, and one must therefore
continue the investigations.

Fallon B, Bershon C (1981). Renal carbuncle: Diagnosis
  and management. Urology 17:303.
Goldman SM, Minkin SD, Naraval DC, Diamond AB, Pion SJ,
  Meringoff BN, Sidh SM, Sanders RC, Cohen SP (1977).
  Renal carbuncle: the use of ultrasound in its diagnosis
  and treatment. J Urol 118:525.
Lang EK (1980). Roentgenologic approach to the diagnosis
  and management of cystic lesions of the kidney: is cyst
  exploration mandatory? Urol Clin North America 7:677.
Marshall FF (1980). The role of selective exploration in
  ambiguous renal cystic lesions. Urol Clin North America
  7:689.
Murphy JB, Marshall FF (1980). Renal cyst versus tumor: a
  continuing dilemna. J Urol 123:566.
Sanders RC (1981). Practical value of diagnostic ultrasound in Urologi. J Urol 126:283.
Steg A (1975). Les affections kystiques de rein de l'adulte
  Paris: Mason p. 179.

Renal Tumors: Proceedings of the First International Symposium on Kidney Tumors, pages 425–432
© 1982 Alan R. Liss, Inc., 150 Fifth Avenue, New York, NY 10011

CYTOLOGIC DIAGNOSIS OF RENAL CELL CARCINOMA

Sixten Franzén and Eva Brehmer-Andersson

Departments of Cytology and Pathology
Karolinska sjukhuset, Stockholm, Sweden

In the late 1940's we started to use the needle
aspiration technique after intravenous pyelography to
differentiate between solid and cystic lesions. A rather
thick needle was used. The diagnostic accuracy improved
significantly when selective renal angiography was introduced in the middle 1950's. In the middle 1960's the
fine needle aspiration biopsy technique was launched,
which provided a means of differentiating between cystic
and solid lesions, and obtaining specimens from a solid
mass for cytologic investigation.

Today, the puncture is usually done with the aid of
ultrasonography. If the lesion is small it is preferable
to use fluoroscopy in two planes under television control.
The patient is placed in a prone position. A guiding
needle, 1-2 mm in diameter, with a stylet, is inserted
in the abdominal wall from behind. When the needle
touches the renal capsule the stylet is replaced by a
thin needle, 0.7 mm in diameter. Material is then
aspirated with a syringe in a special one-hand grip
(Zajicek, 1974). It is important during aspiration to
pierce the tumour mass in different directions to get
representative material. Immediate quick-staining and
microscopy is performed at the X-ray laboratory to make
sure that diagnostic material has been obtained. The
main part of the aspirate is used for smears. Some of
them are air-dried and stained according to May-Grünewald-
Giemsa, other smears are wet-fixed in methanol and stained
according to Papanicolau. According to the cytologic
picture the type and grade of differentiation of the tumor

are determined. Tumour grades are described as well, moderately well or poorly differentiated. The grading is based on the size of the nuclei and nucleoli and the chromatin pattern (Figs. 1, 2, 3). It is also noted if the cell picture is monotonous or pleomorphic.

In 1967 we evaluated the conformity between aspiration biopsy and histopathologic grading in 47 patients (Schreeb et al. 1967). In 36 there was agreement, whereas there was a disparity in 11 cases, usually of one grade (Table I). Rather frequently renal cell carcinomas display more than one histological pattern, which may be the cause of disagreement.

TABLE I

COMPARISON BETWEEN THE CYTOLOGIC AND HISTOLOGIC EVALUATION OF THE DEGREE OF DIFFERENTIATION (H: HIGH, M: MODERATE, P: POOR) IN 47 CASES IN RENAL ADENOCARCINOMA

	Histology		
Cytology	H	M	P
H	4	3	1
M	–	13	6
P	–	1	19

In the last few years an additional small part of the cytologic material has been used for flow-cytometric DNA-analysis (Rönström, et al. 1981). Fig. 4 demonstrates the DNA pattern in normal renal parenchyma, in a case of renal oncocytoma and in renal cell carcinoma of high grade malignancy. Smear from an oncocytoma is shown in Fig. 5.

Patients with renal cell carcinomas, cytologically classified as poorly differentiated, have been given pre-operative X-ray treatment. Recently we have started to evaluate the cumulative experience of about 200 cases from which we have received preoperative cytologic material and some of which have received preoperative irradiation as well. The intention is to find out if preoperative X-ray treatment enhances survival in high grade malignancies and if DNA-analysis of cytologic material will contribute to a more objective grading and improve the possibility to predict the prognosis.

Rönström L, Tribukait B, Esposti, PL (1981). DNA pattern and cytological findings in fine-needle aspirates of untreated prostatic tumors. A flow-cytofluorometric study. The Prostate 2:79.

Schreeb von T, Franzén S, Ljungqvist A (1967). Renal adenocarcinoma. Evaluation of malignancy on a cytologic basis: A comparative cytologic and histologic study. Scand J Urol Nephrol 1:265.

Zajicek J (1974). Aspiration biopsy cytology. Part 1. Basel:Karger, p. 3.

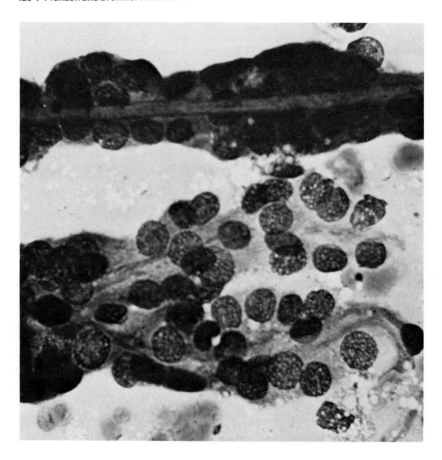

Fig. 1. Smear from very well differentiated renal cell
carcinoma with tubular structures. MGG (10 x 40).

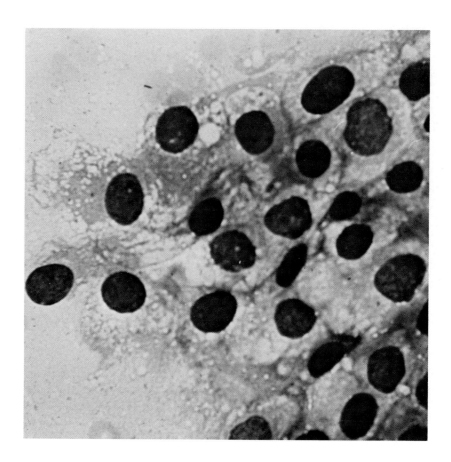

Fig. 2. Moderately well differentiated carcinoma of clear cell type. MGG (10 x 40).

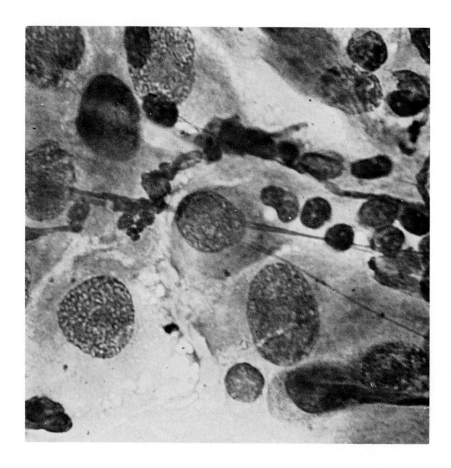

Fig. 3. Poorly differentiated carcinoma. Some lymphocytes are located between the tumour cells. MGG (10 x 40).

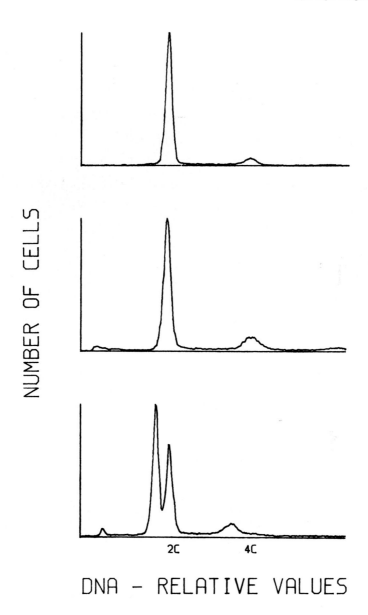

Fig. 4. DNA histograms from normal kidney tissue (above), oncocytoma (middle) and poorly differentiated renal cell carcinoma (below).

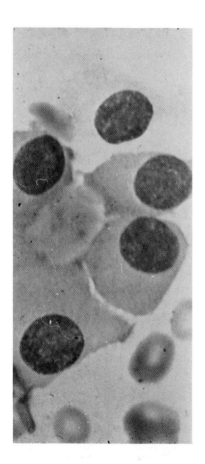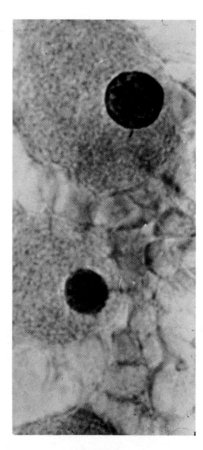

Fig. 5. Smear from a case of renal oncocytoma. MGG left.
Pap-stain right. (10 x 40).

Renal Tumors: Proceedings of the First International Symposium on
Kidney Tumors, pages 433–434

DIAGNOSTIC VALUE OF LIPID CONTENT IN CYST FLUID

S. Pettersson, H. Kleist, O. Jonsson, S.
Lundstam, J. Nauclér & A.E. Nilson
Departments of Urology, Surgery I and Diagnostic
Radiology I, Sahlgrenska sjukhuset, University
of Goteborg, S-413 45 Göteborg, Sweden

Benign renal cysts are of importance mainly as a differential diagnosis to malignant tumours of the renal
parenchyma. The differential diagnosis would be easy if
all malignant tumours were solid. Unfortunately, about
4 per cent of renal carcinomas are cystic (Emmet et al,
1963). Cystic renal tumours may not be possible to differentiate from benign cysts even with modern methods of
investigation including computed tomography and ultrasound.
The percutaneous puncture of cystic lesions therefore remain an important tool in the differential diagnosis
between benign cysts and cystic renal tumours. The fluid
recovered is then generally subjected to macroscopic and
cytologic examinations. To increase the safety in the
differential diagnosis, Lang suggested that the aspirated
fluid should be examined histochemically with regard to its
lipid content, an examination which, however, is only semi-
quantitative (Lang, 1966).

To obtain a quantitative determination of the lipid
content in renal cystic lesions, we examined biochemically
cyst fluid from 18 cystic renal tumours and 42 benign
cysts with regard to the total lipid and cholesterol content and the presence of atypical or malignant cells
(Kleist et al, 1981). The fluid was in 40 of the benign
lesions obtained by percutaneous puncture and in 2 by
puncture during surgery. Fluid from the 18 malignant
lesions was obtained in 12 at surgical exploration of the
kidney and in 6 by percutaneous puncture.

The total lipid and the cholesterol content was low in

the benign cysts (0.30±0.07 and 0.18±0.07 mmol/l, respectively) while it was high in the cystic tumours (13.2±3.3 and 8.5±2.4 mmol/l, respectively). No cystic tumour had a total lipid value of <1.6 mmol/l and 29 of 30 benign cysts had a value of <0.8 mmol/l. Cytological examination of the cyst fluid from 11 cystic tumours showed normal cells in 9 and atypical cells in 2. At renewed cytological examination of cyst fluid recovered during operation normal cells were found in the last 2 patients. The macroscopic appearance of the fluid from the malignant lesions was turbid in 9 and clear in 8 while the benign cysts contained clear fluid in 40 and cloudy fluid in 2.

The results suggest that analysis of the lipid content may greatly increase the accuracy in the differential diagnosis between benign renal cysts and cystic renal tumours. A low lipid value strongly indicates the presence of a benign cyst. A high lipid value suggests that the cystic lesion is a malignant tumour, though a false positive lipid test may be obtained by inflammatory or hemorrhagic cysts. The reliability of the cholesterol and the total lipid determination was equal in this study and it therefore seems sufficient to analyze the cholesterol content of the aspirated cyst fluid, a technique which is available in most clinical chemical laboratories.

Emmet JL, Levine SR, Woolner, LB (1963). Co-existence of renal cyst and tumour: Incidence in 1007 cases. Brit J Urol 35:403.

Lang EK (1966). The differential diagnosis of renal cysts and tumours. Radiology, 87:883.

Kleist H, Jonsson O, Lundstam S, Nauclér J, Nilson AE, Pettersson S (1981). Quantitative lipid analyses in the differential diagnosis of cystic renal lesions. Brit J Urol (in press).

Renal Tumors: Proceedings of the First International Symposium on Kidney Tumors, pages 435–436
© **1982 Alan R. Liss, Inc., 150 Fifth Avenue, New York, NY 10011**

IS EXPLORATIVE LUMBOTOMY STILL INDICATED AS A MEANS OF
DIAGNOSING A KIDNEY TUMOR?

G. Arvis

Department of Urology
Hôpital Saint-Antoine
75012 Paris

Twenty years ago, when complementary exams were not yet
able to determine whether a kidney tumor was benign or
malignant, and when these same exams were unable to
determine the etiology of an hematuria (maybe in relation
with a supposed tumor), it was not rare to propose an explorative lumbotomy. There were two purposes for explorative lumbotomy:

1) diagnostic i.e.
     - to discover a tumor invisible to X-ray analysis
     - to determine the precise nature (benign or
       malignant) of a tumor which had been previously
       discovered.

2) possible therapeutic i.e.
     - ablation of the tumor, or more often, the kidney.

Such rationale seemed reasonable in cases of small
tumors which modified only very slightly the shape of the
kidney or calices. Unfortunately the kidney is not very
easy to explore manually even when it is completely dissected. That is, one cannot distinguish intraparenchymatous
features by palpation, except for those tumors located in
the renal cortex. Too often, when in doubt, the surgeon
would complete the operation by performing a so-called
"security" nephrectomy. In many such cases one only found
either a small benign tumor, as an "angiomatous" lesion or a
subacute focal nephritis or only a big pyramid.
These findings, of course, did not warrant the surgical procedure and nephrectomy was even less justified.

Presently, the limits of our diagnostic accuracy have been improved significantly through developments in early nephrotomography, echotomography, kidney puncture, scanners, arteriography and urine cytology. Thus, it is now rare that the tumor diagnosis (and its presumed nature) is not established prior to surgery. Moreover, these procedures can reveal the slowly evolving renal cancer in the beginning before it reaches a size which can be recognized by the earlier investigative procedures mentioned above. These advances raise questions as to whether explorative lumbotomy is still indicated and, if it is, under what circumstances can it be used as such. It is suggested that when one wants to know whether or not there is a renal tumor, more particularly in case of recurring hematuria, lumbotomy is no longer indicated provided that:

1) one first has to make certain that the hematuria is of renal origin,
2) one has to know the sequence in which to prescribe the exams to be able to reach the correct diagnosis, and
3) these exams are prescribed again after six months or one year later, if the results are negative.

Explorative lumbotomy may be justified as a means of determining the tumor when the echographic picture is not clear, when arteriography shows a negative picture (papillary adenocarcinoma, for example), when the scanner picture is uncertain (tumor smaller than 2 cm) and when urine cytology shows class III cells. Under these circumstances explorative lumbotomy may alleviate concern of not recognizing a malignant tumor. However, one must know the difficulties inherent in this type of exploration and that it must be combined with a concurrent anatomopathological examination. Bearing these concepts in mind, one may conclude that explorative lumbotomy has become the exception amongst the various diagnostic procedures for renal tumors.

Renal Tumors: Proceedings of the First International Symposium on Kidney Tumors, pages 437–438
© **1982 Alan R. Liss, Inc., 150 Fifth Avenue, New York, NY 10011**

RENAL TUMOUR SYNDROME: HIERARCHY OF INVESTIGATIONS

J. Auvert, C.C. Abbou, V. Lavarenne

Service d'Urologie

Hôpital Henri Mondor, 94010 - Cedex Creteil
France

Since non-invasive new explorations have been introduced in the last few years, evaluation of renal tumour
lesions has dramatically changed.

In 106 patients with gross hematuria checked by computerized tomography (C T Scan) in Hôpital Henri Mondor, 75
renal tumour lesions were present.

According to our experience, the assessment of a suspected renal tumour lesion should be based on the results
of intravenous pyelogram (IVP).

(1) Normal IVP.
Renal ultrasound (US) and urine cytology seemed reliable enough to rule out a renal tumour. When gross
hematuria is present cystoscopy should be carried out at
the time of this hematuria. C T Scan did not disclose any
tumour when the other investigations were normal.

(2) IVP shows a renal tumour lesion.
US will separate typical cyst lesions from solid
lesions that are most often carcinomas. C T Scan will
provide proper evaluation of renal solid lesions, sustain-
ing a cancer diagnosis with high reliability and accurately
checking neoplastic intra-abdominal extension. Invasive
investigations should then take place in peculiar cases
only. Transcutaneous cyst puncture should be carried out
only for benigh cystic lesion on US, not for doubtful
lesions. Venacavography is still widely used when venous

involvement is suspected, though it could be progressively ruled out by C T Scan advancer. As for arteriography, it is used only in a few cases (for preoperative renal arterial embolization or before conservative surgery).

(3) IVP shows a pelvic or calyceal defect
C T Scan will accurately separate an X-ray transparent calculus from excretory tract tumours. The distinction between excretory tract tumours and clots may be difficult, thus C T should not be carried out at the time of hematuria. The study of urine pH and urine cytology are useful, since the diagnosis of excretory tumor is well advanced at this stage. Retrograde uretero-pyelography is generally carried out during intra operative cystoscopy.

(4) IVP shows a non-functioning kidney
US is the best method that allows distinction between a kidney lesion and a hydronephrotic kidney. C T Scan is necessary in cases of parenchymal tumour and obstruction. It checks the level and nature of obstruction and that status of renal parenchyma. Yet retrograde investigations as well as cystoscopy may still be necessary.

In conclusion, our indications for the use of ultra-sound and C T Scan evaluation of suspected kidney tumour lesions are summarized in the preceding paragraphs.

Renal Tumors: Proceedings of the First International Symposium on Kidney Tumors, pages 439–445
© **1982 Alan R. Liss, Inc., 150 Fifth Avenue, New York, NY 10011**

STAGING OF RENAL CELL CARCINOMA

Charles J. Robson, M.D., F.R.C.S.(C), F.A.C.S.

Professor & Chairman, Division of Urology
University of Toronto
Toronto, Ontario, Canada

It is generally accepted that staging is an important factor in the continuing study of malignant tumours. Renal cell carcinoma is no exception. Staging should fully describe the profile of the growth itself plus the presence or absence of distant metastases and any features peculiar to that growth, e.g. macroscopic involvement of the renal vein. Staging is important in the estimating of prognosis, the comparison of other series, and in the assessment of therapy. It should also describe the pathology, e.g. microscopic invasion of lymph nodes.

In the prognosis of renal cell carcinoma besides the unmeasurable host to tumour response there are the following five measurable features: 1) The local extent of the tumour. A complete assessment of this preoperatively is most important to the surgeon in planning his procedure. These tumours are notorious for direct extension to the liver, spleen, colon, diaphragm and posterior abdominal wall, and at operation 42 per cent of them will be found extending into the perirenal fat. Angiography may be of some help in this by showing tumour vessels involving the liver and spleen. Presacral injection of carbon dioxide (CO_2) to outline the retroperitoneum may also be used but by far the greatest aid at present is the computerized tomography or c.t. scan (Skinner, Colvin, Vermillion et al 1979), (Robson, Churchill, Anderson 1969). This will delineate or note the absence of planes between the posterior abdominal musculature and the tumour, and between the tumour and the liver and surrounding structures.

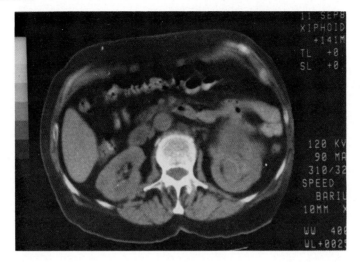

Fig. 1. C.T. scan showing extension of renal cell carcinoma into perinephric fat Stage II.

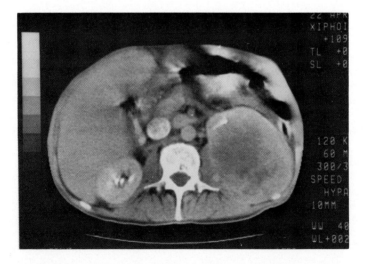

Fig. 2. Large left renal tumour still contained by Gerota's fascia with clear lines of demarcation between posterior abdominal wall and peritoneum Stage II.

2) The presence or absence of distant metastases. This is a most important part of the investigation of this tumour.

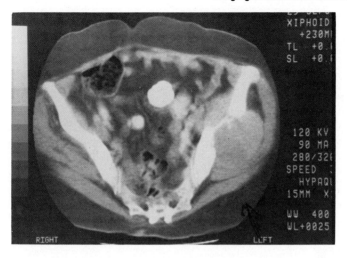

Fig. 3. Destruction of left ilium by metastases Stage IV.

Whereas a single, resectable metastasis will not in our opinion preclude nephrectomy, the presence of multiple secondaries almost certainly precludes cure except in the rare case of spontaneous regression and may indeed save the patient a nephrectomy except in the case where it is felt necessary for paliative reasons, e.g. continuous hematuria, clot colic, etc. Renal cell carcinoma metastasizes by hematogenous spread largely to the skeletal system and to the lungs. Until recently a radiological skeletal survey was the accepted method of assessment of the bones. This has been supplanted by skeletal scan augmented by x-ray studies of any hot spots picked up. Whole lung tomograms are still a very important part of the assessment of renal cell carcinoma. The importance of this examination was brought into focus by a case in which routine posterior-anterior and lateral films of the chest showed two coin lesions in the left lower lobe. The remainder of the left lung and right lung appeared to be clear of any metastases. At operation the two lesions were identified and following radical nephrectomy the left lower lobe was removed by a member of the thoracic surgical unit. On the first post-operative day a chest film was taken to determine the degree of expansion on the operated side and, due to a slightly different exposure, this film showed several pulmonary metastases which were not apparent on the

preoperative film. C.T. scan of the chest is considered
by our radiologists to be much too sensitive and will pick
up small fibromas, etc., which may be misdiagnosed as pulmonary secondaries. Special investigative procedures such
as barium enema or brain scan may also be indicated by a
history of localizing symptoms or findings on physical examination. 3) Involvement of regional lymph nodes. In a
series published in 1968, regional lymph nodes were found
involved in 22.7 per cent of 88 patients on pathological
section. In the present series of 162 cases, lymphadenopathy was found in 34 or 21 per cent. It has been found
that these are only evident on angiography in about 33 per
cent of cases where they show a tumour blush. More recently,
however, they have been picked up by c.t. scanning with an
accuracy of about 88 per cent.

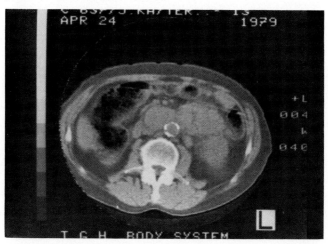

Fig. 4. Large masses of paravertebral nodes Stage III.

Microscopic metastases obviously can only be picked up by
the pathologist. Complete lymphadenectomy from the crura
of the diaphragm to the bifurcation of the iliacs and
junction of the iliac veins not only is important in staging but apparently has a therapeutic effect as well, in
certain cases, with a five year survival of approximately
40 per cent in our series. It also will be important in
the future to decide, when an effective adjuvant therapy
is developed, as to which cases should be so treated.
Mediastinoscopy (Robson, Churchill, Anderson 1969) was

carried out for several years in the belief that if media-stinal glands were positive for tumour on section biopsy the patient was surgically incurable thus a nephrectomy was not performed. It became apparent, however, that the yield of positive cases was very small indeed, being less than 2 per cent, and did not justify this procedure which, even in the most skilled hands, still requires prolongation of the anes-thetic for approximately an hour and is not without some morbidity. 4) Intrarenal involvement of veins and/or vena cava. Renal cell carcinoma is notorious for its hematogen-ous spread either by direct extension into the renal vein and thence to the vena cava and into the right heart or by tumour emboli. Sir Eric Riches believed that macroscopic involvement of main branches of the renal vein or the renal vein itself and the vena cava had a poor prognostic outlook (Riches 1964). Recently with more aggressive surgery this opinion has been questioned (Skinner, Pfister, Colvin 1972), however, the surgeon should be aware of this involvement, i.e. the renal vein or vena cava, prior to the operation so that he may be prepared to deal with it. Angiography, al-though being supplanted by the c.t. scan in demonstrating involvement of the vena cava and renal vein particularly with pedal injection of dye which differentiates between intraluminal and extraluminal narrowing of the cava, is still a most useful prognostic aid. Aortography shows the number and position of the renal arteries, thus allowing early interruption of the blood flow which is most important. It also shows parasite vessels and is a must in using the T.N.M. classification for staging. It will also show whether the opposite kidney is involved by tumour, a rare but possible situation.

Because the above is essential in an attempt to accurately stage renal cell carcinoma, we have continued to use a modified version of staging as proposed by Flocks and Kadesky (Flocks, Kadesky 1958) and Petkovic (Petkovic 1959). The modification has been to group cases showing lymph node and/or vein involvement into one group Stage III. The T.N.M. staging as approved by the International Union Against Cancer is considered to be somewhat unwieldy but this may change with the increased use of computerization. Stage I: The tumour is confined to the kidney parenchyma. Although the pseudocapsule around the tumour may have ruptured, the true renal capsule is intact. Stage II: The renal capsule has been broken through and the perirenal fat is involved by tumour which, however, is still contained

within the envelope of Gerota's fascia. Stage III: Gross
renal vein or main renal vein tributaries or inferior vena
cava involvement and/or lymphatic involvement or a combination of the above. The reason for this change is shown in
Fig. 5,

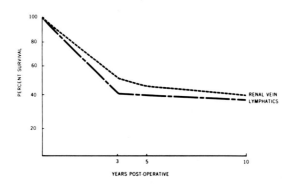

Fig. 5.

where it is noticed that the five and ten year survival are
almost identical. Stage IV: There is involvement of the
adjacent organs other than the adrenal or distant metastases.

Table 1.

     Renal Cell Carcinoma - Staging of Tumours

Stage I
  Confined to kidney
Stage II
  Perirenal fat involvement but confined to
  Gerota's fascia
Stage III
  A - Gross RV or IVC involvement
  B - Lymphatic involvement
  C - Vascular + lymphatic involvement
Stage IV
  A - Adjacent organs other than adrenal involved
  B - Distant metastases

SUMMARY

An attempt has been made to outline the important features concerned in the staging of renal cell carcinoma and some of the procedures that may be carried out to implement this staging. A simple, modified staging is proposed.

REFERENCES

Flocks RH, Kadesky MC (1958). Malignant neoplasms of the kidney: an analysis of 353 patients followed five years or more. J Urol 79:196-201.

Petkovic SD (1959). An anatomical classification of renal tumors in the adult as a basis for prognosis. J Urol 81:618-623.

Riches E (1964). Surgery of renal tumors, in, Riches E. Ed: Tumors of the kidney and ureter, Baltimore, Williams and Wilkins Chap 23, pp.275-289.

Robson CJ, Churchill BM, Anderson W (1969). The results of radical nephrectomy for renal cell carcinoma. J Urol 101:297-301.

Skinner DG, Colvin RB, Vermillion CD et al (1979). Diagnosis and management of renal cell carcinoma: A clinical and pathologic study of 309 cases. Cancer 28: 1165-1177.

Skinner DG, Pfister RF, Colvin R (1972). Extension of renal cell carcinoma into the vena cava: the rationale for aggressive surgical management. J Urol 107:711-716.

Renal Tumors: Proceedings of the First International Symposium on Kidney Tumors, pages 447–452
© **1982 Alan R. Liss, Inc., 150 Fifth Avenue, New York, NY 10011**

THE NATURAL HISTORY OF RENAL CELL CARCINOMA

Charles J. Robson, M.D., F.R.C.S.(C), F.A.C.S.

Professor & Chairman, Division of Urology
University of Toronto
Toronto, Ontario, Canada

Renal cell carcinoma or hypernephroma is the masquerader of the retroperitoneum. In 30 to 45 per cent of cases there are no presenting symptoms referable to the primary tumour and its presence is only manifested by changes in biochemistry or endocrine disorders or by the common symptoms of most tumours, i.e. cachexia, malaise, fever, and anemia, etc. The triad of gross hematuria, flank pain and mass, which for years has been copied from one textbook to another as being the classical presenting symptoms, occur only in about 10 to 15 per cent of patients. Any one of these features is present in only about 65 per cent of cases.

The true natural history of renal cell carcinoma is as varied as its many presenting manifestations. We know that the highest incidence is during the sixth decade, that the ratio of male to female is two to one and that it is a disease of urban dwellers. It took sixty plus years after the initial description of the tumour in 1826, to prove that the basic cell was that of the adult convoluted tubule but there still is discussion as to whether renal cortical adenoma or adenomatous hyperplasia, frequently found in association with renal cell carcinoma, are indeed precursors or intermittent stages in the development of the tumour. The rate of growth may be extremely indolent, as shown by many papers in the literature citing patients who have lived a very long period of time after diagnosis. These cases have recently been classified as oncocytoma, and attempts have been made to differentiate these from true renal cell carcinoma. Riches (Riches 1964) reported a series of 443 untreated patients deemed inoperable

because of the extent of tumour or other conditions pre-
cluding operation. The crude survival rate was 4.4 per
cent at three years and 1.7 per cent at five years.

METHOD AND SITE OF SPREAD

Between 30 and 45 per cent of patients already have
metastatic spread of their renal cell carcinoma at the time
of admission to hospital (Middleton 1967). Renal cell carcinoma spreads by direct extension to the perinephric fat
(42 per cent), to the adrenal (6 per cent), to the liver
either by direct extension or by invasion of the portal
system of veins (Robson, Churchill, Anderson 1969). Hematogenous spread is by invasion of the intrarenal veins. An
unbroken tumour thrombus may extend from the renal vein to
the vena cava and right atrium, thereby setting the pattern
for tumour emboli to the lungs and also to other sites as
well. Pulmonary metastases are usually endobronchial and
may cause hemoptysis. Bony metastases are seen in about
32 per cent of patients dying of renal carcinoma. They are
typically osteolytic and frequently solitary. Tumour cells
may enter the plexus of Batson and involve bones of the
lumbar spine and pelvis (Bennington, Kradjian 1967). There
is free communication between the lymphatic plexus of the
kidney parenchyma and the perinephric fat and eventually
with the lymph nodes lying on the lateral or medial side of
the great vessels. From there most efferents drain into
the cysterna chyli although some may join the thoracic duct
directly. Occasionally the thoracic duct divides into two
branches, the right one emptying into the right subclavian
vein, thus both supraclavicular areas must be examined for
suspicious nodes in preoperative staging (Gray 1966).
Adjacent organs such as colon, spleen and diaphragm are
also involved in about 9 per cent of cases.

PRESENTING SIGNS AND SYMPTOMS

Local Signs and Symptoms

1) Hematuria. This is caused by tumour involving the
calyces or pelvis. It is usually painless but clot colic
may occur. It is usually intermittent and occurs in about
60 per cent the patients. 2) Renal mass. This is found

in about one-third of the patients. It is a late finding
and has no prognostic value. 3) Loin pain. This occurs
in about 50 per cent of patients. It is usually dull and
aching in nature although it may be colicky due to passage
of clots. It has a grave prognosis. 4) Acute varicocele.
This usually occurs on the left side due to thrombus blocking the entry of the left spermatic vein into the left renal,
however, it may occur on the right side due to involvement
by tumour growth. 5) High output cardiac failure. This
may be caused by massive arteriovenous fistula and manifested by hypertension and a bruit. The increased cardiac
output returns to normal after nephrectomy (DeWeerd 1965).

Systemic Signs and Symptoms

1) Fever. This is of the swinging recurrent type and
is of variable degree. The fever usually abates with the
nephrectomy (Bottiger 1956-57). It is caused by an endogenous pyrogen and renal cell carcinoma tissue taken from a
febrile patient will cause a fever in laboratory animals in
contradistinction to tissue from a normal kidney or the
tumour from an afebrile patient (Rawlins, Luff, Cranston
1970). 2) Anemia. This is not due to bleeding or marrow
metastases but probably is a toxic effect on the marrow by
a circulating substance. 3) Hepatic Dysfunction. This is
reversible. It is not associated only with renal cell
carcinoma (Walsh, Kissane 1968) but has been reported in
connection with zanthogranulomatous pyelonephritis
(Vermillion, Morlock, Bartholomew, Kelalis 1970) and gastrointestinal malignancies (Abels, Rekers, Binkley, Pack,
Rhoads 1942) and is not the result of metastases. The exact
mechanism of this hepatorenal axis is not known but the
abnormal liver function tests, which include an elevated
alpha-2 globulin, elevated serum alkaline phosphatase and
prothrombin time, usually return to normal after nephrectomy. If they do not, it usually is a manifestation of
a metastatic growth. Their re-elevation after nephrectomy
also is of grave prognostic value. 4) Amyloidosis. This
occurs in a small percentage of cases with renal cell carcinoma and frequently involves the kidney, liver, spleen and
adrenal, and is not reversed by nephrectomy (Cline, Williams
1968). 5) Neuromyopathy. This may be another rare manifestation of renal cell carcinoma with reversible neurological disorders resembling peripheral myopathy or
polyneuritis (Thrush 1970). 6) Polycythemia. This occurs

in about 2 per cent of cases and differs from polycythemia rubra vera in that there is no splenomegaly, nor is there elevation of the leucocytes or platelet count. It is due to increase in the erythropoeitin and renal cell carcinoma has been shown to secrete this hormone (Pennington 1966). The erythrocytosis returns to normal value after nephrectomy unless metastases are present, and its re-appearance after a period of time following operation is a grave prognostic sign. 7) Hypertension. Theoretically this may occur as a result of compression of renal tissue by tumour with the release of renin and indeed recently Sufrin et al reported elevated peripheral renin blood levels in patients with high stage and anaplastic lesions with a subsequent fall in plasma renin level following nephrectomy (Sufrin, Mirand, Moore, Chu, Murphy 1977). 8) Hypercalcemia. This finding in the absence of bone metastases may be associated with other tumours of the liver, breast, pancreas, and lung as well as renal cell carcinoma. Again, the value of the calcium falls with nephrectomy and it has been shown that a parathyroid hormone-like material has been secreted by renal cell carcinoma (Buckle, McMillan, Mallinson 1970).
9) Enteropathy. Enteropathy with a protein loss has been described in a patient with renal cell carcinoma. Intestinal function and x-ray appearance returned to normal after nephrectomy, and the tumour was shown to be producing glucagon (Gleeson, Bloom, Polak, Henry, Dowling 1970).
10) Gonadotropin production. This has been reported with gynecomastia areolar pigmentation and diminished libido. Urine and plasma gonadotropins were elevated. Amenorrhoea is present in the female (Case Records of the Massachusetts General Hospital 1972).

SPONTANEOUS REGRESSION

Copious documentation in the literature of spontaneous regression of the primary and more notably metastases, although there are only sixty-nine recorded cases, has led to the unfounded belief that it is a frequent occurrence. Some authors have actually advocated nephrectomy in the presence of multiple metastases in the hope that this would result in regression. Statistics do not bear this out and to subject an individual to a nephrectomy for a surgically incurable disease certainly is not warranted.

REFERENCES

Abels JC, Rekers PE, Binkley GE, Pack GT, Rhoads CP (1942).
  Metabolic studies in patients with cancer of gastroin-
  testinal tract - II. Hepatic dysfunction. Ann Intern
  Med 16:221-240.
Bennington JL, Kradjian RM (1967). Distribution of Metasta-
  ses from renal cell carcinoma. In Renal Carcinoma.
  Philadelphia, W.B. Saunders Co. pp.156-179.
Bottiger LE (1956-57). Fever of unknown origin - IV. Fever
  in carcinoma of the kidney. Acta Med Scand 156:477-485.
Buckle RM, McMillan M, Mallinson C (1970). Ectopic secre-
  tion of parathyroid hormone by a renal adenocarcinoma in
  a patient with hypercalcemia. Br Med J 4:724-726.
Case records of the Massachusetts General Hospital (Case 13-
  1972) (1972). New Engl J Med 286:713-719.
Cline MJ, Williams HE (1968). Extra-renal manifestations of
  hypernephroma. Calif Med 109:35-40.
DeWeerd JH (1965). Arteriovenous fistula in hypernephroma.
  J Urol 93:666-668.
Gleeson MH, Bloom SR, Polak JM, Henry K, Dowling RH (1970).
  An endocrine tumor in kidney affecting small bowel
  structure, motility and function. Gut 11:1060.
Gray H (1966). The lymphatic system. In Anatomy of the
  Human Body, CM Goss, Ed. Philadelphia, Lea & Febiger
  pp. 735-780.
Middleton RG (1967). Surgery for metastatic renal cell
  carcinoma. J Urol 97:973-977.
Pennington DG (1966). The relation of erythropoietin to
  polycythemia. Proc R Soc Med 59:1091-1094.
Rawlins MD, Luff RH, Cranston WI (1970). Pyrexia in renal
  carcinoma. Lancet 1:1371-3.
Riches E (1964). The natural history of renal tumors. In
  Tumors of the Kidney and Ureter. Edinburgh and London,
  E & S Livingstone Ltd pp.124-134.
Robson CJ, Churchill BM, Anderson W (1969). The results of
  radical nephrectomy for renal cell carcinoma. J. Urol
  101:297-301.
Sufrin G, Mirand EA, Moore RH, Chu TM, Murphy GP (1977).
  Hormones in renal cancer. J Urol 117:433-437.
Thrush DC (1970). Neuropathy, IgM paraproteinemia, and
  autoantibodies in hypernephroma. Br Med J 4:474.
Vermillion SE, Morlock CG, Bartholomew LG, Kelalis PP (1970).
  Nephrogenic hepatic dysfunction - Secondary to tumefac-
  tive xanthogranulomatous pyelonephritis. Ann Surg 171:
  130-136.

Walsh PN, Kissane JM (1968). Nonmetastatic hypernephroma with reversible hepatic dysfunction. Arch Intern Med 122:214-222.

Renal Tumors: Proceedings of the First International Symposium on Kidney Tumors, pages 453–455
© 1982 Alan R. Liss, Inc., 150 Fifth Avenue, New York, NY 10011

THORACOPHRENOLAPAROTOMY

W. Grégoir, M.D.

University of Brussels

Department of Urology, Brugmann Hospital, Brussels

The aim of renal cancer surgery is to remove "en bloc" the tumour, the kidney, and the perinephric fat, after having ligated the vessels, to avoid intra-operative spreading of tumour cells. The incision must also allow for the possibility of performing a periaortic lymphadenectomy. It was well to be expected with the development of anaesthesia, that the kidneys, as well as the lower part of the oesophagus, would be approached through a transthoracic incision. Both kidneys are covered on the major part of their posterior surface by the thoracic wall.

The classic thoracophrenolaparotomy is centered on the 11th, the 10th or the 9th rib when the approach is done through the periosteum, after resection of the rib. If the incision is intercostal, it runs in the 10th, 9th or 8th space. Rib resection is never mandatory. The incision starts on the outer aspect of the sacro-lumbar muscular mass and follows the direction of the rib or the intercostal space, and is carried on anteriorly in the direction of the umbilicus to the external aspect of the rectus sheath. If necessary, the incision can be prolonged downwards on the edge of the sheath or simply extend across the rectus to the midline. This approach is very wide, it places the kidney and its vessels in the center of the operative field, gives access to any adjacent organ which may be involved, and places the surgeon in such a position as to gain control of the pedicle directly by dissecting from top to bottom, which is a big advantage and a real safety.

On the right side, primary exposure of the inferior
vena cava can be achieved by a technical modification.
After opening the chest in the 8th or 9th intercostal space,
the diaphragm is incised in a radial direction down to the
right atrium. The right colonic angle is freed. The liver,
liberated on its right aspect by cutting the triangular
and coronary ligament, is then tilted to the left. This
manoeuver gives a direct access to the sub-phrenic segment
of the vena cava; it further allows dissection upwards to
the atrium. It also gives greater safety in ligating the
suprarenal vessels and the renal pedicle. It is thus
particularly useful with big tumours of the upper pole on
the right side and even more so when neoplastic thrombi or
direct invasion of the vena cava demand its opening or
partial resection as a necessary complement to nephrectomy.
The same manoeuver can be done on the left side for big
tumours of the upper pole, it facilitates the dissection
of the suprarenal pedicle and the approach to the renal
artery.

Large thoracophrenolaparotomy has limited indications.
It is particularly indicated in very big tumours where
safety requires a large approach or in tumours of the upper
pole where ablation "en bloc" of the whole renal space
and of the suprarenal gland is necessary.

A far less aggressive approach is the thoraco-subcostal
incision in the 10th space. The thoracic segment of the
incision can be limited to the anterior half of the 10th
intercostal space; the pleural opening is thus limited and
the thoracic closure is particularly easy. The abdominal
segment of the incision is subcostal and runs to the rectus
sheath and eventually to the midline. The approach is quite
wide, extending on the right side to the high aspect of
the vena cava after lifting the liver, and on the left side
to the splenic pedicle, the tail of the pancreas and the
renal artery. This approach finds its best indications in
the medium sized tumours. Pleural drainage is usually not
necessary, in contrast to the large classical thoracophrenolaparotomy.

For gigantic tumours, particularly those which develop
from the upper pole of the kidney, classic thoracophrenolaparotomy is certainly the best approach. It is evident that
in left kidney tumours with caval invasion, thoracophrenolaparotomy is contra-indicated; a bilateral subcostal

incision or a xypho-pubic incision is then preferable.

If thoracophrenolaparotomy provides comfortable safety and a large approach which has no equivalent, it should be proportional to the difficulty and the magnitude of the operation. It is contra-indicated in pulmonary lesions, in respiratory failure and in poor risk patients, although one is often amazed by the ease of the postoperative course in the great majority of the cases.

Essential to surgery of renal cancer are the ease and directness of approach to the pedicle and resection "en bloc" of the renal mass. It does not matter whether these are achieved through a transthoracic incision, a xypho-pubic approach or a subcostal incision. Personal routine, the surgeon's preferences, the pulmonary status of the patient and the size and localization of the tumour determine the choice of approach. Large thoracophrenolaparotomy still has an established advantage in big tumours of the upper pole, particularly on the right side when there is actual or suspected invasion of the renal vein or vena cava.

Renal Tumors: Proceedings of the First International Symposium on
Kidney Tumors, pages 457–459
© 1982 Alan R. Liss, Inc., 150 Fifth Avenue, New York, NY 10011

LUMBAR FLANK APPROACH

Saad Khoury

Clinique Urologique, Hopital de la Pitié,
Paris

The lumbar flank approach for renal cancer is carried
out through a classical flank lumbotomy with wide resection of the 11th rib. The technique of this approach
is quite familiar to urologists and we shall only recall
its main features. The patient is positioned on his or
her side with the appropriate kidney exposed. The line
of incision is made on the body of the 11th rib and
extends to the abdomen. The periostium is incised along
the body of the rib and a periosteal elevation is used
to develop the subperiosteal plane. The doyen instrument
is used to develop the subperiosteal space behind the
rib and free it for the next surgical maneuvre. The
proximal end of the rib is transected and lifted from
the underlying subperiosteal bed. The distal portion of
the rib is similarily transected. After the rib has
been removed, the distal periosteal bed can be used to
develop an avascular blunt plane of dissection beneath
the medial abdominal muscles. This maneuvre also allows
the peritoneal wall located near the rib to be pushed
medially by several fingers to increase tension
anteriorly on the muscles for further dissection and
hemostatic control.

The bed of the rib is dissected backwards along the
intercostal nerve. Care is necessary to avoid tearing the
underlying pleura. The localization of the pleura is
facilitated by hyperinflation of the lungs. The pleura
must be freed carefully from its attachement to the
diaphragm to avoid tearing when the retractor is put in
place. Once this is done the flank muscles are incised

exposing the retroperitoneal fat. In the surgery of renal
cancer Gerota's facia should not be opened. The ascending
colon and duodenum on the right side and the descending
colon on the left side are freed and retracted medially.
It may be helpful to open the peritoneal cavity to achieve
better control of the abdominal organs. The renal
pedicule is exposed and the renal artery is isolated and
ligated first. This is followed by ligation of the renal
vein.

In cases where the renal artery is hidden by an inter-
mingling of veins, one may ligate the renal artery between
the aorta and the vena cava on the right side. In other
cases one should not hesitate to free the posterior face
of the kidney behind Gerota's facia to expose from behind
the renal artery. There is no need to expose oneself to
venous bleeding and the hypothetical risk of disseminating
cancer cells by manipulating the tumor. The vessels are
doubly ligated and the kidney with perinephric fat and
the adrenal are taken out "en bloc." We do not believe
that periaortic lymph nodes should be dissected as a
complement to radical nephrectomy. The advantages of this
approach are twofold:

(1) the technique is familiar to urologists
(2) it is not debilitation. The main inconvenience
is that it does not expose sufficiently the upper pole
in a case of a large tumor.

The ideal indication for this approach is a tumor
of the lower pole at the local stage I or II. Indications
could be extended to larger tumors of the lower pole or
even tumors of the upper pole if it is known beforehand
that the pedicule area is free and its dissection will
present no major problems. The preoperative work up
especially with CT scan provides accurate information
relevant to local resectability of tumor and to the
condition of the hilus. This makes it possible to use
with more confidence the lumbar approach without fear of
bad surprises.

CONCLUSION

In conclusion nearly 50% of kidney tumors can be safely removed through a lumbar approach with resection of the 11th rib with or without opening the peritoneal cavity. The morbidity of this approach is very low and the hospitalization time is relatively short.

Renal Tumors: Proceedings of the First International Symposium on Kidney Tumors, pages 461–464
© 1982 Alan R. Liss, Inc., 150 Fifth Avenue, New York, NY 10011

THE ABDOMINAL APPROACH IN KIDNEY TUMORS OF THE ADULT

Herbert Brendler, M.D.

Professor and Chairman, Department of Urology
Mount Sinai Medical Center
New York, New York

Most urologic surgeons today favor radical nephrectomy as the operation of choice for renal malignancy. This consists of en bloc removal of the kidney and adrenal, perinephric fat and Gerota's fascia in its entirety. Controversy still exists as to the value of concomitant lymphadenectomy.

The abdominal, i.e. transperitoneal, approach offers important advantages, principally excellent exposure and early access to the renal pedicle. Additionally, exploration for tumor spread to other structures is facilitated, and the opposite kidney may be examined. Exposure is more than adequate for total removal of lymphatic tissues down to the aortic bifurcation. In the event of tumor invasion of the vena cava, increased mobilization of the great vessels can readily be accomplished.

Several incisions are available for transperitoneal exposure of kidney tumors.

Midline or paramedian: This approach is favored by a number of urologic surgeons. Either incision is satisfactory in the presence of a wide subcostal angle. It is essential, however, that the incision be of sufficient length and extend to or above the xiphoid. The midline approach is more prone to postoperative hernia formation, whereas in the paramedian the anterior and posterior rectus fascial layers provide a stronger, 2-layer closure. The midline incision can be extended superiorly, should it become necessary to perform a sternotomy preparatory to cardiopulmonary bypass.

By incorporating a transverse component, the exposure can be considerably improved, an important consideration in stocky or obese individuals. The old Cabot and Young incisions described more than 50 years ago often afford satisfactory visualization and access to the renal vessels. In dealing with tumors of the lower pole, the upper limb of the Young T-incision can be eliminated without compromising the exposure.

Anterior subcostal: This incision is made with the patient in the supine position and the flank slightly elevated. It extends from the tip of the 12th rib in a curved manner 1-2 cm below the costal margin across the midline. It usually terminates midway over the opposite rectus, but can be extended further. The anterior abdominal muscles, including the ipsilateral rectus, are divided, and the opposite rectus as well, if necessary. The peritoneal cavity is entered in the midline and the ligamentum teres divided. Increased exposure for right-sided tumors may be obtained by extending the incision laterally into the flank, or by incorporating a vertical component.

For tumors on the left side which are not overly large, a bilateral subcostal ("chevron") incision is especially advantageous. The patient is placed in the supine position with the back slightly arched. The incision extends from one anterior axillary line to the other, curving gradually toward the xiphoid 1-2 cm below the costal margin. As with the unilateral subcostal, the peritoneum is opened in or near the midline.

11th rib extrapleural: For large tumors on either side, especially those arising from the upper pole, this incision provides optimal exposure without the necessity of entering the chest. The patient is placed in the semi-oblique position with some elevation of the flank. The incision extends along the 11th rib, beginning as far posteriorly as possible, then is carried midway between the xiphoid and umbilicus across the midline. The 11th rib is resected and the retroperitoneal space entered through the periosteal bed and by incising the underlying diaphragm. Care is taken not to injure the pleura which can be visualized in the posterior angle of the incision. The incision is then deepened anteriorly through the abdominal muscles, including

both recti, and the peritoneal cavity opened. Either a
Finochietto rib retractor or Smith ring retractor are
satisfactory for maintaining exposure.

Of all the approaches in current use for kidney tumors,
the writer has found the combined 11th rib extrapleural
transperitoneal route the most satisfactory by virtue of
its ability to provide wide exposure and ready access to
the vascular pedicle and great vessels. This approach
offers exceptional versatility in dealing with very large
tumors on either side, tumors arising from the upper poles,
those which extend across the midline and obscure the renal
vessels, and those which have already invaded contiguous
structures such as bowel.

On the left, the splenic flexure can be clearly
visualized and dealt with through this approach, something
usually quite difficult through any of the anterior longitudinal incisions, and even in the subcostal approach in
those individuals with narrow subcostal angles due to the
marked overhang of the rib cage. The attachments of the
splenic flexure are divided sharply so as to avoid injury
to the spleen. Following this the spleen and pancreas are
retracted upward and packed off. The lateral parietal
peritoneum is incised next, permitting the splenic flexure
and descending colon to be retracted medially off the surface of the tumor without opening Gerota's fascia, until
the aorta comes into view. Exposure of the renal vessels
follows.

On the right side, mobilization of the colon is easier.
After incising the parietal peritoneum along the border of
the bowel, the hepatic flexure and ascending colon are freed
and retracted medially off the surface of the tumor. The
second portion of the duodenum is identified, liberated and
retracted medially by the Kocher maneuver. Progressive retraction exposes the vena cava and permits isolation of the
renal vessels.

Closure is straightforward. The peritoneum is sutured
with continuous 2-0 chromic catgut. The muscles are closed
in layers, using interrupted figure-of-eight 2-0 chromic.
No attempt is made to re-approximate the intercostal muscles.
Should the pleura have been inadvertently entered, it is
closed under positive pressure, using continuous 2-0 chromic
catgut sutures. Occasionally, with large openings, under-

water tube drainage may be required for 24 hours. Placement of drains is largely a matter of personal preference. In certain situations, none may be required, but usually one or more penrose drains are left indwelling, to be removed in stages postoperatively.

Renal Tumors: Proceedings of the First International Symposium on Kidney Tumors, pages 465–469
© **1982 Alan R. Liss, Inc., 150 Fifth Avenue, New York, NY 10011**

THE ANTERIOR TRANSABDOMINAL TRANSVERSAL SUB-COSTAL APPROACH
FOR REMOVAL OF RENAL CANCER

Dufour B., Choquenet Ch.

Service d'Urologie
Hôpital Necker, Paris

The choice of incision for removal of a tumorous
kidney depends on the location, volume and extent of the
tumor itself (invasion of the colon, of the renal vein
and above all of the vena cava), as well as the anatomic
and physiologic condition of the patient. The surgeon's
skill and preference are also critical factors.

When the tumor is small, without any distal or veinous
invasion, any route can be chosen, even a simple and
direct lumbar approach, because the operation is easy;
but it may be difficult if the tumor is very large with
extensive invasion (and especially veinous).

The majority of surgeons agree that to properly remove a tumorous kidney it is necessary to have a generous
transabdominal exposure, in order to divide the renal
pedicle from the beginning before handling the tumor, and
to be able to cope with any invasion which may be en-
counted.

None of the numerous incisions which we used satisfied
us entirely; not even the thoracoabdominal nephrectomy,
which is generally considered as the best route in difficult cases.

For 5 years we have been using systematically an
anterior transabdominal transversal incision; it runs
2 cm parallel and below the costal margin, from below
the xyphoid down to the tip of the XIth or XIIth rib;
depending on the anatomy of the patient and the size and

location of the tumor, the incision can be extended to the other side making a "chevron-like" incision.

The patient lies on his back; the upper lumbar spine is elevated by means of a cushion and the body is slightly turned so that the operative site is a little higher than the rest of the abdomen.

Full exposure is provided and held by a self-retaining sub-costal retractor which lifts up the thoracic edge and makes the diaphragm vertical, exposing all the sub-diaphragmatic area.

This approach that we have personally used more than 40 times satisfied us entirely; exceptionally it might be enlarged towards the thorax by adding a thoracic incision and excision of the 8th rib, opening the pleura and cutting the diaphragm. We did it just once.

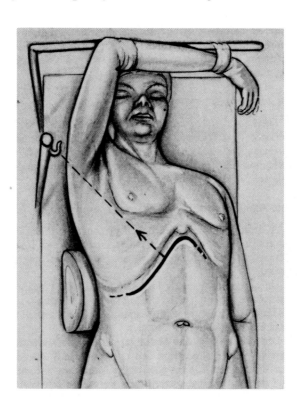

The advantages of this procedure are as follows:

Anatomic
This approach leads directly to the initial part of
the abdominal aorta, vena cava and the source of the renal
artery, because the incision is directly above the xyphoid
at the level of the XIIth dorsal vertebra. (The anterior
projection of the renal artery is located about 1.5 cm
above a horizontal line joining the tips of the 9th ribs.)

On the left side, access to the aorta and the renal
artery can be obtained either by retracting the left
flexure of the colon or by direct incision of the
posterior peritoneum in front of the aorta, by retracting
the 4th duodenum. If the renal vein and even if the vena
cava itself is invaded, it is easy, by a complete
"chevron," to check and to explore from the beginning the
vena cava by retraction of the right flexure of the colon
and the duodenopancreas.

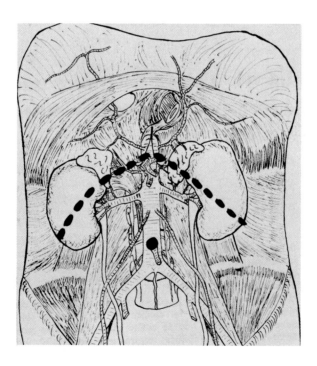

On the right side, the renal artery can be found and divided either on the right side of the vena cava or between the vena cava and the aorta.

The invasion of the vena cava itself, whether the cancer is on the right or on the left, can necessitate the dissection and possibly the taping off of the vein under and above the liver. The liver can be retracted medically after having been detached from the diaphragm by dividing the triangular and coronar ligaments in order to expose the vena cava behind the liver. All the infra-diaphragmatic part of the vena cava can be exposed by this approach (without having to open the thorax).

The intrapericardic part of the vena cava and the right atrium could be exposed if necessary either by a thoracic enlargement or through a simple incision of the diaphragm.

Follow-up

The mortality and morbidity of the enlarged nephrectomy by this approach is low. This purely abdominal approach is very well tolerated by the patient from a respiratory point of view; the absence of diaphragmatic incision, the absence of pleural opening, and the absence of lateral decubitus facilitate the ease of respiratory function during and after the operation.

These physiologic advantages, which are already important for a patient in a normal pulmonary condition, become of paramount importance when the patient is old or has some respiratory trouble.

A comparative study of 88 enlarged nephrectomies done either by this approach or by a thoracoabdominal incision has shown that the sub-costal approach causes less mortality and less morbidity. In addition, the duraction of hospitalization is shorter and the cost lower.

The wound suture is strong and there is a minimal risk of herniation.

The incision described herein is not new. E. Poutasse in the early sixties advocated this route, and used it for all kinds of renal surgery. Subsequently,

R. Chute and J. A. Baron in the U.S.A., and J. Ducassou
and A. Ponthieu in France also advised its use.

In fact, on the whole, even though it is used regularly
for surgery of the upper part of the abdomen (stomach,
hiatus, pancreas), this approach is not often used by
urologists and yet it is, undoubtedly in my opinion, one
of the best if not the best.

Chute B, Baron JA (1968). The transverse upper abdominal
    incision in urological surgery. J Urol 99:528.
Poutasse E (1961). Anterior approach to upper urinary
    tract surgery. J Urol 85: 199.
Ponthieu A, Ducassou J (1971). About the anterior
    approach to kidney, the transverse subcostal approach.
    J Urol and Nephrol 77:307.
Dufour B, Choquenet Ch (1980). The anterior trans-
    abdominal subcostal approach of the tumorous kidney.
    Chirurgie - T. 106:441. Edit. Masson.

Renal Tumors: Proceedings of the First International Symposium on Kidney Tumors, pages 471–473
© 1982 Alan R. Liss, Inc., 150 Fifth Avenue, New York, NY 10011

THE CHOICE OF SURGICAL INCISION

Philip H. Smith[1], M.B., F.R.C.S., and
David F. Green[2], M.D.

1. Head, Dept. of Urology, St. James's University
   Hospital, Leeds, U.K.
2. Tutor in Urology and Clinical Research Fellow,
   St. James's University Hospital, Leeds and
   The University of Leeds, Leeds, U.K.

Any analysis of the different incisions available for
nephrectomy must take account of the variations in tumour size
and extension and allow for such individual views as a surgeon
may have because of his training and personal preferences.
The problems to be considered include those of access, morbidity and survival.

It is obvious that a 10 cm tumour of the upper pole of
the right kidney perhaps with extension to the inferior vena
cava demands greater access than a 2 cm lesion in the lower
pole of the same kidney. It is equally clear that a patient
treated by a long paramedian incision is usually in more dis-
comfort than one treated using a subcostal or loin approach,
and not as ill as the patient with a thoraco-abdominal
incision.

The point we would like to consider however is whether
the incision, which is to some degree determined by the extent
of the surgery which is proposed, is related to the survival
of the patient. If lymph node dissection is contemplated or
exploration of the inferior vena cava (IVC) considered mandatory, the exposure will be greater than that required for
simple nephrectomy or that for partial nephrectomy or enucleation of a lesion in a solitary kidney.

Relevant to this consideration is the paper given by
Dr. Hellsten who made several important observations based on

the post mortem study in Malmö. He noted that:-

1.   approximately two-thirds of all patients with renal cell cancer (RCC) died of some other condition and without their RCC being recognised.

2.   of the 256 patients with unrecognised RCC lymph node invasion was found in 37. The retroperitoneal nodes were involved in 25 and nodes at the pulmonary hilum in 24. This means that at least half the patients with retroperitoneal node involvement have involved nodes in other sites.

3.   the size of the tumour was related to the incidence of metastases, tumours of 8 cm diameter or larger being associated with metastases in two-thirds of all patients.

If these findings can be confirmed and represent facets of the natural history of the disease as it appears in other countries, it becomes necessary to think again about the whole concept of treatment of renal cancer.

The implication is that, in the elderly patient at least, RCC is associated with the ageing process from which two-thirds of such patients will die before their cancer develops to such a stage that it threatens life. This observation lends support to the view put forward at the NATO ASI on cancer of the kidney and prostate in Erice, Sicily in 1981 that "patients with asymptomatic lesions over the age of 75 should not be treated" (Denis 1981). In patients in this age group who do develop symptoms, embolectomy may be the best initial therapy, possibly followed by surgery at a later date if necessary - a policy of "deferred treatment" which has been advocated at intervals over the years for patients with carcinoma of the prostate.

The findings in patients with lymph node involvement together with the recognition that metastases are already present in the majority of those with larger tumours suggest that formal lymphadenectomy must have a limited role whatever the size of the primary and that for the larger primary tumour the operation is likely to achieve a "cure" only until the metastases, which may lie dormant for up to 25 years, (Bradham et al 1973), declare themselves.

The increasing use of partial nephrectomy or tumour enucleation for patients with RCC in a solitary kidney is also a point of importance in this general discussion. A localised enucleation or partial nephrectomy inevitably breaches the perinephric fat to allow access to the kidney and is not routinely associated with lymph node dissection.

Brosman (1982) has recently reviewed the published figures on local excision in patients with a solitary kidney and in patients with bilateral tumours. This approach in patients with one kidney from birth (or after nephrectomy for benign disease) and in those with asynchronous or synchronous cancer is, in each group, followed by a 60 - 70% five year survival. Such an unexpected finding again calls into question the accepted wisdom of radical nephrectomy with node dissection.

The following papers consider the place of lymph node dissection, management of extension to the inferior vena cava, and the treatment of RCC in the solitary kidney. Unless new evidence becomes available from these contributions, one is inevitably led to consider a conservative approach requiring limited access until a randomised study proves the superiority of some more extensive technique, or until some other more effective therapy becomes available.

Bradham RR, Wannamaker CC, Pratt-Thomas HR (1973). Renal Cell Carcinoma Metastases 25 Years After Nephrectomy. JAMA 223: 921.

Brosman SA (1982). Adenocarcinoma Occurring in a Solitary Kidney. In Smith PH, Pavone-Macaluso M (eds): "Cancer of the Prostate and Kidney," London and New York: Plenum Press (in press).

Denis L (1981) Personal communication.

Renal Tumors: Proceedings of the First International Symposium on Kidney Tumors, pages 475–480
© **1982 Alan R. Liss, Inc., 150 Fifth Avenue, New York, NY 10011**

RESULTS OF RADICAL NEPHRECTOMY WITHOUT LYMPHADENECTOMY IN
RENAL CELL CARCINOMA

C. Chatelain

Urological Clinic
La Pitié Hospital
Paris, France

From October 1968 to October 1978, 222 patients with
renal cell carcinoma were operated at our center. Two
hundred and four had a radical nephrectomy (Table 1). The

TABLE 1

SURGICAL TREATMENT OF 222 PATIENTS WITH RENAL CELL CARCINOMA
BETWEEN OCTOBER 1968 – OCTOBER 1978*

	Number of Patients
Radical Nephrectomy	204
Partial Nephrectomy	4
Exploration Laparotomy	14
Bilateral Surgery	2
Renal Arterial Embolization	32
Surgical Treatment of Metastasis	28
Additional Treatments	
Radiotherapy	16 post. + 6 preop.
Chemotherapy	13
Hormonal Therapy	32
(Progesterone)	

*La Pitié Hospital, Paris

operative mortality was 3.9%. Complete information and
follow-up were available in 164 of these patients and we
shall in this study analyze their evaluation. Staging of
the patients (Robson's classification) is summarized in
Table 2. Our series contains relatively more advanced

TABLE 2

STAGING OF PATIENTS (ROBSON'S CLASSIFICATION)
(168 CASES)

			Number of Patients
Stage I			45
Stage II			20
Stage III	A	27	
	B	5	
	C	8	40
Stage IV	A	10	
	B	53	63
Total			168

cases than in other series published in the literature. The
most commonly used surgical approaches were thoracoabdominal
and the abdominal incision. Sternotomy was added in a few
cases when the control of the vena cava and the right atrium
was necessary. Our technique of radical nephrectomy consisted of an "en bloc" removal of the kidney with perinephric
fat and occasional tumor extensions after primary control of
renal vessels. The additional removal of the adrenals was
carried out in 55% of cases and in nine cases various procedures were done on the vena cava and the right atrium
(Table 3).

TABLE 3

SURGICAL PROCEDURES ASSOCIATED TO RADICAL NEPHRECTOMY

	Number of Cases
Adrenalectomy	91
Splenectomy	8
Caudal Pancreatectomy	1
Partial Duodenectomy	2
Right Colectomy	2
Left Colectomy	1
Partial Hepatectomy	2
Orchidectomy	1
Cavectomy (± right atrium)	9
Partial Lymphadenectomy	13

Lymphadenectomy extending to all regional lymphatics and periaortic lymph nodes was not associated with radical nephrectomy. Only lymph nodes of the Hilius were removed. Preoperative embolization was done in 15% of cases. The treatment of metastasis will be analyzed elsewhere in this symposium.

RESULTS

Results are summarized in Figure 1.

Five-year survival was 71% at Stage I, 77% at Stage II, 48% at Stage III and 23% at Stage IV. Results in Stage II were slightly better than than in Stage I. We have no explanation for this finding encountered also in other series.

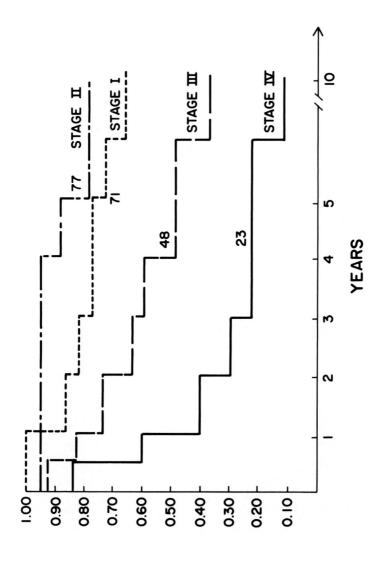

Fig. 1. Cumulative actuarial survival of 168 patients after radical nephrectomy.

TABLE 4

SURVIVAL RATE IN SOME PUBLISHED SERIES

	Years	Lymphadenectomy			
		Lymph + ROBSON 1969 86 cases	Lymph + CUKIER 1979 120 cases	Lymph ± BOXER 1979 96 cases	Lymph − Present Series 1980 168 cases
		%	%	%	%
STAGE I	1 to 3	(3) 73	(2) 92	(1) 94	(2) 81
	5	66	83	56	71
	10	60	59	20	(65)
STAGE II	1 to 3	67	84	100	95
	5	64	84	100	77
	10	67	−	66	(77)
STAGE III	1 to 3	59	62	89	62
	5	42	53	50	48
	10	38	−	25	(38)
STAGE IV	3	25	27	68	31
	5	11	−	8	23
	10	0	−	0	(12)

Boxer et al. 1979.
Chatelain et al. 1980.
Cukier et al. 1979.
Robson et al. 1969.

Two main conclusions could be drawn from our results:

1) Our results are similar to those obtained
   in other comparable series published in
   the literature whether lymphadenectomy
   was associated or not to radical nephrectomy
   (Table 4). This additional lymphadenectomy
   appears to have no effect on survival.
   Table 4 compares evalution in some published
   series. Results are particularly uniform in
   Stage III.

2) The relatively good survival obtained in
   our series in Stage IV patients is due to
   the fact that a good number of these patients
   had solitary metastasis. Detailed analysis
   of evalution of patients with metastasis
   is done elsewhere.

REFERENCES

Boxer RJ, Waisman J, Lieber MM, Mampase FM, Skinner DG (1979).
  Renal carcinoma computer analysis of 96 patients treated
  by nephrectomy. J Urol 122:598.
Chatelain C, Richard F, Carvalho R, Le Gall D (1980). Traitement chirurgical de l'adénocarcinome renal. Etude de 222
  5e Congrès Assoc Urol du Québec. Montréal, Nov 27-30, 1980.
Cukier J, Amiel JL, Bronstein M, Droz JP. Cancer du rein
  chez l'adulte; resultat du traitement actuel. 120 cas.
Robson CJ, Churchill BM, Anderson W (1969). The results of
  radical nephrectomy for renal cell carcinoma. J Urol 101:
  297.

Renal Tumors: Proceedings of the First International Symposium on Kidney Tumors, pages 481–488
© 1982 Alan R. Liss, Inc., 150 Fifth Avenue, New York, NY 10011

RESULTS OF RADICAL THORACO-ABDOMINAL NEPHRECTOMY IN THE TREATMENT OF RENAL CELL CARCINOMA

Charles J. Robson, M.D., F.R.C.S.(C), F.A.C.S.

Professor & Chairman, Division of Urology
University of Toronto
Toronto, Ontario, Canada

By definition radical thoraco-abdominal nephrectomy means a transpleural, transdiaphragmatic and transabdominal approach to the kidney usually through the bed of the ninth or tenth rib with removal of the kidney within an intact Gerota's capsule containing the perinephric fat and a meticulous dissection of the lymph field from the crus of the diaphragm to the bifurcation of the aorta or the junction of the common iliac veins. It should include the lymphatics between the great vessels and the lymph field on the lateral side of the great vessel on the side of the involved kidney.

In the period 1954 to 1978, there have been 162 radical thoraco-abdominal nephrectomies done by the staff of the Toronto General Hospital by the above procedure. These cases all had a standard workup for their preoperative staging consisting of a complete skeletal technetium scan or a complete skeletal survey by radiography, whole lung tomograms, the importance of which has been emphasized in a previous presentation, aortography performed routinely by the Seldinger technique with flush and selective catheterizations of the renal arteries usually with adrenalin perfusion. This procedure not only confirms the diagnosis by showing up tumour vessels in most cases but also shows the position and number of the renal arteries, thus enabling the surgeon to interrupt the arterial blood supply at an early stage of the operation and thus reduce the hazard of tumour embolization. Recently all have had c.t. scans. Although computer scanning will show tumour involvement of the main renal vein and vena cava, particularly if combined with pedal insertion of dye, direct inferior cavography is

still more accurate in showing the extent of the thrombus
and allowing for preoperative planning for thrombectomy.

MORTALITY

The hospital mortality rate of the 162 patients was 4.4
per cent. One patient died of cardiac arrest. There were
two coronary occlusions. One patient died of hemorrhage on
the operating table due to involvement of the lateral wall
of the vena cava and tumour involving the wall above the
right renal vein, the tumour being on the left side. This
was in the period prior to dialysis and transplantation.
Sepsis was the cause of one patient's demise due to septic
shock, and one patient died of unknown causes when an
autopsy was not obtained.

Morbidity has not been a serious factor in this series.
We have not used chest drainage unless there were significant pleural adhesions requiring division, and thoracentesis
was required in eight cases. Non-fatal pulmonary embolus
occurred in three cases and empyema in one. Postoperative
hemorrhage requiring re-operation occurred in one patient.
Prolonged ileus requiring periods of nasogastric suction
occurred in two cases. Postoperative atelectasis occurred
in four cases, two of whom required bronchoscopic suction.
One case had acute gastric dilatation.

Table 1.

Thoraco-abdominal nephrectomy

1981

Morbidity	No.Cases
Pulmonary embolus	3
Empyema	1
Pleural effusion requiring thoracentesis	8
Postoperative hemorrhage - re-operation	1
Prolonged ileus	2
Atelectasis	4
Gastric dilatation	1

PROGNOSIS

The prognosis for renal cell carcinoma is dependent
upon five factors and/or a combination of these (Robson CJ,
Churchill BM, Anderson W 1969). 1) Involvement of the
adjacent structures by direct extension. 2) The presence
or absence of distant metastases. 3) Involvement of the
regional lymph nodes. 4) Gross invasion of the renal vein
or its main tributaries. 5) Histological grade of the
tumour. In our series of 162 cases 17 or 10.6 per cent
showed an intact pseudocapsule and the growth was confined
to the kidney per se in 51 cases or 31 per cent, 68 or 42
per cent had perinephric fat invasion by direct extension,
9 had involved ipsilateral adrenal or 5 per cent, 34 or
21 per cent showed regional lymphadenopathy, 52 or 31 per
cent showed invasion of the renal vein and 17 or 9 per cent
had involvement of the vena cava. Distant metastases were
present in 9 per cent.

Table 2.

Analysis of 162 cases of

renal cell carcinoma

17 - Intact pseudocapsule	- 10.6%
51 - Confined to kidney	- 31%
68 - Involved perinephric fat	- 42%
9 - Involved ipsilateral adrenal	- 5%
34 - Regional lymphadenopathy	- 21%
52 - Macroscopic invasion of renal vein	- 31%
17 - Involved the vena cava	- 9%

These tumours were staged according to the extent of their
spread, as proposed by Flocks and Kadesky (Flocks RH,
Kadesky MC 1958) and by Petkovic (Petkovic SD 1959) with
slight modifications in Stage III. The reason for the
minor change in Stage III is shown in Fig. 1, which shows
that at the end of ten years the survival rate of these
cases with renal vein involvement and lymphatics was
practically identical. That the staging has a very definite
prognostic value is shown in the figures in Table 3 & Fig.2.

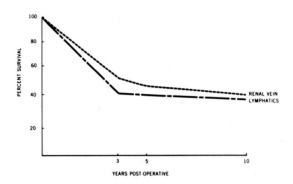

Fig. 1.

Table 3.

Survival in renal cell ca. with radical nephrectomy

162 cases

	3 yrs.	5 yrs.	10 yrs.
Stage I	48/66 73%	31/48 65%	18/30 60%
Stage II	20/30 65%	12/20 64%	6/11 54%
Stage III	32/54 55%	13/30 43%	4/10 40%
Stage IV	3/12 25%	1/3 33%	0
Total	103/162 65%	57/101 56%	28/51 40%

Here are shown the survival rates of the various stages for

three, five and ten year periods. The overall survival of all stages in three years was 65 per cent, 56 percent at five years and 40 per cent at ten years. The survival rate

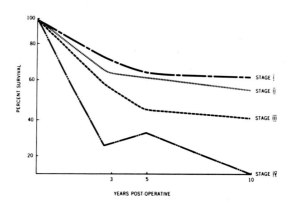

Fig. 2.

of this series compared to other published series is shown in the composite graph (Fig. 3). Three large series of

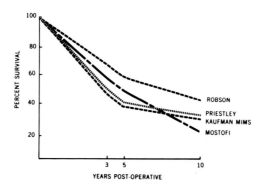

Fig. 3.

simple nephrectomy have been reported by Priestley
(Priestley 1939), by Mostofi (Mostofi 1967), and Kaufman
and Mims (Kaufman, Mims 1966). The statistically significant improvement in survival following radical nephrectomy
is, we believe, due to three factors. 1) Early ligation of
the renal artery, thus minimizing the chance of vascular
tumour emboli. 2) Removal of the entire perinephric fat
envelope without its incision, thereby decreasing the
chance of local tumour implantation and of leaving tumour
in the renal bed. The perinephric fat was involved in 42
per cent of cases. 3) Removal of the lymphatic drainage
system, which was involved by tumour in 21 per cent.

There is general agreement in the literature that
lymphadenectomy has a definite place in the staging and
prognosis of renal cell carcinoma. Of some import and a
factor not known is how often the lymphadenectomy is a
meticulous one in the case where several large nodes are
seen and perhaps sampled. The therapeutic value of lymphadenectomy, however, has been and continues to be questioned
(deKernion 1980) on several aspects, the first being the
anatomy of the lymphatic range of renal cell carcinoma.
Hulten (Hulten, Rosencrantz, Wahlquist et al 1969) has published a complete study on the distribution of the lymphatic metastases. As might be prophesied, most of the involved nodes were in the region of the hilum, however, there
was involvement of the nodes on the opposite side of the
great vessel involved and one patient had the ipsilateral
iliac nodes as the only site of lymphatic spread. Parasitic vessels, which are usually seen with this tumour, may
drain anywhere in the retroperitoneum from the iliacs to
the crus of the diaphragm but it is believed that they all
will eventually go into the para-aortic or paracaval nodes.
In our series we did not split the lymphatic chain wishing
to remove it as carefully as possible, however, in the
future the various areas will be marked. It is our belief
that lymphadenectomy has a definite therapeutic value.
There have been positive lymphatics in 34 out of 162 or 21
per cent. We have a ten year survival rate of 33 per cent,
and it is interesting that most deaths occurred within two
years of operation. Of interest also is that where there
was only microscopic involvement of the lymph nodes the
prognosis was much better than when the lymph nodes were
grossly involved with a ratio of 2:1. Peters (Peters,
Brown 1980) gives a five year survival of Stage III of 43
per cent with lymphadenectomy versus 26 per cent without.

Local recurrence has been a large factor in the later
mortality of people with renal cell carcinoma and in this
series it only occurred in 10 per cent of cases, probably
largely because of the intact Gerota's fascia, but I think
lymphadenectomy also contributed to this. There has been no
morbidity or mortality directly associated with lymphadenectomy.

TUMOUR GRADE

The importance of grading in the prognosis of renal
cell carcinoma has been emphasized continually particularly
by Riches (Riches 1964), and we have used the criteria as
advocated by Thackeray in the grading and have not used the
method of grading of the nuclei only as reported by Skinner
and deKernion (Skinner, deKernion 1978). Grade I, as might
be expected, had the best prognosis with a 64 per cent
three year survival, 57 per cent at five years and 58 per
cent at ten years. Grade II showed 58 per cent at three
years, 47 per cent at five years and 33 per cent ten year
survival, whereas Grade III showed 53, 51 and 46 per cent.

Table 4.

Renal cell carcinoma - survival by grade

	3 yrs.	5 yrs.	10 yrs.
Grade I	64%	57%	58%
Grade II	58%	47%	33%
Grade III	53%	51%	46%

Recently there has been an attempt made to differentiate renal cell carcinomas into so-called oncocytoma
which with their different staining properties suggest a
much improved prognosis. They have been separated off from
the main group of tumours and would correspond to a grade
of I according to Thackeray. As most of these tumours are
pleomorphic and with disagreement amongst pathologists regarding their grade, perhaps we should be satisfied to call
them, as Mostofi does (Mostofi 1967), simply good tumours
and bad tumours.

SUMMARY

A series of 162 cases of renal cell carcinoma treated by radical thoraco-abdominal nephrectomy is presented, together with the three, five and ten year survival. The increase in survival rate is probably due to three factors. 1) Early ligation of the renal artery and vein. 2) Complete removal of the perinephric envelope. 3) Surgical extirpation of the lymphatic field. Prognosis in renal cell carcinoma is directly related to the stage and grade of the tumour and as yet nephrectomy offers the only hope of cure.

REFERENCES

de Kernion JB (1980). Lymphadenectomy for renal cell carcinoma. Urol Clinics of NA Vol 7 No 3.

Flocks RH, Kadesky MC (1958). Malignant neoplasms of the kidney: An analysis of 353 patients followed five years or more. J Urol 79:196-201.

Hulten L, Rosencrantz T, Wahlquist L et al (1969). Scand J Urol Nephrol 3:129-133.

Kaufman JJ, Mims MM (1966). Tumors of the kidney. In: Current problems in surgery.

Mostofi FK (1967). Pathology and spread of renal cell carcinoma. In King JS Jr (ed): Renal neoplasia, Boston, Little, Brown and Co. p.41.

Peters PC, Brown GL (1980). The role of lymphadenectomy in the management of renal cell carcinoma. Urol Clinics of NA Vol 7 No 3.

Petkovic SD (1959). An anatomical classification of renal tumors in the adult as a basis for prognosis. J Urol 81:618-623.

Priestley JT (1939). Survival following the removal of malignant renal neoplasms. JAMA 113:902.

Riches E (1964). Surgery of renal tumors, in, Riches E. Ed: Tumors of the kidney and ureter, Baltimore, Williams and Wilkins Chap 23, pp 275-289.

Robson CJ, Churchill BM, Anderson W (1969). The results of radical nephrectomy for renal cell carcinoma. J Urol 101:297-301.

Skinner DG, deKernion JB (1978). Clinical manifestations and treatment of renal parenchymal tumors. In Skinner DC, deKernion JB (eds): Genitourinary Cancer, Philadelphia, W.B. Saunders Co. p.127.

Renal Tumors: Proceedings of the First International Symposium on Kidney Tumors, pages 489–492
© **1982 Alan R. Liss, Inc., 150 Fifth Avenue, New York, NY 10011**

COMPARATIVE STUDY OF ACTUARIAL SURVIVAL RATES IN STAGE II AND III RENAL CELL CARCINOMAS MANAGED BY RADICAL NEPHRECTOMY ALONE OR ASSOCIATED WITH FORMAL RETROPERITONEAL LYMPH NODE DISSECTION

A. Gilloz and J. Tostain

Department of Urology

University of Saint-Etienne, Hopital Bellevue, 42100 Saint-Etienne

In order to appreciate whether retroperitoneal lymph node dissection associated with radical nephrectomy improved the prognosis of renal cell carcinoma, we conducted a retrospective study of 157 patients with renal cell carcinoma seen over 15 years (from January 1965 to December 1979), 145 of whom were managed by radical nephrectomy. Forty radical nephrectomies performed after January 1975 were associated with formal retroperitoneal lymph node dissection; 12 patients were not eligible for radical nephrectomy.

METHODS

Firstly, this series has a great homogeneity: all the surgical procedures were indicated and performed by the same surgeon, or sometimes with his help. The current status of these 145 operated patients has been confirmed in July and August 1980. We know the accurate date of every death, and no patient was lost to follow up. Secondly, surgical adjunct to radical nephrectomy did not consist of simple lymph node picking, but in formal retroperitoneal lymph node and cellular tissue dissection between the inferior mesenteric artery and diaphragm. When the left kidney was involved a complete dissection of the cellular tissue of the anterior wall of the vena cava and around the aorta was performed. In cases of carcinoma of the right kidney a dissection of the cellular tissue of the anterior wall of the aorta and around the vena cava was performed. Thirdly, a previous study of this series (Gilloz et al. 1981) using Robson's classification (Robson et al. 1969) showed that retroperitoneal lymph node dissection did not improve prognosis of Stage I (tumor confined to the kidney parenchyma, the true renal capsule is intact) or Stage IV (involvement of the adjacent organs other than the adrenal or distant metastases not accessible to surgery) carcinomas.

Consequently, renal cell carcinoma survival was analyzed in the remaining group of 73 patients with Stage II (renal capsule has been broken through and the perirenal fat is involved by the tumor which, however, is still contained within the envelopes of Gerota's fascia) or Stage III (gross renal vein or inferior renal cava involvement or lymphatic involvement or combination of the above). Of these 73 radical nephrectomies, 25 were associated with lymph node dissection during the last five years, witn no postoperative death. To compare favorably the long term survival of patients managed anteriorly by radical nephrectomy alone, 8 postoperative deaths which had occurred within this group prior to 1974 (6 deaths between 1965-69; 2 deaths between 1970-1974) have been excluded. The statistical analysis included standard actuarial methods with a statistically significant cut off level at p   0.05.

RESULTS

The results are presented in Figures 1 and 2. In Figure 1, survival rates are compared in two 5-year successive periods. Note:

Curve B, which is 1970-74 when 26 radical nephrectomies without lymphadenectomy were performed (2 postoperative deaths excluded).

In Curve A cases performed between 1975-1979, 25 radical nephrectomies were associated with lymphadenectomy (no postoperative death).

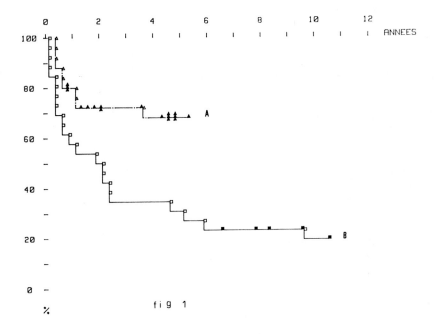

Fig. 1. The 5-year survival rate for the 2 groups receiving radical nephrectomy with and without lymphadenectomy.

In Figure 2, survival rates of all Stage II and III renal carcinomas surgically managed during 15 years are compared. Note that in Curve D, 40 radical nephrectomies without lymphadenectomy (8 postoperative deaths excluded) were performed whereas in Curve C 25 radical nephrectomies were associated with lymphadenectomy (no postoperative deaths). In our series, the 5-year survival rate of Stage II and III renal carcinomas improved from 30% with radical nephrectomy alone (postoperative death excluded), to 68% when lymphadenectomy was performed (no postoperative death observed). (Confidence level: 15-20%, p 0.05). Since no secondary treatment (chemotherapy or radiotherapy) has yet been proved to be effective, we shall continue to manage Stage II and III renal cell carcinomas by radical nephrectomy associated with formal retroperitoneal lymph node and cellular tissue dissection. The same management is applied to Stage I, since accurate staging (histopathologic) is otherwise impossible at the time of operation.

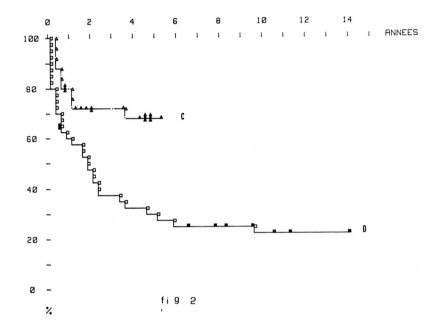

fig 2

Fig. 2.   The 15-year survival rate for the 2 groups receiving radical nephrectomy with and without lymphadenectomy.

We thank the Department of Medical Statistics, (J.C.
Healy, Prof.) University of Saint-Etienne Medical School.

Gilloz AP, Tostain J, Rusch PH (1981).   L'association d'une
    cellulo-lymphadenectomie à la néphrectomie élargie est-elle
    justifiée dans le traitement du cancer du rein?   (S the
    formal retroperitoneal cellular tissue and lymph nodes
    dissection a valuable adjunct to radical nephrectomy in
    renal cell carcinoma management?)   Société Francaise
    d'Urologie 16 mars 1981.   A paraître in Annales d'
    Urologie.
Robson CH J, Churchill BM, Anderson W (1969).   The results
    of radical nephrectomy for renal cell carcinoma.   J
    Urol 101:297.

Renal Tumors: Proceedings of the First International Symposium on
Kidney Tumors, pages 493–495
© 1982 Alan R. Liss, Inc., 150 Fifth Avenue, New York, NY 10011

SHOULD LYMPHADENECTOMY BE ASSOCIATED TO RADICAL NEPHRECTOMY
IN RENAL CELL CARCINOMA?

C. Chatelain
Urologic Clinic, Hôpital de la Pitié
Paris, France

Radical nephrectomy has replaced simple nephrectomy in
the treatment of renal cell carcinoma. There is a large
consensus at present among urologists that radical nephrectomy
should remove "en bloc" the tumor, the kidney and the perinephric fat after primary ligation of renal pedicule. There
is no doubt that this technique is beneficial. Additional
lymphadenectomy extending to the regional lymphatics and
lumbo-aortic lymph nodes is still controversial. It it
necessary? Is it useful? Does it have a favorable impact
on survival? Opinions are unsettled. Some authors perform
systematically a large lymphadenectomy when doing a radical
nephrectomy (Series 1, Table 1). Others and ourselves do
not perform systematic lymphadenectomy. If we compare
results especially concerning Stage III, we see no significant differences in the series whether lymphadenectomy
was done or not (Series 4 and 8, Table 1). Some authors had
two periods in their practice: a period without lymphadenectomy and a period with lymphadenectomy. In Series 2
(Table 1), looking at 5-year survival we see that at Stage I
there was no difference between radical nephrectomy with or
without lymphadenectomy. At Stage II, radical nephrectomy
with lymphadenectomy give a 10% amelioration of survival and
at Stage III, there was no statistical proof that lymphadenectomy gave better survival.

Series 3 in Table 1 indicates that there was no
statistical difference between nephrectomy with or without
lymphadenectomy. In Series 6, there was no proof of
prognostic amelioration by lymphadenectomy, and in Series 7,
lymphadenectomy was useful for staging, but it had no impact

TABLE 1

COMPARISON OF SURVIVAL IN DIFFERENT SERIES PUBLISHED IN THE
LITERATURE OF RADICAL NEPHRECTOMY WITH OR WITHOUT
LYMPHADENECTOMY (5 Years Survival)

Series	Lymphadenectomy		Stages			
			I	II	III	IV
1 (86 cases) Robson et al., 1969	+		66	64	42	11
2 (309 cases) Skinner et al., 1972	±		65	47	51	8
3 (96 cases) Boxer et al., 1979	±		56	100	50	8
4 (178 cases) Oliver et al., 1979	-		80	44	38	10
5 (120 cases) Cukier et al., 1979	+		83	84	53	-
6 (130 cases) Waters and Richie, 1979	±		51	58.5 (+vein)	12.3 (lymph)	0
7 (143 cases) Sullivan et al., 1979	±	NS NE	74 31	66 43	20 29	0 21
8 (168 cases) Our Series, 1980	-		71	77	48	23
9 (499 cases) McNichols et al., 1981	±		67	51	33.5	13.5

on long term survival. Finally, in Series 9, lymphadenectomy
was not found to be useful.

In conclusion, we should admit that at the present time,
we have no objective proof of the efficiency of lymphadenectomy
in the treatment of renal cell carcinoma. Further prospective
comparative studies may not yield results that are much
different.

Lymph nodes are invaded in renal cell carcinoma in
about 20 to 25% of cases. In most of these cases, extension
has already spread to the lymphatics of the mediastinum and
even a larger lymphadenectomy would still be incomplete.
In 75% of the remaining cases, where lymph nodes are not
invaded, lymphadenectomy is at best useless and might be
harmful. It may remove a physiologic barrier against
dissemination of cancer cells and depress local immunological
reactions. For all these reasons, we do not advise the
association of lymphadenectomy to radical nephrectomy in the
treatment of renal carcinoma.

Renal Tumors: Proceedings of the First International Symposium on Kidney Tumors, pages 497–507
© **1982 Alan R. Liss, Inc., 150 Fifth Avenue, New York, NY 10011**

LOCALLY EXTENSIVE RENAL CELL CARCINOMA – CURRENT SURGICAL
MANAGEMENT OF INVASION OF VENA CAVA, LIVER, OR BOWEL

Ruben F. Gittes, M.D.

Professor of Urological Surgery
Harvard Medical School
Boston, MA 02115

The continuing delay in the availability of effective
adjuvant therapy in renal cell carcinoma has encouraged the
trial of extended radical surgery in those cases that demonstrate involvement of the lumen of the vena cava, or the
adjacent liver parenchyma, the psoas muscle, intestinal wall
of the duodenum or colon, all by direct growth invasion.
Such non-metastatic involvement invites en bloc excision with
the distant hope of curing the patient and with the immediate
expectation of palliation from eliminating the bulky tumor.
Our personal experience of 15 years at 2 medical centers provides the basis for our retrospective conclusions.

PREOPERATIVE EVALUATION OF EXTENT OF TUMOR

The still-improving technology of computerized abdominal
tomographic (CAT) scanning is now the first and often the
only preoperative diagnostic procedure to define the local
direct extent of the tumor. If intact perirenal fat and a
normal vena cava (and often even a normal renal vein) are
shown, we proceed with surgery. The same test offers optimal
scanning of the liver and the lungs and less than adequate
definition of the retroperitoneal nodes.

Venography of the vena cava is added at our center only
if the CAT scan suggests widening of the cava or renal vein.
Both AP and lateral views must be obtained. At other centers,
routine use is made of a drip of intravenous contrast into a
leg vein during the CAT scan for renal masses. This technique
separates the caval lumen from adjacent soft tissue on the
tomograms.

Arteriography is no longer used in most cases. It becomes necessary and important when the CAT scan fails to define a separation between the kidney tumor and either liver or the psoas muscle. Parasitic hepatic and lumbar vessels can be defined supplying the tumor. In tumors with duodenal or colonic compression mesenteric angiography is similarly helpful.

The advent of computerized digital subtraction angiography which provides an outline of large vessels after intravenous contrast, may soon return to us the relative advantage of routine definition of the renal arteries without the invasiveness of arteriography. We have abandoned the use of preoperative embolization after concluding that the pain and the systemic fever, malaise, and anorexia complicated the patient's preoperative course and anesthesia tolerance to a degree that was not outweighed by the possible reduction in tumor bulk and intraoperative blood loss. While it is true that tumor extension into the caval lumen is supplied by end-branches of the renal artery and its bulk or protrusion might retract or "shrink" with embolization we worry that the surface tumor is kept alive by venous blood and central necrosis of the tumor "thrombus" may facilitate the breaking off of pieces of viable tumor from its surface. We are sure that in the cases of liver, bowel, or psoas involvement there is no role for embolization because of abundant parasitic collaterals in the critical area and, again, the increased danger of tumor breakage during surgery if some of its non-critical bulk is acutely necrotic.

INTRAOPERATIVE TECHNIQUES

Thoracoabdominal exposure is most valuable for large tumors, planning to cut across the costal margin at the 8th to 10th rib (depending on how cephalad the tumor extends) and to carry the diagonal part of the incision to the midline and then turn downward to below the umbilicus. The rectus is divided. The diaphragm is divided to the central tendon.

When the vena cava or the posterior surface of the liver is involved we expose and divide the small lower hepatic veins and we mobilize the liver towards the left side, by dividing the avascular peritoneal and diaphragmatic attachments of the right lobe and dome of the liver. The liver and right kidney thus can be rotated <u>en bloc</u> on the axis of the cava and three dimensional exposure of the tumor's extension is achieved. The renal artery is ligated in situ at its origin from the aorta early in the dissection.

Liver Invasion by Direct Extension

When the tumor is attached to the liver we will divide all other attachment's first and as a last step, with three-dimensional access, fracture across the right hepatic lobe in such a way as to minimize the raw cut surface to be left behind. Long blunt-typed needles threaded with large-caliber absorbable suture material are useful to place large horizontal mattresses sutures just deep to the cut liver edge. We have not had to dissect the porta hepatis for any of these cases - and have never had a bile fistula or significant delayed bleeding.

Vena Cava Extension

When the tumor intrudes into the lumen of the cava, without extension above the diaphragm, the right liver is mobilized from the diaphragm as described above and rotated to the left out of the way to expose the cava. Gentle palpation, and often direct incision through the semitransparent cava determines the portion of the cava well above the tumor. Being careful to spare the large superior hepatic vein, the cava is gently freed up enough to place a partially-occlusive plastic clip across it. Such clips are usually used for surgical prevention of pulmonary emboli. We use them transiently intraoperatively to prevent a disastrous large embolus of tumor during the dissection of the involved cava. Now again we free the tumorous kidney from all attachments first and free-up the cava and opposite renal vein more than enough to allow the exclusion of the tumor by cross clamping vascular clamps. If the tumor does not reach across the full lumen of the cava, so that the opposite wall is free of attachment of the tumor. Then we cross-clamp to avoid backflow and we incise the cava in a long elliptical incision, using Potts scissors and great care not to touch the intraluminal tumor. The specimen is then lifted out to take the vena caval extension en bloc with the renal tumor and the unopened renal vein, sacrificing only a cuff of free caval wall. The residual caval wall in situ is rolled up into a tube of decreased diameter, protecting the venous drainage of the opposite kidney. This technique applies to either right or left lesions protruding into the cava.

When the tumor <u>fills</u> the cava with complete obstruction and multiple collaterals are seen on the inferior vena cavagram, then a superior retrograde cavagram is done to define the upper end of the tumor in the cava lumen. The usual case of this sort is a right-sided tumor and the left renal vein has already developed collaterals. As a result it can be ligated with impunity and the entire trunk of cava removed, with its stuffing of tumor in a closed manner <u>en</u> <u>bloc</u> with the kidney. When the left kidney has tumor extending to fill the cava the right renal vein still drains superiorly and does not have as many collaterals available as the left. In the three such extensive left cases we have operated on, we have either preserved a free strip of the right side of the cava to keep the right renal vein in continuity with the upper cava (2 cases) or we interpose a free graft of superior mesenteric vein between the right renal vein and the portal vein (1 case).

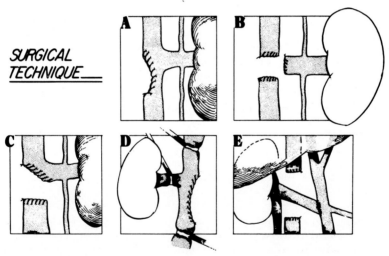

SURGICAL
TECHNIQUE___

Fig. 1 Surgical techniques used in inferior vena caval resection for renal cell carcinoma. A, venacavotomy with tumor extraction with open or closed technique - used for tumor originating in right kidney and extending to level of renal veins. B, ligation of left renal vein and inferior vena cava - done in cases with tumor on right side and extensive involvement at level of renal or lower hepatic veins. C, ligation of inferior vena cava distal to renal veins

with maintenance of continuity of left renal vein and proximal inferior vena cava – used for tumor originating in
right kidney with extensive involvement of inferior vena
cava at level of renal veins in non-collateralized patients.
D, venacavotomy with tumor extraction using open technique –
performed in cases with tumor originating in left kidney.
E, ligation of inferior vena cava with maintenance of venous
drainage of right kidney by renal vein-to-portal vein interposition graft – used in cases with tumor on left side and
extensive involvement of inferior vena cava.

When the tumor thrombus extends above the diaphragm and
into the right atrium we extend our incision higher in the
right chest and work with a cardiac surgeon keeping a bypass
pump team on standby. Rummel-type tourniquet tapes are
loosely placed around the cava above and below the hepatic
inflow. A Foley catheter with a 30 cc balloon is used to
draw back the entire thrombus still attached to the kidney
tumor. To accomplish that the catheter is slipped through
a purse-string suture in the free side wall of the cava above
the renal vein and advanced with care until the tip is in
the atrium. The hepatic inflow is controlled by the Pringle
maneuver (Pringle 1908; Yellin 1971) – placing a vascular
clamp transiently across the porta hepatis. The balloon is
filled and drawn back like an embolectomy balloon except
that it is done in tandem slowly while lifting out the kidney and the cuff of adherent cava just cut free. The blood
loss is still significant. Tumor fracture must be antici-
pated so that the Rummel clamps are tightened sequentially
during the tandem lift-out. Liver blood flow is restored
rapidly after the tumor is out – before the closure of the
cavotomy – and backflow controlled by the tourniquet just
above the cavotomy.

Intestinal Extension

Direct extension into the intestines – duodenum or
colon – is most unusual and indicates a very aggressive tumor
which is certain to reappear in lymph nodes or distant metastases. More likely to happen is a compromise of the vascularity of the colon which results in colonic ischemia when
a large tumor is resected and the mesenteric vessels damaged.
This is particularly likely to happen in the older patients

with vascular disease in whom the inferior mesenteric artery
may be involved intimately by the tumor but still be essential for appropriate perfusion of the sigmoid colon.

In any case in which the preoperative evaluation suggests
large tumor impinging on the intestine or on its mesentery,
preoperative preparation of the bowel as for large bowel
surgery should be carried out routinely. We use a 36 hour
regimen of Erythromycin and Neomycin by mouth along with
mechanical cleansing of the bowel.

The surgical technique of resection of an attached segment of bowel or of a window of mesentery involved by the
tumor is unremarkable. It should be mentioned that the peritoneum should always be opened primarily in these cases so
that any involvement of the posterior peritoneum and the
mesentery can be seen directly and the resection attempted
en bloc, avoiding the separation of the involved posterior
peritoneum and the tumor surface. The large thoracoabdominal
incision with primary entry into the perineal cavity is
important in these cases.

RESULTS

From the experience of this author and of various other
publications that have appeared recently (Abdelsayed 1978;
Scheft 1974; Beck 1977; Cole 1975) it is clear that the
results are not as dismal as they appeared from the very
extensive cases reviewed by Marshall (Marshall 1970) nor as
optimistic as the review of cases by Skinner (Skinner 1972).
The continuation of this author's personal series initially
reported in 1974 (McCullough 1974) of cases operated on with
a chance for cure, the 5 year survival is 25% (3/12). A
combined series made up of several surgeons with a larger
number was recently published (Kearney 1981) has a 5 year
survival of 16%.

Immediate mortality and morbidity for the operation
included one postoperative death (4%) and 6 cases requiring
temporary dialysis (25%). The dialysis was temporary in all
of them, with the maximum duration of 6 weeks.

The long term results for invasion of the liver or the
bowel are quite unfavorable, as expected. There were no
survivors in a personal series of 6 cases with liver invasion

and only one survivor (8%) in a combined series of 12 cases. In a combined series of 9 cases of bowel invasion (4 to the duodenum, 5 to the colon wall) there were no 5 year survivors.

DISCUSSION

Vena cava invasion remains potentially curable by en bloc resection but the long term survival is overall probably less than 20%. Skinner's survival of 6 of 11 patients with vena cava involvement (55%) in a retrospective series did not itemize the level of involvement as we did for our combined series (Kearney 1981) and may have been skewed in terms of the number of patients with involvement at the insertion of the renal vein only.

Excellent palliation with minimum mortality and morbidity is afforded by the radical procedure that involves resection of the vena cava. In the absence of effective adjuvant chemotherapy, such radical surgery will remain advisable in patients who are good surgical risks.

Invasion of the liver or the bowel, either duodenum or colon, represents a dismal prognostic factor. It must be presumed that some palliation is afforded by the nephrectomy that includes the effected bowel. These cases are usually demonstrated to have the invasion of the bowel only at the operating table and if the patient has had a previous bowel preparation, resection of a small piece of bowel is a small added burden in return for the palliation of removing the large primary tumor. Clearly long term cure is not a realistic goal when the disease demonstrates such aggressive behavior with invasion of the liver or the bowel.

SUMMARY

Review of a personal and combined experience in cases of renal cell carcinoma invading the vena cava, liver, or bowel, has been carried out. The methodology in each of these situations is described.

The long term results for survival after vena cava invasion are less than 20% at 5 years - lower than previous optimistic estimates. The long term survival with invasion of the liver or bowel is negligible. However, excellent palliation is achieved and the urological surgeon should be prepared to carry out the additional resection of adjacent invaded liver or bowel to achieve palliative nephrectomy in such cases when the invasion is found at the operating table.

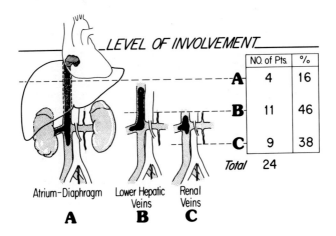

	NO. of Pts.	%
A	4	16
B	11	46
C	9	38
Total	24	

Fig. 2   Levels of tumor extension in inferior vena cava and number of patients in this series with tumor at various levels.

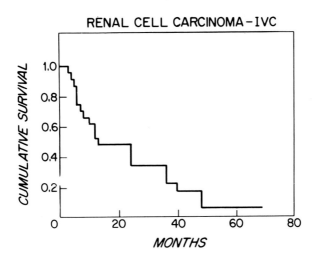

Fig. 3   Cumulative survival of 24 patients who underwent removal of renal cell carcinoma from inferior vena cava.

Abdelsayed MA, Bissada NK, Finkbeiner AE, Redman JF (1978).
Renal tumors involving the inferior vena cava: plan for
management. J Urol 120:153.

Beck AD (1977). Renal cell carcinoma involving the inferior
vena cava: Radiologic evaluation and surgical management. J Urol 118:533.

Cole AT, Julian WA, Fried FA (1975). Aggressive surgery for
renal cell carcinoma with vena cava tumor thrombus.
Urology 6:227.

Duckett JW, Lifland JH, Peters PC (1973). Resection of the
inferior vena cava for adjacent malignant diseases.
Surg Gynecol Obstet 136:711.

Esho JO, Owoseni AA (1977). Vena cava resection with renal
cell carcinoma. Eur Urol 3:111.

Freed SZ, Gliedman ML (1975). The removal of renal carcinoma
thrombus extending into the right atrium. J Urol 113:
163.

Gleason DM, Reilly RJ, Anderson RM, O'Hara JE, Kartchner MM,
Komar NN (1972). Removal of hypernephroma and inferior
vena cava. Arch Surg 105:795.

Goldstein HM, Green B, Weaver RM (1978). Ultrasonic detection of renal tumor extension into the inferior vena cava.
Am J Roentgenol 130:1083.

Kearney GP, Waters WB, Klein LA, Richie JP, Gittes RF (1981).
Results of inferior vena cava resection for renal cell
carcinoma. J Urol 125:769.

Lome LG, Bush IM (1972). Resection of the vena cava for
renal cell carcinoma: an experimental study. J Urol 107:
717.

Marks WM, Korobkin M, Callen PW, Kaiser JA (1978). CT
diagnosis of tumor thrombosis of the renal vein and
inferior vena cava. Am J Roentgenol 131:843.

Marshall VF, Middleton RG, Holswade GR, Goldsmith EI (1970).
Surgery for renal cell carcinoma in the vena cava. J
Urol 103:414.

McCullough DL, Gittes RF (1974). Vena cava resection for
renal cell carcinoma. J Urol 112:162.

Pathak IC (1971). Survival after right nephrectomy, excision
of intrahepatic vena cava and ligation of left renal vein:
a case report. J Urol 106:599.

Paul JG, Rhodes DB, Skow JR (1975). Renal cell carcinoma
presenting as right atrial tumor with successful removal
using cardiopulmonary bypass. Ann Surg 181:471.

Pringle JH (1908). Notes on the arrest of hepatic hemorrhage
due to trauma. Ann Surg 48:541.

Schefft P, Novick AC, Straffon RA, Stewart BH (1977). Surgery for renal cell carcinoma extending into the inferior vena cava. J Urol 120:28.

Skinner DG, Pfister RF, Colvin R (1972). Extension of renal cell carcinoma into the vena cava: the rationale for aggressive surgical management. J Urol 107:711.

Yellin AE, Chaffee CB, Donovan AJ (1971). Vascular isolation in treatment of juxtahepatic venous injuries. Arch Surg 102:566.

Renal Tumors: Proceedings of the First International Symposium on Kidney Tumors, pages 509–517
© **1982 Alan R. Liss, Inc., 150 Fifth Avenue, New York, NY 10011**

BENCH SURGERY IN RENAL TUMORS

Ruben F. Gittes, M.D.

Professor of Urological Surgery
Harvard Medical School
Boston, MA 02115

Extracorporeal or "bench" surgery developed as a logical extension of renal transplantation and autotransplantation, with pioneering contributions by Gelin and Calne (1,2). This author has used it in highly selected cases in the past 10 years, only in renal cell carcinoma.

INDICATIONS

Only large or multicentric renal adenocarcinoma in a functionally solitary kidney constitutes a clear indication for bench surgery. It is illustrative to tabulate this author's experience with tumors of the solitary kidney, cases without demonstrable metastases in which surgery was done for cure. Of 25 such patients only 7 had bench surgery.

Table 1.   Selection of Operation in Tumors of the Solitary
Kidney Treated for Cure (1970-1980)*

	Tumor Histology	
	Adenocarcinoma	Transitional Cell
In-situ Partial Nx	8	9
Extracorporeal Surg.	7	0
Total Nephrectomy	1	0

*Author's personal series

And all eight with transitional cell carcinoma were managed in situ: with exclusion of the affected calyx and nephroscopic exam of the residual calyces. Bench surgery is an alternative

to nephrectomy and dialysis for those patients whose tumors
have an indistinct central margin, in whom dissection is
likely to cut across a tumor margin. On the bench the pathologist can check margins and the chance of gross spillage
of tumor into the renal bed is eliminated. Not included in
this review are palliative cases done to preserve residual
renal function in the presence of known metastases.

TECHNIQUE

A small adjustable-height instrument stand (Mayo stand)
is the "bench". It is attached to the edge of the incision
after the kidney is freed up except for its vessels and the
ureter (Figure 1). The main artery or arteries are divided
close to the aorta and the renal vein right at the cava.
The kidney is lifted onto the "bench" and a soft cannula
already connected to a suspended ice-cold bottle of a high-
potassium, intra-cellular type solution (Gittes, McCullough

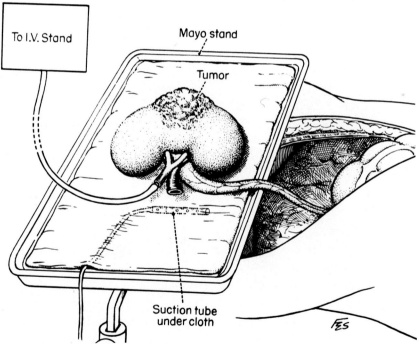

FIGURE 1. "Bench" technique. Kidney is cooled by gravity
perfusion. Retrograde vascular supply of ureter is maintained.

1975) is hand held in the artery and then tied in place for
the duration of the ex-vivo dissection. The effluent from
the vein(s) is not recirculated, but drawn off by suction.
With constant orientation from the angiogram, the perirenal
fat is dissected away from the normal portions of the kidney
and left attached to the surface of the tumorous part. When
palpation and direct vision outline the limits of the tumor,
the arterial and venous branches are carefully identified
in the renal hilus. Those identified as feeding the tumor
are directly injected with indigo carmine or methylene blue
due to confirm their identification. Venous branches from
the tumor are ligated in situ and may require longitudinal
excision of part of the main renal vein if tumor is protruding into it from a branch. Repair of veins is done with
running 6-0 proline suture.

Then the normal parenchyma is transected at a 0.5 to
1 cm distance from the edge of the tumor and the contour of
the tumor or tumors is followed by sharp dissection within
tissue which is putatively and grossly visible as normal.
Either a large crater is left behind in the side of the kidney, or a full thickness wedge of the kidney containing the
isolated tumor is removed and polar remnants with intact
blood supply remain to be repaired and joined together. Fine
catgut or polyglycollic sutures (6-0) are used to close any
calyces opened. The kidney is reimplanted with the ureter
having been kept intact, into the pelvic vessels in the manner used for a kidney transplant except that the remnant is
inverted to place the vessels posteriorly (Figure 2). The
ureter is carefully inspected for any ischemic damage and
to insure a gentle curvature without obstruction. The patient
may require postoperative dialysis support for temporary ATN -
but most have not.

The pathologist has ample time to confirm that the edges
of excised tissue are free of tumor invasion. In two cases
the pathological exam during the case suggested the need for
excision of additional margin of normal kidney.

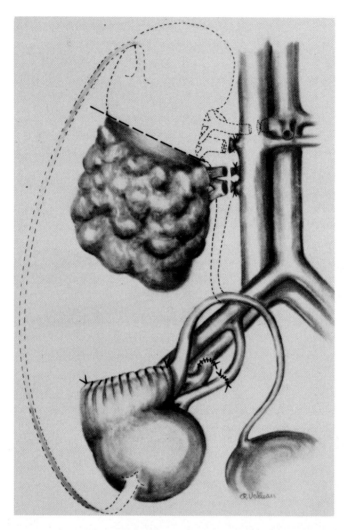

FIGURE 2. Inversion maneuver for ipsilateral autotransplantation of renal remnant after "bench" surgery. The renal vessels are thus placed posteriorly next to the recipient vessels and the intact ureter makes a gentle hairpin turn anteriorly.

RESULTS

Numbers are sparse because of the limited indications. Only 7 of our 25 operations for tumor in solitary kidney were on the "bench". Our own 7 cases are tabulated in Table 2. We have not lost a patient from local recurrence or from metastatic disease.

Table 2. Extracorporeal Renal Surgery for Adenocarcinoma
        (1970-1980)

Total cases	7
Age range	42-74
Deaths	1
(74 yo diabetic c̄ sepsis at 1 mo)	
Distant mets	1
(lung nodule excised 1977)	
Living with no evidence of tumor	6
Follow up (yrs)	2-10

One case did demonstrate a solitary pulmonary metastases in 1977, 3 years after bench surgery. It was removed and no further tumor has appeared.

Another case (CB) had a second tumor appear in the substance of the autotransplanted renal remnant, well demonstrated by CT tomography and poorly by angiography. It was removed by repeated bench surgery 3½ years after the first. A third tumor, separate in its location and subcapsular, appeared 5 years after the first and was removed by in situ excision with renal cooling (Figure 3).

One patient died of sepsis and secondary renal failure 1 month after bench surgery. He was the oldest attempted at 74 years of age and a diabetic. All others are alive and putatively free of tumor (84%). One is a 10 year survivor and 2 others are 8 and 7 years respectively.

DISCUSSION

Various authors have added to the early case reports of surgery for tumor in the solitary kidney (Gittes, McCullough 1975; Puigvert 1976; Gil Vernet 1975; Palmer 1978; Straffon 1980). Many cases are well suited for in situ surgery, either simple polar amputation (Puivert 1976) or by

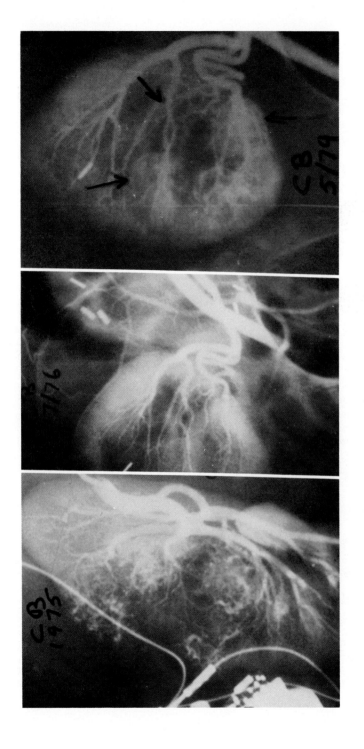

FIGURE 3. (A) Angiogram of solitary kidney in 1975 showing a large vascular tumor. (B) Angiogram after the first bench procedure demonstrating that the renal remnant is free of the vascular tumor. (C) Angiogram in 1979 demonstrating the presence of a new lesion in the renal cortex of the remnant.

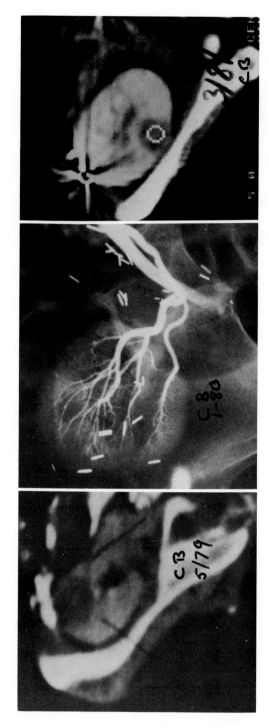

FIGURE 3. (D) CAT scan in 1979 showing the anterior location of the new lesion and the feasibility of repeat "bench" surgery. (E) Angiogram 6 months after repeat bench surgery with repeat autotransplantation. (F) CAT scan of 3/81 with yet another small renal cell carcinoma. This one is well defined and superficial and was removed <u>in situ</u> with cooling.

in situ clamping of the pedicle and cooling as used for staghorn surgery (Straffon 1980). We agree that the bloodless field achieved with clamping and cooling in situ is adequate for well-defined cortical tumors that do not encroach on the renal sinus. Such tumors can be excavated from the under-lying cortex without need to dissect any hilar vessels and with minimal risk of tumor spillage.

But large tumors replacing one half of the kidney or its mid portion require hilar dissection of vessels and carry a high risk of inadvertent transection of tumor margin. By careful dissection, with optimal exposure and ample time for repair of the remnant and with the security of being able to avoid tumor spillage in the patient if tumor is transected during the dissection, highly selected cases have been successfully treated and apparently cured. These would otherwise have required nephrectomy and dialysis, not an easy alternative. Since we are not paying a price of local or wound recurrence, the experience encourages further appli-cation of the technique for palliation in solitary kidneys with metastases and possibly the increased use of "en bloc" partial nephrectomy in non-solitary kidneys in propitious cases with peripheral polar lesions.

SUMMARY

Extracorporeal or "bench" surgery is useful in highly selected cases of renal cell carcinoma in a solitary kidney, those with large tumors involving the center third of the kidney or multiple tumors. This author reports on its use in 7 patients out of 25 operated for cure for tumor in a solitary kidney. Except for 1 postoperative non-cancer death, all are now alive and free of tumor between 2 and 10 years after surgery.

Calne RY (1971). Tumor in a single kidney: nephrectomy, excision and autotransplantation. Lancet p. 761.

Gelin E, Goran C, Gustafsson A, Bengt S (1971). Bloodlessness for extracorporeal organ repair. Rev Surg 28:305.

Gil-Vernet JM, Caralps A, Revert L, Andreu J, Carretero P, Figuls J (1975). Extracorporeal renal surgery. Urology 5:444.

Gittes RF, McCullough DL (1975). Bench surgery for tumor in a solitary kidney. J Urol 113:12.

Novick AC, Stewart BH, Straffon RA (1980). Extracorporeal renal surgery and autotransplantation: indications, techniques and results. J Urol 123:806.

Palmer JM, Swanson DA (1978). Conservative surgery in solitary and bilateral renal carcinoma: indications and technical considerations. 120:113.

Puigvert A (1976). Partial nephrectomy for renal tumor: 21 cases. Eur Urol 2:70.

Renal Tumors: Proceedings of the First International Symposium on
Kidney Tumors, pages 519–527

CONSERVATIVE SURGERY IN RENAL CELL CARCINOMA

René Küss

Clinique Urologique, Hôpital de la Pitié

Paris, France

The optimal surgical treatment for renal cell carcinoma
is radical nephrectomy because renal function is satisfactorily
maintained by the other kidney. However, this is not always
the case, as when the neoplasm develops in a solitary kidney,
or, obviously, in the case of a bilateral tumor, noted in
1.5 to 3% of cases (Krumbach, Ansell 1959; Novick et al, 1977;
Shaad et al, 1970; Small et al, 1968; Steg et al, 1969; Svab
1956; Wickham 1965). In these cases, partial nephrectomy or
tumorectomy may appear as a viable solution. While this may
not be in keeping with strictly orthodox views on cancer
surgery, it is justified on the basis of the particular
nature of renal cell carcinoma and the good results achieved.
The following features of renal cell carcinoma help to make
partial surgery possible:

1. The lesion usually develops near the renal
    cortex, far removed from the hilum.

2. It is frequently well encapsulated and can
    therefore be shelled out.

3. In 60-70% the lesion is localized at one
    kidney pole. This is extremely favorable
    to partial nephrectomy.

4. Renal function can be maintained at normal
    or near normal limits when only 20% of the
    nephron is present.

Partial nephrectomy has been further enhanced by the development of new diagnostic methods such as selective arteriography and CT scanning, which permitted more precise definition of tumor extension. Also of importance was the development of new operative techniques such as pedicle clumping or kidney cooling, with the concomitant use of mannitol, frusemide or dopamine. Another important development was bench surgery and implantation of the kidney once the tumor has been removed.

The development of partial surgery resembles that of renal dialysis in some respects. Between 1950 and 1960, 21 cases were reported in the literature; between 1960 and 1970 there were 83; since 1970 more than 218 cases have been reported. Temporary dialysis may be required after surgery, and in very rare cases involving localized problems such as haemorrhage, infarction, or extension, permanent dialysis may be needed (Goldstein, Abeshouse 1937; Küss, Guillou 1972).

Indications

Partial surgery in renal cell carcinoma can be considered as an acceptable alternative when the tumor is bilateral, or when it presents in a solitary kidney. This type of surgery is contraindicated in very old patients and those in poor general health. It is well known that renal cell neoplasm grows slowly. If there is tumor extension, that is, if the tumor has become locally invasive outside the kidney, if it has invaded adjacent lymph nodes, or if it involves more than 50% of the renal parenchyma, then this surgery is contraindicated. Similarly, this procedure is not indicated when there are multiple metastases. Such contraindications may be present in 30-50% of cases (Malek et al, 1976; Novick et al, 1977; Wickham 1975).

In terms of the operation itself, either a hemi-nephrectomy can be performed or a wedge nephrectomy if the tumor is situated in the middle of the kidney. The choice here depends on the clinical state ascertained either before or during the procedure. In cases of bilateral tumor, a bilateral partial nephrectomy can be carried out, or a unilateral nephrectomy with a contralateral partial nephrectomy. The presence of a solitary metastasis is not a contraindication if it can be treated surgically.

When local extension is not amenable to partial resection the alternatives are no treatment in the hope that the growth will expand slowly, selective arterial embolization and radical nephrectomy and dialysis. Renal transplantation is not considered in patients in whom immunosuppressive treatment can accelerate the developemnt of metastases which otherwise may remain quiescent (Personal case, 1960).

RESULTS AND PERSONAL EXPERIENCE

Between 1961 and 1977, we carried out 19 partial nephrectomies for renal cell neoplasm. Of these, 13 were for lesions of solitary kidneys, and five were for bilateral tumors. In one case, partial nephrectomy was carried out on a lesion, thought to be tuberculous, which turned out to be neoplastic (Table 1). The survival rates for this group are as follows:

Two patients have survived more than ten years.
Seven patients have survived more than two years.
Four patients for more than one year.
Three patients died in the first six months following surgery.
Three other deaths occurred at two and one-half years, three years and five months, and five years.

The three year survival rate is 68%.

Review of the Literature

In a review of 148 cases followed since 1965, it was shown that there had been a fall in the operative mortality from 4-7% in 1967 to between 1.5 and 3% (Novick et al, 1977). Long term results appear to be favorable. The three-year survival is estimated between 45% and 56%, and the five-year survival between 33% and 48% (Kaufmann et al, 1968). This is similar to the overall survival rate for renal cell carcinoma treated by radical nephrectomy, but the comparison really is invalid, since partial surgery is done only in cases where cancer is limited to the kidney (Stage I).

A further comparison was made between patients having had a partial nephrectomy for renal cell carcinoma on a

TABLE 1

CLINICAL DATA ON 19 PARTIAL NEPHRECTOMY CASES BETWEEN 1961 AND 1977

Case No.:	1	2	3	4	5
Age:	26	61	54	70	54
Condition of Opposite Kidney	Normal	Nephrectomy for T.B. 15 years earlier	Agenesia	Nephrectomy for lithiasis 11 years earlier	Nephrectomy for cancer 12 years earlier
Surgery	Partial nephrectomy	Partial nephrectomy	Partial nephrectomy	Shelling out of lesion	Partial nephrectomy
Date	11/10/61	09/21/67	12/16/68	03/28/71	01/23/75
Pathology	Adeno-carcinoma	Adeno-carcinoma	Adeno-carcinoma	Leiomyo-sarcoma	Adeno-carcinoma
Adjuvant	0	0	Testosterone chemotherapy	0	0
Survival	Living without metastases 20 years	Living without metastases 14 years and 2 months	Dead - Lung metastases at 41 months	Dead - cerebral vas. acc. at 5 months	Dead at 5 years with brain metastases

TABLE 1 - continued

CLINICAL DATA ON 19 PARTIAL NEPHRECTOMY CASES BETWEEN 1961 AND 1977

Case No.:	6	7	8	9	10
Age:	73	73	58	53	72
Condition of Opposite Kidney	Simultaneous bilateral cancer	Nephrectomy for lithiasis 40 years later	Agenesis	Simultaneous bilateral cancer	Nephrectomy for cancer 7 years later
Surgery	Partial nephrectomy	Partial nephrectomy	Partial nephrectomy	Shelling out of lesion + radical nephrectomy with caval thromb.	Shelling out of lesion
Date	03/26/75	05/23/75	10/05/76	10/05/76	04/08/77
Pathology	Adeno-carcinoma	Adeno-carcinoma	Adeno-carcinoma	Adeno-carcinoma	Adeno-carcinoma
Adjuvant	0	0	0	0	Progesterone
Survival	Dead with metastases at 30 months	Dead of scepticemia and pulmonary embolism at 17 days	Living without metastases 5 years and 5 months	Living without metastases 5 years	Living without metastases 4 years

TABLE 1 - continued

CLINICAL DATA ON 19 PARTIAL NEPHRECTOMY CASES BETWEEN 1961 AND 1977

Case No.:	11	12	13	14	15
Age:	76	64	39	51	72
Condition of Opposite Kidney	Simultaneous bilateral cancer	Agenesia	Simultaneous bilateral cancer	Nephrectomy for cancer 4 years earlier	Agenesia
Surgery	Shelling out of lesion + radical nephrectomy	Partial nephrectomy	Shelling out of lesion + radical nephrectomy	Shelling out of lesion	Shelling out of lesion
Date	10/03/78	05/31/78	09/28/78	02/01/79	04/03/79
Pathology	Adeno-carcinoma	Adeno-carcinoma	Adeno-carcinoma	Adeno-carcinoma	Adeno-carcinoma
Adjuvant	Progesterone	0	0	Progesterone	0
Survival	Living without metastases 2 years	Dead at 6 days pulmonary embolism	Living without metastases 3 years	Living 30 months but radical nephrectomy I. 1981 for reduction	Living without metastases 30 months

TABLE 1 - continued

CLINICAL DATA ON 19 PARTIAL NEPHRECTOMY CASES BETWEEN 1961 AND 1977

Case No.:	16	17	18	19
Age:	59	58	68	81
Condition of Opposite Kidney	Agenesia	Agenesia	Simultaneous bilateral cancer	Deficient
Surgery	Partial nephrectomy	Shelling out lesion	Partial nephrectomy + radical nephrectomy	Shelling out of lesion
Date	02/03/80	07/16/80	08/26/80	03/25/81
Pathology	Adeno-carcinoma	Adeno-carcinoma	Adeno-carcinoma	Adeno-carcinoma
Adjuvant	0	0	0	0
Survival	Living without metastases 18 months	Living without metastases 15 months	Living without metastases 12 months	Living without metastases 7 months

solitary kidney, the other kidney being either congenitally
absent or removed because of a benign lesion, and patients
who had a radical nephrectomy for a renal cell carcinoma
less than 5 cm in diameter. There was no significant
difference between the two groups (Novick et al, 1977;
Wickham 1975). For this reason, some urologists have
extended the indication for partial nephrectomy to cover
cases of renal carcinoma in which the other kidney is present,
and functioning (Babics; Puigvert 1969; Szendroi, Babics
1955; Vermooten 1950). We do not share this view.

In conclusion, we consider that patients who have a
renal cell carcinoma on a solitary kidney or who have
bilateral tumors should not be regarded as "untouchable".
The treatment of choice is resection of the tumor. Their
survival rate is nearly the same as that of patients of the
same stage undergoing radical nephrectomy.

REFERENCES

Babics A. Directeur de la Clinique d'Urologie de Budapest.
    Communication personnelle.
Goldstein AE, Abeshouse BS (1937). Partial resection of
    the kidney. Report of 6 cases and review of the literature.
    J Urol 38:15.
Krumbach RW, Ansell JS (1959). Partial resection of the
    right kidney and radical removal of the left kidney in a
    patient with bilateral hypernephroma. Surgery 45:585.
Küss R, Le Guillou M (1972). Chirurgie conservatrice dans
    les cancers du rein de l'adulte. A propos de 5 observations
    personnelles. J Urol Nephrol 7-8:599.
Malek RS, Utz DC, Culp GS (1976). Hypernephroma in the
    solitary kidney: experience with 20 cases and review of
    the literature. J Urol 116: 553.
Novick AC, Stewart BH, Straffon RA, Banowsky LM (1977).
    Partial nephrectomy in the treatment of renal adenocarcinoma.
    J Urol 118:932.
Puigvert A (1969). Chirurgie conservatrice dans les tumeurs
    de l'appareil urinaire superieur. Lyon chir 65:285.
Schaad P, Brizard CP, Bonnet C (1970). Tumeur de Grawitz
interessant les deux reins, traitee en un seul temps par
    nephrectomie gauche elargie et nephrectomie droite partielle.
    Bull Mem Soc Chir Paris 60:302.
Small MP, Everett Anderson E, Atmill WH (1968). Simultaneous
    bilateral renal cell carcinoma case report and review of the

literature. J Urol 8:100.

Steg A, Benassayag E, Gallan Ph (1969). Cancer du rein bilateral. Nephrectomie elargie droite et nephrectomie partielle gauche en un temps. Ann Urol 3:211.

Svab J (1956). Zewi Seltene falle von Neirengeschwulstein: Kasuistischer Beitrag zur Gravwitzschen geschwulst in solitarer niere and zu den Beiderseitigen nieren geschwulsten. Z Urol Nephrol 49:241.

Szendroi, Babics A (1955). Urologia 22:1.

Vermooten V (1950). Indication for conservative surgery in certain renal tumors. A study based on the growth pattern of the clear cell carcinoma. J Urol 64:200.

Wickham JEA (1975). Conservative renal surgery for adeno-carcinoma. The place of bench surgery. Br J Urol 47:25.

Renal Tumors: Proceedings of the First International Symposium on Kidney Tumors, pages 529–531
© **1982 Alan R. Liss, Inc., 150 Fifth Avenue, New York, NY 10011**

RENAL CELL CARCINOMA EXTENDING INTO THE INFERIOR VENA CAVA.
TECHNICAL PROBLEMS.

J. Cinqualbre, J.M.PY, C. Bollack

Department of Urology (Pr Claude Bollack)
Hôpital Central, 67005 Cedex Strasbourg, France

Renal adenocarcinoma very often develops in the venous
system. Even in cases where the extension reaches the inferior vena cava or surpasses it, the long-term prognosis
is not significantly altered, provided that resection of
the neoplastic tissue is complete. Our purpose is to
present the technical surgical aspects, without discussing
indications, based on a personal series of 12 cases
including:

> 5 cases where the neoplastic bud extended
> to the inferior (infra-hepatic or retro-
> hepatic) vena cava
> 4 cases of complete obstruction of the
> inferior vena cava where a right angio-
> cardiography determined the upper limit
> to be in the auricle
> 3 cases of a floating thrombus extending
> into the right auricle.

There were no operative mortalities. Three out of
twelve patients died half a year or more post surgically:
one, after six months, of acute hepatic insufficiency,
probably from post-transfusional hepatitis, and the two
others after six and nine months, of generalised metastasis.
The remaining nine patients are still alive with one to
three years of follow-up.

Based on this experience, we herein discuss several
technical aspects related to the surgical procedures
performed.

The surgical approach

Instead of a thoraco-phrenolaparotomy, we advocate an abdominal approach, through a subcostal incision, patient tolerance to which is much better both during surgery and in the post-operative period.

Vascular control

Arterial control by preoperative renal embolisation is systematic. Venous control must be complete and includes the renal vein on the healthy side and on the pathological side, the hepatic pedicle (Pringle manoeuver), and control of the infra-renal and supra-hepatic inferior vena cava. Regarding the latter, it is occasionally difficult and dangerous to control the inferior vena cava downstream from the tumour under the liver. In the same way, it appears to be excessive to open the pericardium. For our part, we achieved in all cases supra-hepatic, but sub-diaphragmatic control, according to the technique developed by Starzl for hepatic transplantations.

Inferior vena cava resection

Resection of the inferior vena cava wall is always limited. Neoplastic adhesions stick together easily and either a simple lateral resection or a larger resection with plasti between the inferior vena cava and the renal vein remaining on the unaffected side can be achieved. This re-establishment of continuity is imperative if the right kidney stays in place; the procedure is optional if it concerns the left kidney.

Correction of haemodynamic disorders

A severe collapse was observed when the vena cava was clamped, particularly when the bud was not obstructive, because there was no collateral circulation. The manoeuver suppresses all the return from the inferior limbs and splanchnic vessels and is accompanied by an 80% reduction in venous return to the heart. A massive compensation only provokes an increase in the central venous pressure, without avoiding a significant drop in arterial blood pressure. We find it very effective to coordinate the clamping of the aorta above the iliac bifurcation, excluding the inferior limbs and therefore ensuring in all cases the restoration of a satisfactory arterial pressure.

In conclusion, discovery of an extension of a renal cell carcinoma should no longer be reason to preclude therapy. Surgery is not always easy, but it should remain simple, notably by a strict abdominal approach, systematic control of the distal vena cava above the liver and by the prevention of collapse during surgery, which relies as much on an adequate vascular filling as on the aortic clamping.

Renal Tumors: Proceedings of the First International Symposium on
Kidney Tumors, pages 533–540
© 1982 Alan R. Liss, Inc., 150 Fifth Avenue, New York, NY 10011

IS RADICAL NEPHRECTOMY USEFUL WHEN METASTASES ARE PRESENT?

C. Chatelain

Clinique Urologique, Hôpital de la Pitié,
Paris

From 1968 to 1978, 222 patients with a renal cell
carcinoma underwent surgical treatment at our Center. Within this group 76 (34.2%) patients had clinically demonstrable
metastatic disease at the time of initial diagnosis (Table 1).
For the purpose of our analysis, the 76 patients were
divided in two groups. Group I was comprised of 8 patients
whose tumors were considered unresectable at laparatomy.
There were 68 patients in Group II in whom the primary
tumor was removed by radical nephrectomy.

RESULTS

Evaluation of Group I. There were eight patients in this
group with unresectable primary tumor. These patients
had extensive local disease with wide spread metastasis.
Their survival was poor. Two died in the immediate postoperative period. Five died in less than 6 months from
disseminated metastasis and only one survived one year
(Table 2).

Evaluation of Group II. The 68 patients in this group
underwent radical nephrectomy. The operative mortality
rate was 5.8%. This rate is higher than the overall
mortality rate for all our radical nephrectomies. Four
patients were lost for follow-up and 60 patients were
followed and reported in this study (Table 3). Survival
was better in cases with solitary metastasis than when
multiple metastasis were present. Thirty patients had
multiple metastasis at diagnosis. Survival is summarized
by Table 4. Fifty-six of the patients died before 6 months,

90% died before 2 years and only 3 patients survived between 2 and 3 years.

Thirty patients had a solitary metastasis (Table 5). Thirty-three per cent were dead within the first 2 years after radical nephrectomy. The other cases survived between 2 and 7 years. Six patients were still alive with a follow-up period of 3 to 6 years. One patient who had a metastasis to the thyroid gland died 7 years after nephrectomy from brain metastases.

A solitary bony metastasis was the most frequent in our series and the prognosis was relatively favourable. Out of 11 patients with solitary bony metastasis, only 1 died before 1 year. Six survived between 2 and 6 years and 4 are still alive with a follow-up extending from 3.5 to 6 years.

Solitary metastases were resected surgically in 15 of our 30 patients. In the remaining 15 patients, the solitary metastasis was not operated upon either because multiple metastasis appeared quickly after diagnosis (especially when the solitary lesion was in the lungs) or because the lesions were considered completely asymptomatic and stable. Table 6 indicates that surgical treatment of solitary metastasis did not influence survival significantly.

DISCUSSION

We asked ourselves whether radical nephrectomy should be performed in presence of metastasis. A randomized prospective study comparing the survival of patients with metastatic renal cell carcinoma who either had their primary tumor removed or left in situ is ethically difficult to justify and has not been performed. Nevertheless, in our series, patients with multiple metastasis have such a poor prognosis that one can safely assume that radical nephrectomy had no significant effect on survival.

However, in the presence of multiple metastasis, radical nephrectomy may be justified in rare cases where control of local symptoms (pain or hematuria) is necessary.

Spontaneous regression of metastasis following radical nephrectomy is quite infrequent and justification of nephrectomy purely in hope of spontaneous regression of metastatic disease is difficult to defend in view of an operative mortality rate in this group of 5.3%.

Things are different in the case of solitary metastasis. These patients have a relatively long life expectency (Table 5). The early deaths in our series occurred in patients with lung metastasis which were presumed to be solitary but were in fact multiple. Survival depends also on the site of metastasis. Patients with bony metastasis had the longest survival. All our patients with solitary bony metastasis except one lived more than 2 years. The results of the treatment of the solitary metastasis itself when present at the time of radical nephrectomy are still to be defined. If we compare a group of 15 patients in our series who had their solitary metastasis excised with another group of 15 patients in whom solitary metastases were not treated, we found no difference in survival (Table 6), though no firm conclusion could be drawn from this retrospective study and we continue to remove solitary metastasis whenever it is technically possible. In conclusion, we believe that we can say that in case of metastasis, radical nephrectomy is justified only if a solitary metastasis is present and when therapy is directed at controlling local symptoms, providing emotional support to the patient, and reducing tumor bulk as part of a controlled clinical trial using chemotherapy or immunotherapy.

Table 1 STAGING OF 222 PATIENTS WITH RENAL CELL CARCINOMA
OPERATED AT CLINIQUE UROLOGIQUE DE L'HOPITAL DE LA PITIE.

CLASSIFICATION *

Stage I (kidney)	53

Stage II (Perinephric fat)	24

Stage III

A	(RV and IVC)	38
B	(Nodes)	5
C	(V + N)	<u>11</u>
		54

Stage IV

A	(local)	15
B	(Metastasis)	<u>76</u>
		91

* C. Robson

Table 2 SURVIVAL OF 8 PATIENTS HAVING METASTATIS RENAL CELL
CARCINOMA WITH UNRESECTABLE PRIMARY TUMOR

Post-operative death	2
Death in less than 6 months	5
Death in one year	1

Table 3 60 PATIENTS WITH METASTATIC RENAL CELL CARCINOMA
HAVING RADICAL NEPHRECTOMY AND FOLLOW-UP

Multiple Metastases	30
Single Metastasis	30

Table 4 SURVIVAL* OF 30 PATIENTS WITH MULTIPLE METASTASES AFTER RADICAL NEPHRECTOMY

SITE	DEAD				LIVING
	6 months	6 to 11 Months	12 to 23 months	2 years and more	
Lungs	4	1		2 years 3 years	
Liver		1			
Brain	2	1			
Bone	3	1	1	2 years	0
Other	1				
Plurivisceral	7	3	2		
TOTAL	17	7	3	3	0

*90% were dead before 2 years

Table 5   SURVIVAL OF 30 PATIENTS WITH SINGLE METASTASIS AFTER RADICAL NEPHRECTOMY

SITE	DEAD				LIVING
	6 months	6 to 11 months	12 to 23 months	2 years and more	
Lungs	3	2		2 years 2 years 2 years 3 months	5 years
Liver			1		
Brain			2	5 years	4 years 1/2
Bone		1		2 years (x3) 4 years 4 years 6 years	3 years 1/2 4 years (x2) 6 years
Other	1		1	2 years 1/2 5 years 7 years	
TOTAL	4	3	4	13	6

Table 6 COMPARISON OF SURVIVAL BETWEEN 15 PATIENTS WITH SINGLE METASTASIS WHETHER THE METASTASIS WAS SURGICALLY TREATED OR NOT

Metastasis	DEAD				LIVING
	6 months	6 to 11 months	12 to 23 months	2 years and more	
Treated (N=15)	1		4	7	3
Nontreated (N=15)	3	3		6	3

Renal Tumors: Proceedings of the First International Symposium on
Kidney Tumors, pages 541–547
© 1982 Alan R. Liss, Inc., 150 Fifth Avenue, New York, NY 10011

THE TREATMENT OF METASTASIS FROM RENAL CELL CARCINOMA

Saad Khoury, M.D.
Clinique Urologique, Hôpital de al Pitié
Paris, France

The presence of metastasis in patients with renal cell
carcinoma is sometimes a difficult and challenging therapeutic
problem. As a matter of fact, these lesions are frequent;
30% of the patients have metastasis at diagnosis, and 95%
at post mortem (Tolia, Whitmore 1975). They are compatible
sometimes with a relatively long survival, the average being
nine months. Metastases occur in relatively young patients,
the mean age being 56 years. These lesions are frequently
associated with symptoms and pain that may force the
clinicians to adopt a therapeutic attitude even if it is
palliative

The distribution of metastasis in renal cancer is given
in Tables 1 and 2. Note that at post mortem the incidence
of metastasis increased from 30% to 95% of the cases. The
distribution of metastasis also varies. In particular, liver
metastasis increases from 8% at diagnosis to 39% at post
mortem.

Several therapeutic modalities are used in the treatment
of metastasis from renal cell carcinoma (Table 3). Radiotherapy is reserved for the treatment of painful bony
metastasis. Chemotherapy and hormone therapy have been
generally discouring. Nephrectomy or arterial embolization
of the primary tumor are not effective treatments for
metastasis as suggested by some. The responses are too rare
and too short duration to be significant. In our opinion,
the multidisciplinary approach which proved useful in the
management of other tumors is not helpful in kidney tumors.
Surgery remains the best palliative treatment of metastasis

from renal cell carcinoma. But although metastasis are
rather frequent at the time of initial diagnosis, indications
for later surgery remain rare. Surgical treatment can
actually only be considered in cases of a solitary metastasis,
as survival is too poor when multiple metastasis are present.
Solitary metastasis represent a very small percentage of the
cases (3-5%) (Tolia, Whitmore 1975).

TABLE 1

RENAL CELL CARCINOMA
METASTASIS AT DIAGNOSIS

30% of patients
70% limited at one organ
47% multiple
 3% single

TABLE 2

RENAL CELL CARCINOMA
SITES AND FREQUENCY OF METASTASIS

Localization	At Diagnosis Percent	At Autopsy Percent
Lung and Mediastinum	50	67
Bone	49	39
Skin	11	13
Liver	8	39
Brain	3	6

TABLE 3

RENAL CELL CARCINOMA
TREATMENT MODALITIES

Surgery
Radiotherapy
Chemotherapy
Hormone Therapy
Immunotherapy
Association

Therapeutic indications vary with the site of metastasis. Lung metastasis are the most frequent problem (Katzenstein et al, 1978). The treatment is generally surgical. The technique and indications are reviewed in Table 4.

TABLE 4

RENAL CELL CARCINOMA
PULMONARY METASTASIS TREATMENT

A) Surgical Procedures:
    Wedge resection
    Lobectomy rarely
    Pneumonectomy exceptionally

B) Indications:
    Solitary
    Multiple if unilateral

The presence of multiple lesions, if they are unilateral and resectable, is not always a contraindication to surgical treatment. Because of the rarity of this lesion, certain possible coincidences must be considered. Sarcoidosis, tuberculosis as well as some collagen and fungal diseases can produce pulmonary lesions that mimic on x-ray metastatic lung lesions. These non-neoplastic lesions may regress spontaneously or after medical treatment. A period of observation may be justified in these situations. Survival after removal of solitary metastasis from lung differs according to whether the lesion is concomitant or secondary to radical nephrectomy. In the first case, the average survival is 18 months; in the second case, it is generally three years.

Bony metastasis ranks second in clinical frequency. The aim of treatment is palliative. The object of treatment is to consolidate a lytic metastasis on a weight bearing bone and to prevent pain. The strategy of the treatment is shown in Table 5. If pain is focal, radiotherapy (800 to 1000 rads) remains the best treatment. Such results against pain are favorable in 70% of cases. This response is generally sustained in 80% of those who survive more than one year. If pain is disseminated, radiotherapy does not

TABLE 5

RENAL CELL CARCINOMA
BONE METASTASES

Pain	Lytic Lesions
A) Localized Radiotherapy 70% subjective response	A) Orthopedic fixation ± Radiotherapy ± Cryosurgery
B) Diffuse Chemotherapy 21% subjective response	B) Total replacement of long bones (experimental)

give good results. Hemi corporeal irradiation has given some results in metastasis from prostatic carcinoma, but has not been successfully tried in metastasis from renal cell carcinoma.

Chemotherapy has had limited success for pain relief. We obtained favorable results (20%) by using a combination of CCNU and hydroxyurea. This response was of short duration, i.e. about four months on the average.

Patients with large lytic lesions in weight bearing bones (especially the femur) should undergo preventive orthopedic fixation if their life expectancy excees three to four months. The orthopedic fixation may be accompanied by a curetage of lesions and local cryotherapy administered by pouring liquid nitrogen into the curated lesions. The method had so far has seen limited use and its utility remains to be determined (Marcone et al, 1972). Orthopedic fixation may be also followed by irradiation of lesions, but is not yet possible to say if this complementary treatment is useful. Total replacement of the involved bone, the femur for instance, has been accomplished in particular by Marcov in New York. Results seem to be interesting in a few selected cases of solitary bony metastasis. When multiple bony metastasis are present, survival is poor. Survival of patients with solitary bony metastasis is relatively favorable as indicated by the series of Professor Küss at la Pitié Hospital. Out of ten patients, six had lived between two and six years and four patients are still living after three to six years.

Brain metastasis can be the most significant from the clinical point of view. In a certain number of cases, they are the first symptom of the disease. The preferred present treatment of a single brain metastasis is surgery. It consists in shelling out the lesion which is often separated by a cleavage zone from normal brain tissue. Surgical treatment of solitary lesions undoubtedly improves prognosis, as we can see in the series published by Paillas. When single brain metastasis was not operated, survival was three months in the average, whereas in a comparable group where the brain metastasis was operated, the mean survival was seven months.

When brain metastasis is the presenting and diagnostic symptom of the disease, survival of patients is less favorable than in the group of patients where metastasis appeared secondarily after radical nephrectomy. In a series of 16 patients reviewed by Van Effenter at la Pitié Hospital in Paris, survival in cases revealing lesions is five months. It is six years on the average when the lesions appeared secondarily after radical nephrectomy. Prognosis of revealing lesions is not as poor in all series and especially in the series presented by Pr. Chatelain.

Liver metastasis are much more frequent at post mortem than at diagnosis. These lesions occur therefore at the latest stage in the natural history of the disease and are an index of poor prognosis. Treatment of solitary metastasis (or clinically apparently solitary) is carried out by an atypical partial hepatectomy. Hemostasis of liver sections is facilitated by the use of denatured collagen that may be left in situ. The results of survival in this struction are undocumented but are believed to be generally very poor.

CONCLUSION

As long as there is not a generally effective systemic treatment of renal cell carcinoma, local treatment of metastasis would have little effect on the evolution of the disease aside from very rare cases.

In cases of multiple metastasis specific treatment is generally only recommended in case of bony metastasis involving pain lytic action on weight bearing bones and fractions. Steroids at high doses may occasionally provide symptomatic relief in end stages of the disease.

For solitary metastasis, treatment is more justified. There are two different groups of solitary lesions of very different prognosis. These are the solitary lesions present at the time of diagnosis and secondard lesions appearing after radical nephrectomy. The latter dgroup has a better prognosis. For metastasis present at the time of diagnosis, the value of treatment and its effects on survival are not obvious as shown in a comparative study of la Pitié Hospital. The 15 patients treated exhibited about the same survival as the untreated group. We can say at present that for metastasis found at diagnosis, treatment is only recommended when it is dictated by a specific clinical necessity, as in the case of brain tumors or in cases of other symptomatic

lesions. For secondary solitary lesions appearing after
radical nephrectomy, treatment may effect survival but it
is difficult to know if these favorable results are due to
treatment or to the fact that these are slow growing lesions.

REFERENCES

Katzenstein AL, Purirs R, Gmelich J, Askins F (1978).
  Pulmonary resection for metastatic renal carcinoma.
  Cancer 41:72.
Marcove RC, Sadrieh J, Huvos AG, Grabstald H (1972).
  Cryosurgery in the treatment of solitary or multiple bone
  metastases from renal cell carcinoma. J Urol 108:540.
Tolia BM, Whitmore WF (1975). Solitary metastasis from
  renal cell carcinoma. J Urol 114:836.

Renal Tumors: Proceedings of the First International Symposium on Kidney Tumors, pages 549–560
© **1982 Alan R. Liss, Inc., 150 Fifth Avenue, New York, NY 10011**

TUMOR RECURRENCE IN THE RENAL FOSSA AND/OR THE ABDOMINAL
WALL AFTER RADICAL NEPHRECTOMY FOR RENAL CELL CARCINOMA

Aurelio C. Uson, M.D.

Department of Urología, Hospital Clínico de
San Carlos, Faculty of Med., Complutensis
University, Madrid, Spain

INTRODUCTION

As reported (Beare, McDonald 1949; Angervall et al,
1969; Mostofi 1967; Angervall, Wahlqvist 1978), both direct
and metastatic tumor spread at the time of necropsy or perifacial nephrectomy alone, or with homolateral adrenalectomy
and, in some cases, with extensive regional lymphadenectomy
as well, have revealed the following:

1)   The renal capsule is invaded in 75% of the investigated
      specimens and the renal fascia in 38%.

2)   There were metastases to hilar and/or regional lymph
      nodes in 22% of cases and to the homolateral adrenal
      gland in 10%.

On the other hand, it has been found (Hulten et al, 1969;
Svane 1969; Thackray 1964) that in renal cell carcinoma which
were less than 6 cm in diameter and, also, in those which
were clinically silent or discovered incidentally, renal
growth was usually confined within the renal capsule and
overall cure rate was 86%.

It is agreed that renal cell carcinomas spread into
adjacent structures by direct extension and to regional or
distant sites by lymphatic, hematogenous or lymphohematogenous
pathways (Fig. 1).

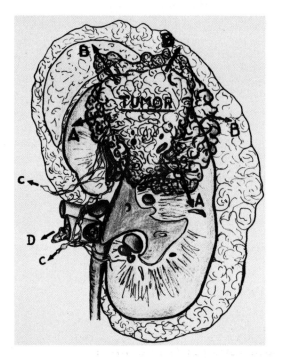

Fig. 1.   A. Intrarenal spread; B. Perirenal invasion;
C. Lymphatic extension; D. Hematogenous spread.

Furthermore, it is believed that local tumor recurrences such
as in the renal fossa, surrounding structures and/or in the
abdominal wall are mainly due to the following parameters:

1)   Size, weight, location and physical integrity of the
     renal tumor.

2)   Histopathological type, grade and stage of the renal
     cell carcinoma.

3)   Thoroughness of the surgical technique employed.

     Other factors which may also partake in the genesis of
local recurrences after radical nephrectomy for renal adenocarcinoma are:

1)   The age and the overall clinical condition, as well as
     the immunological competence of the patient.

2)   Additional postoperative treatments such as radio-
       therapy, chemotherapy and/or immunotherapy.

       As a result of the afore mentioned parameters and/or
factors, we may conclude that any renal cell carcinoma
which cannot be surgically removed or otherwise destroyed
"in toto" will recur, in due time, in the renal fossa,
abdominal wall, regional lymph nodes and/or at distant
sites. Based also on these facts, Robson among others
(Robson et al, 1969; Skinner et al, 1972; Grabstald 1969)
has been one of the pioneers and a staunch defendant of
doing perifacial nephrectomy for renal cell carcinoma, along
with radical retroperitoneal lymphadenectomy from the crus
of the diaphragm above to the aortic bifurcation below,
including the nodes which lie behind and in front of the
greater abdominal vessels. In the opinion of some, this
type of radical nephrectomy offers today a better chance
for complete tumor removal and possible cure. It should be
emphasized that no radical nephrectomy alone, regardless
of its type and/or thoroughness, can possibly cure a patient
whose renal tumor has already spread beyond the surgical
margins of an excised anatomical specimen. Nevertheless,
it is believed that today the changes for local tumor recurrence following surgery have decreased as a result of both
a wider use of the radical nephrectomy and an earlier diagnosis of kidney tumors. However, the true incidence of
local tumor recurrences is not known with total accuracy,
even though we suspect that they occur in clinical practice
much more commonly than they have been reported. In addition
the discovery of distant metastases, at times, may over-
shadow the presence of local tumor recurrences.

METHODS AND RESULTS

       In order to investigate and evaluate, as well as possible,
the incidence, size and extension of the tumor recurrences
at the renal fossa and/or abdominal wall after nephrectomy
for renal cell carcinoma, as well as the follow-up and
final outcome, we submitted a questionnaire to 46 hospitals
throughout Spain. This questionnaire covered the period
from 1976 through 1980. The questionnaire covered the
following points of interest:

a) name of the hospital, city, country and doctor filling the questionnaire

b) types of nephrectomy performed year by year from 1976 through 1980

c) size, number and location of the tumor recurrences

d) dates at which the local recurrences were discovered and dates at which the nephrectomies were performed on these patients

e) size, location, physical integrity and particularly, the grade and stage of the renal cell carcinoma at the time of nephrectomy

f) type and modality of the specific treatment of the local recurrences with periodic follow-up of these patients

g) final results and/or condition of these patients with dates when last seen

h) additional pathogenetic factors and/or surgical details regarding the possible causes and/or reasons accounting for the local recurrences

Of the 46 hospitals to which the questionnaire was sent, we received an answer from 17 Urological Services. The data from each of these hospitals appear in Table 1 and the results from these data are summarized in Table 2.

DISCUSSION

Based on reliable publications (Murphy 1973; Patel, Lavengood 1978) and, also on our own experience, perifacial nephrectomy with ipsilateral adrenalectomy plus hilar and retroperitoneal lymph node dissection, as proposed by Robson and others (Robson et al, 1969; Skinner et al, 1972; Grabstald 1969) can be considered today as the procedure of choice for complete removal of Stage III renal cell carcinomas. On the other hand, local tumor recurrence in the renal fossa and/or the abdominal wall after any type of nephrectomy is undoubtedly due to foci of malignant cells left behind after surgical removal of a renal cell

TABLE 1

THE NATIONAL SPANISH SURVEY OF RENAL CANCER

1   A total of 518 nephrectomies were performed for renal cell carcinoma in these 17 hospitals from 1976 through 1980.

2   A total of 17 patients with local tumor recurrences at the renal fossa and/or abdominal wall were reported from these hospitals during that period.

3   The overall percentage of local recurrences seen during this time was 3.3%.

4   The time between the nephrectomy and the discovery of the local recurrence varied from 3 months to 5 years, although the great majority were found within the first year after nephrectomy.

5   All patients with renal cell carcinomas which were found to have local recurrences after nephrectomy had at least a pathological Stage II or III.

6   About 50% of patients who had local recurrences after nephrectomy died within a year from the time at which the recurrence was discovered, and up to 80% in 2 years.

7   About 60% of these patients with local tumor recurrences showed iso or metachronous metastases elsewhere.

TABLE 2A

TUMOR RECURRENCE IN RENAL FOSSA AND/OR ABDOMINAL WALL AFTER
NEPHRECTOMY FOR RENAL CELL CARCINOMA IN SPAIN

Hospitals	Years	Nephrectomies
Galicia General Hospital Santiago de Compostela	76-80	40 R
Ramon Y Cajal - Madrid	77-80	76 R
Puerta de Hierro - Madrid	77-80	36 R
Instituto Nacional de Oncologia (I.N.O. Madrid	76-80	26 18 R 8 S
Hospital Clinico - Madrid	76-80	48 34 R 14 S
Principes de España Barcelona	76-80	25 20 R 5 S
Hospital Clinico Y Clinica San Jose - Barcelona	76-80	43 R
Licinio de la Fuente Segovia	76-80	11 S
20 de Noviembre - Alicante	76-80	24 R
Nuestra Señora de Aranzazu San Sebastian	76-80	60 R
Montecelo - Pontevedra	76-80	11 R
Hospital Clinico - Sevilla	76-80	20 R
University Hospital Navarra	76-80	25 R
Marques de Valdecilla Santander	76-80	15 R
Virgen de la Vega - Salamanca	76-80	15 R
Virgen del Rocio - Sevilla	76-80	26 R
General Sanjurgo - Valencia	76-80	17 R

TABLE 2B

TUMOR RECURRENCE IN RENAL FOSSA AND/OR ABDOMINAL WALL AFTER
NEPHRECTOMY FOR RENAL CELL CARCINOMA IN SPAIN

Recurrences	Time from Nephrectomy to Recurrence	Type and Stage of Renal Cell Ca
5	Min: 12 months Max: 48 months Aver: 21.4 months	Renal cell Ca and at least Stage III
0	0	Renal cell Ca Some Stage III
0	0	Renal cell Ca Some Stage III
2	Min: 4 months Max: 23 months	Renal cell Ca Some Stage III
0	0	Renal cell Ca Some Stage III
0	0	Renal cell Ca Some Stage III
0	0	Renal cell Ca Some Stage III
3	Min: 4 months Max: 11 months Aver: 7 months	Renal cell Ca All Stage III
1	32 months	Renal cell Ca Stage III
1	36 months	Renal cell Ca Stage III
1	5 months	Renal cell Ca Stage III
2	6 months 9 months	Renal cell Ca at least Stage III
0	0	Renal cell Ca Some Stage III
0	0	Renal cell Ca Some Stage III
1	11 months	Renal cell Ca Stage
0	0	Renal cell Ca Some Stage III
1	5 years	Renal cell Ca Stage III

TABLE 2C

TUMOR RECURRENCE IN RENAL FOSSA AND/OR ABDOMINAL WALL AFTER
NEPHRECTOMY FOR RENAL CELL CARCINOMA IN SPAIN

Location of Recurrence	Treatment	Results
Renal fossa + intra-peritoneum	None	Death in 3 months
Renal fossa - brain	None	Death in 2 months
Renal fossa	Cobalt therapy	Death in 12 months
Renal fossa	Cobalt therapy	Death in 8 months
Renal fossa + lungs	None	Death in 3 months
0	0	0
0	0	0
Thoraco-abdominal scar	Cobalt therapy	Death in 12 months
Renal fossa	Chemotherapy	Death in 5 months
0	0	0
0	0	0
0	0	0
Lumbar wall		
Lumbar wall	0	Death between 9 -
Renal fossa + wall		15 months
Renal fossa	Chemotherapy + Medroxy-progesterone	Alive with tumor after 15 months
Renal fossa + intestinal loops	Surgical excision	Death in 6 months
Renal fossa + abdominal wall	0	Death in 12 and 8 months
0	0	0
0	0	0
Renal fossa	Chemotherapy	Death in 12 months
0	0	0
Renal fossa	Nothing	Lost to follow-up

carcinoma. According to Sufrin and Murphy and others (Sufrin, Murphy 1980; Abrams et al, 1950) the initial site of failure after a nephrectomy done for curative reasons, may either be in the renal fossa or a distant organ. In fact, of those patients who had metachronus metastases, 48% did so within one year after nephrectomy, 57% within two years and 70% recurred within three years (Middleton 1967; Lokich, Harrison 1975). In contrast to those patients who had tumor recurrence in the renal fossa 32% did so within one year, 47% within two years and 58% within three years (Rafla 1970). As mentioned earlier, the collective experience gathered from the hospitals in Spain that reported local tumor recurrences after nephrectomy for renal cell carcinoma varied from three months to five years, although the great majority were discovered within the first two years.

In my opinion, the single most important factor responsible for local tumor recurrence after radical nephrectomy, either at the renal fossa or in the surgical scar, is miscalculation and the enigmatic pathological grade and stage of the renal growth prior to surgery. Obviously, other interrelated factors are also involved in influencing tumor recurrences as well as survival and final outcome in patients with renal cell carcinoma who "a priori" are considered to be curable by radical nephrectomy. However, it is impossible, as yet, to measure preoperatively with sufficient accuracy some of those factors, nor can the final results be predicted with certainty after radical nephrectomy for renal cell carcinoma. On the other hand, the lack of medical reports based on properly designed protocols and/or well controlled studies with adequate follow-up in many patients after radical nephrectomy for renal cell carcinoma, makes it very difficult to derive any reasonable answer. Because of this and the scanty information gathered in the questionnaire used in this study, some of the findings and the interpretations expressed in this report are open to important criticism. Therefore, we plan to continue this clinical research project in hopes of obtaining better and more reliable information and to clarify, in the near future, the question of "tumor recurrences in the renal fossa and/or abdominal wall, after radical nephrectomy for renal cell carcinoma."

SUMMARY AND CONCLUSIONS

The true incidence of tumor recurrences in the renal
fossa and/or the abdominal wall after radical nephrectomy
for renal cell carcinoma remains, as yet, an unknown question.
However, it seems that local tumor recurrences is much lower
today than 15 years ago. This improvement is mainly due
to an earlier and more precise diagnosis of kidney tumors,
a better selection of patients for surgery and, particularly,
to a wider use of the radical nephrectomy.

From a theoretical view point only Stage III and IV
renal cell carcinomas can recur locally at the renal fossa
and/or surgical scar after radical nephrectomy. In this
regard, it stands to reason that recurrence is due to tumor
implants or foci of tumor cells left behind. Obviously,
patients with Stage IV renal cell carcinoma will also show
metastases elsewhere, alone or with evidence of local tumor
recurrences.

The urologist at the time of radical nephrectomy must
look and be aware of the possibility of neoplastic spread
beyond the surgical margins of the anatomical specimen and,
in such cases, he should leave a few metallic clips at the
sites of tumor spread. In addition, the entire operative
field should be thoroughly irrigated with sterile water or
a saline solution. Furthermore, during the postoperative
period these patients should be treated adequately either
with external radiotherapy alone, delivered to the renal
fossa, or combined with parenteral chemotherapy, hormonal
or immunotherapy in a precise and correct manner.

In conclusion, as long as the etiopathogenesis of renal
cell carcinoma remains unknown, the best chances for achiev-
ing a complete cure, and avoidance of local recurrences and/
or distant metastases as well, rely first on an early
diagnosis of these tumors and second on complete surgical
removal not only of the main renal growth but also of its
local and regional tumor spread, if possible.

Beare JB, McDonald JR (1949). Involvement of the renal capsule in surgically removed hypernephroma: a gross and histopathologic study. J Urol 61:857.

Angervall L, Carlstrom E, Wahlqvist L, Ahren C (1969). Effects of clinical and morphological variables on spread of renal carcinoma in an operative series.Scand J Urol Nephrol 3:134.

Mostofi FK (1967). Pathology and spread of renal cell carcinoma. In: International Symposium on Renal Neoplasia. Edited by J.S.King, Jr. Boston: Little , Brown&Co. 41.

Angervall L, Wahlqvist L (1978). Follow-up and prognosis of renal carcinoma in a series operated by perifascial nephrectomy combined with adrenalectomy and retroperitoneal lymphadenectomy. Eur Urol 4:13.

Hulten L, Rosencrantz M, Seeman T, Wahlqvist L, Ahren C (1969). Occurrence and localization of lymph node metastases in renal carcinoma. Scand J Urol Nephrol 3:129.

Svane S (1969). Tumor thrombus of the inferior vena cava resulting from renal carcinoma. A report on 12 autopsied cases. Scand J Urol Nephrol 3:245.

Thackray AC (1964). The pathology and spread of renal adenocarcinoma. In: Tumours of the Kidney and Ureter. Edited by E. Riches.Baltimore: The Williams&Wilkins Co 72.

Robson CJ, Churchill BM, Anderson W (1969). The results of radical nephrectomy for renal cell carcinoma. J Urol 101:297.

Skinner DG, Vermillion CD, Colvin RB (1972). The surgical management of renal carcinoma. J Urol 107:705.

Grabstald H (1969). Renal cell tumors. Surg Clin N Amer 49:337.

Murphy GP (1973). Proceedings: current results from treatment of renal cell carcinoma. Proc Natl Cancer Conf 7:751.

Patel NP, Lavengood RW (1978). Renal cell carcinoma natural history and results of treatment. J Urol 119:722.

Sufrin G, Murphy GP (1980). Renal adenocarcinoma. Urol Surv 30:129.

Abrams HL, Spiro R, Goldstein N (1950). Metastases in carcinoma, analysis of 1000 autopsied cases. Cancer 3:74.

Middleton RG (1967). Surgery for metastatic renal cell carcinoma. J Urol 97:973.

Lokich JJ, Harrison JH (1975). Renal cell carcinoma; natural history and chemotherapeutic experience. J Urol 114:371.
Rafla S (1970). Renal cell carcinoma. Natural history and results of treatment. Cancer 25:26.

**Renal Tumors: Proceedings of the First International Symposium on
Kidney Tumors, pages 561-567**
© **1982 Alan R. Liss, Inc., 150 Fifth Avenue, New York, NY 10011**

REFLECTIONS ON THE TREATMENT OF TRANSITIONAL-CELL TUMOURS
OF THE UPPER URINARY TRACT.

Etienne MAZEMAN

Professeur d'Urologie

Centre Hospitalier   Lille   France

The principle of routine nephroureterectomy for all
transitional-cell tumours of the upper urinary tract is
often questioned, and recently there have been further articles published advocating conservative surgery, especially
for tumours of low histological grade (Blandy 1981;
Murphy et al. 1980, 1981).

Why, indeed, should one sacrifice a healthy kidney,
together with its collecting system, for a small and relatively benign tumour of the pelvis or ureter, when one does
not perform total cystectomy for benign papillomas of the
bladder ?

This argument is brought up repeatedly but, in fact,
it is very debatable because the two situations are not
strictly comparable for the following reasons :

1) First and foremost because a person has two kidneys but
only one bladder. In fact it is likely that if extirpation
of the bladder were not accompanied by the inevitably distressing disabilities of urinary diversion, total cystectomy would be indicated far more often for recurrent
tumours, even for those of low-grade malignancy.

2) Moreover, it is clear that the upper urinary tract cannot be investigated as easily and with as much accuracy as
the bladder :
    - with the bladder, cystoscopy does not as a rule
leave one in any doubt as to the existence of the tumour
and whether it is solitary or multiple.

- in contrast, with the upper urinary tract it is
sometimes difficult to confirm or exclude a small tumour,
which may for example be hidden at the bottom of a calix,
or to diagnose accurately (and this is essential in choo-
sing the correct treatment - whether it is solitary or
multifocal (Cukier 1981 : 130 cases, 11 % inaccurate
diagnosis).

Of the early recurrences after conservative surgery
of the upper urinary tract, how many are in reality only
more extensive tumours than were first recognized ?

3) In the same way, unlike bladder tumours where biopsy is
not a problem, it is never easy to confirm that a tumour
of the upper urinary tract is benign, which is the correct
indication for conservative surgery.

4) Directly recurrence occurs one can no longer compare
the bladder with the upper urinary tract.

The consequences with regard to treatment are so
different : in the bladder, as long as the lesion is of
low histological grade, repeated transurethral resection is
easy, whereas secondary nephroureterectomy is a much more
difficult undertaking in a patient who is frequently aged.

5) Finally, there is always the risk of disseminating malignant cells outside the urinary tract, a risk which is
inherent in all conservative surgery for tumours of the
upper urinary tract. Different people attach different
importance to this risk, but it is indisputable.

It is impossible, therefore, to draw any conclusions
from the treatment of bladder tumours to decide how to treat
similar tumours of the upper urinary tract.

The practicalities of the situations created are far
too different even though the urinary tract is one system
and though the pathogenesis, histology and evolution of
tumours which develop within it are the same.

To obtain, therefore, an objective idea of the value
of conservative surgery we must stick to the facts.

From the outset two facts emerge:

1) Apart from the very special experience of Petkovic with regard to tumours associated with Balkan nephropathy, reports on tumours of the renal pelvis and ureter treated conservatively and followed for an adequate length of time are rare.

So, we find among the latest series to be reported:

D. Murphy and H. Zincke 1980-81: 224 tumours, 11 conservative procedures of which 5 were necessitated because the lesions were bilateral or the opposite kidney was diseased.

J. Cukier 1981: 130 tumours, 6 conservative procedures, all made necessary by the circumstances.

D. Werth 1981: 35 ureteric tumours, no conservative procedure.

2) Experience with conservative surgery, therefore, is as yet limited. Besides, one cannot deny that its results are, to put it mildly, questionable, even if the histological grade of the tumour is low, at least for the tumours of the renal pelvis and calices:

1 - In Murphy and Zincke's series, of 48 patients who had a tumour of grade 1, only 2 were treated conservatively and 1 of these who had a partial pyelectomy died 4 years later of disseminated malignant disease.

2 - Autotransplantation of the kidney with pyelovesical anastomosis is an original and interesting technique which was proposed several years ago (Pettersson et al. 1981). It has already enabled him to confirm cystoscopically caliceal recurrence in 3 of his original 5 cases and the period of follow-up is still short.

3 - In the report which I presented in 1972 to the Congress of the French Urological Association and which reviewed 1118 cases of transitional-cell tumour of the renal pelvis and ureter, 151 tumours were treated conservatively and of these 117 had been followed-up for more than one year. The results were all very significant.

- In 23 tumours of the renal pelvis or calices. 65.2% recurred and of these one third were of higher histological grade than the original tumour. These figures, impressive though they are, are nevertheless an underestimate. In fact one of the "good results" is a personal case, that of a young woman 30 years old who died 10 years after conservative surgery for a benign tumour of the renal pelvis from multiple, poorly differentiated recurrences.

- In contrast, the results are much better for ureteric tumours (27 recurrences among 94 cases - an incidence
of 28%) and similar findings have been published recently
(Babaian, Johnson 1980) 44 tumours of the ureter; (Heney
et al. 1981) 60 tumours of the ureter; (Giulani 1981) 15
tumours of the pelvic ureter.

There seem to be two possible reasons which could
explain this difference in evolution which at first sight
appears illogical, since it concerns the same disease:

The first reason is the very great preponderance of
tumours in the lower third of the ureter. Given the fact
that urothelial tumours propagate chiefly by descent,
excision of the lower third of the ureter together with
a cuff of bladder provides almost as much security as total
nephrectomy.

The second reason is a purely technical one,
conservative surgery being, in effect, much better established as regards the ureter than it is in the interior
of the renal pelvis or calices, where the procedure is
less well tried.

This means that, except in cases of necessity
(absence or destruction of the opposite kidney, renal
insufficiency, bilateral lesions) and in cases of tumours
of the lower third of the ureter, total nephroureterectomy
with removal of a cuff of bladder around the ureteric
orifice remains the procedure of choice. This decision
can be difficult to take especially if the tumour is of
low grade malignancy, but it is, nevertheless, a reasonable
one because the risk of conservative surgery is considerable, and is it right to take this risk in a patient
whose opposite kidney is normal when the chances of a
similar tumour in the opposite side is less than 2%?

REMARKS

1 - From the moment one decides to remove the kidney,
it seems illogical to leave any of the ureter below it
in place. In our experience, the longer the length of
ureter left, the greater the chances of recurrence.

Nevertheless, simple nephrectomy may be justified in
certain circumstances:

- for a malignant tumour of the renal pelvis invading
so widely that nephrectomy can only be palliative,

- for a squamous tumour because ureteric recurrence is so rare,
- when the precarious general condition of the patient does not allow one to prolong the operation.

In these cases the technique of ureteric stripping can prove useful.

2 - Moreover, it is prudent, as the results obtained by Cukier et al. 1981 and Skinner 1981 prove, to extend the excision to the whole area around the kidney and ureter, and to complete it if there is the least doubt by a regional lymphnode dissection.

3 - As regards radiotherapy and chemotherapy, they have not yet proved their efficacy.

Even the most powerful antimitotic agents, such as Cis-platinum, have no significant effect (Peters, Oneill 1980).

Certain people have recently based great hopes in the combination of conservative surgery and topical chemotherapy, but the latter has proved so disappointing as regards the bladder that there is bound to be a certain skepticism about its possible efficacy in the upper urinary tract.

4 - A special case: that of transitional-cell tumours of the upper urinary tract appearing after treatment of a bladder tumour.

In more than 50% of these cases ureteric reflux can be demonstrated by micturating cystography. Even if it is not demonstrated, one can very well imagine in a patient who has had multiple endoscopic resections the possibility of a transient reflux, secondary to damage to the ureteric orifice, secondary to inflammation of the trigone which may have been accentuated by topical chemotherapy or, much more simply, due to the waves of high pressure produced within the bladder when it is being washed out with the Ellik evacuator.

Such reflux could easily be missed on a subsequent micturating cystogram. Reflux, then, is common and its danger is proven. When there is evidence of it during or after treating a bladder tumour, the patient has a 25% chance of developing a transitional-cell tumour of the renal pelvis or ureter (Martinez Pineiro et al. 1981; Sole Balcells, Zungri 1981).

Should one then do a preventative, anti-reflux operation? This might appear excessive, especially with the risks of reimplantation into a tumour-bearing bladder.

- On the other hand, it seems logical to advise resection of the bladder neck or prostate if there is dysectasiant factor, which will be certain to make the reflux worse.

- Finally, one must emphasize the need for a particularly careful follow-up of all patients whose bladder lesions require repeated resection or those who have had partial or total cystectomy. The follow-up regime should include at least an intravenous urogram, and perhaps eventually a micturating cystogramm, annually.

In conclusion, except in cases of necessity, the indications for conservative surgery are rare and essentially limited to tumours of the lower third of the ureter.
When circumstances dictate that the kidney must be preserved, one has the choice between a local excision, which could be called "radical conservative surgery." These techniques include the removal of almost all the upper urinary tract followed by uretero-ileoplasty or, preferably autotransplantàtion of the kidney with pyelo-vesical anastomosis, of which the early results seem encouraging.

Babaian RJ, Johnson DE (1980). Primary carcinoma of the ureter. J Urol 123:357.

Blandy JP (1981). Tumeurs du haut appareil urinaire. J Urol Nephro 87:3, 139.

Cukier J, Abourachid H, Pascal B, Sueur JP, Merimski E (1981). Tumeurs de la voie excrétrice haute. J Urol Nephro 87:2, 57.

Giulani L (1981). Traitement chirurgical des tumeurs de la voie excrétrice supérieure. Journées Urologiques de Necker. Masson Edit.

Heney NM, Nocks BN, Daly JJ, Blitzer, Parkhurst EC (1981). Prognostic factors in carcinoma of the ureter. J Urol 125:632.

Martinez Pineiro JA, Pertusa C, Torronteras J, Armero AH (1981). Tumeurs urothéliales du haut appareil urinaire apparaissant après traitement d'une tumeur de vessie. Journées Urologiques de Nicker. Masson Edit.

Mazeman E (1972). Rapport au Congrès de l'Association Francaise d'Urologie. Masson Edit. Paris. 1976. Tumours of the upper urinary tract. Report of 1118 cases. Eur Urol 2:120.

Murphy DM, Zincke H, Furlow WL (1980). Primary grade
1 transitional cell carcinoma of the renal pelvis
and ureter. J Ruol 123:629

Murphy DM, Zincke H, Furlow WL (1981). Management of
high grade transitional cell cancer of the upper
urinary tract. J Urol 125:25.

Peters PC, O'Neill, MR (1980). Cis-diamminedichloropla-
tinum as a therapeutic agent in metastatic transitional
cell carcinoma. J Urol 123:375.

Pettersson S, Aamot P, Brynger H, Johansson S (1981).
Extracorporeal renal surgery, autotransplantation and
calicoverisoctomy for renal plevic and ureteric
tumours. Scand J Urol 60:33.

Skinner G (1981). Traitement des tumeurs bu bassinet.
Journées Urologiques de Necker. Masson Edit.

Sole Balcells F, Zungri E (1981). Tumeurs de la voie
excrétrice haute. Journées Urologiques de Necker.
Masson Edit.

Werth DD, Weigel JW, Mebust WK (1981). Primary neoplasm
of the ureter. J Urol 125:628.

Renal Tumors: Proceedings of the First International Symposium on
Kidney Tumors, pages 569-571
© 1982 Alan R. Liss, Inc., 150 Fifth Avenue, New York, NY 10011

AUTOTRANSPLANTATION WITH DIRECT PYELOVESICAL ANASTOMOSIS IN
RENAL PELVIC AND URETERIC TUMOURS, A NEW APPROACH

S. Pettersson, H. Brynger, Ch. Henriksson, S.
Johansson, A.E. Nilson, and T. Ranch
Departments of Urology, Surgery I, Pathology II,
and Diagnostic Radiology I, Sahlgrenska sjukhuset,
University of Göteborg, S-413 45 Göteborg, Sweden

The standard surgical procedure in patients with pelvic
and ureteric tumours has for many years been nephroureterectomy including resection of a bladder cuff (Grabstald et al,
1971). The propensity of the urothelium to develop tumours
throughout the urinary tract has, however, made other
authorities advocate more conservative treatment, i.e. local
excisions and segmental resections (Gibson, 1966). Our
ambition has been to combine an agressive surgical attitude
towards both the tumour itself and the urothelium of the
ipsilateral ureter and pelvis with conservative surgery
with regard to the renal parenchyma (Pettersson et al, 1979).

Eight patients, one female and seven males, with pelvic
and/or ureteric tumours were operated upon according to
this principle. The mean age was 63 years with a range of
51-77 years. Two patients had bilateral pelvic tumours,
one had tumours in the pelvis and ureter of a solitary
kidney and 5 had unilateral pelvic or ureteric tumours.
One of the two patients with bilateral tumours had been
treated for recurrent transitional cell tumours with
squamous cell differentiation in the bladder for several
years.

Transabdominal perifascial nephrectomy, complete
ureterectomy and retroperitoneal lymphadenectomy were performed. The kidney was perfused cold with Sack's solution,
and on a work bench the whole ureter and most of the renal
pelvis were resected extracorporeally. Additional tumours
of the collecting system were excised and the calyces reconstructed. The calyces were also examined endoscopically

by means of a resectoscope for children (14.5 F); any additional tumours were electroresected or coagulated. Grading and staging of the tumours were performed by examination of frozen sections during the operation. The kidney was autotransplanted to the ipsilateral iliac fossa and the revascularization was performed end to side to the external iliac artery and vein. A direct anastomosis was performed between the remnant of the renal pelvis and the fundus of the mobilized urinary bladder.

The patients were followed with cytological, bacteriological, endoscopic and radiologic examinations and with regard to renal function.

In the two patients with bilateral tumours only one kidney was autotransplanted, and the other was discarded. Five patients had grade I tumours (WHO), another two had grade III tumours, and one had both grade II tumours and inverted urothelial papillomas. In 6 patients no infiltration was observed in the autotransplanted kidney, in one the tumours infiltrated the lamina propria and in one a microscopic lymph node metastasis was found in the paraffin-embedded specimens. No postoperative complication were encountered. One patient died in an accident one year postoperatively but no residual tumour was found post mortem. One patient died in metastasis from his squamous cell carcinoma of the bladder, the kidney and renal pelvis being without recurrence. In three patients small recurrent tumours were discovered in the calyces at postoperative endoscopic follow-up. All tumours were coagulated transurethrally. The current observation time is 17 months (range 2-43 months). No significant reduction of renal function was observed postoperatively and recurrent urinary tract infections were no serious problem.

The method presented has several advantages over previously described surgical procedures. Compared to radical nephroureterectomy the method spares the renal parenchyma. There is no evidence that the radicality of the treatment for a ureteric or a non-infiltrating pelvic carcinoma is increased by discarding the kidney. Compared to local excisions the risk of development of subsequent tumours of the ipsilateral pelvic and ureter is strongly reduced with the presented method. Furthermore, the method provides facilities for postoperative endoscopic control and treatment of recurrent pelvic tumours.

Gibson TE (1966). Local excision in transitional cell tumours of the upper urinary tract. Trans Am Ass Gen-Ur Surg, 58:179.

Grabstald H, Whitmore WF, Melamed MR (1971). Renal pelvic tumours. JAMA, 218:845.

Pettersson S, Brynger H, Johansson S, Nilson AE (1979). Extracorporeal surgery and autotransplantation for carcinoma of the pelvis and ureter. Scand J Urol Nephrol 13:89.

Renal Tumors: Proceedings of the First International Symposium on
Kidney Tumors, pages 573-580
© 1982 Alan R. Liss, Inc., 150 Fifth Avenue, New York, NY 10011

RENAL ANGIOMYOLIPOMA

Alain Jardin, M.D.

Professor of Urology
Clinique Urologique de la Pitié, Paris

Renal angiomyolipoma was described a century ago and
over the last 20 years it has been the subject of more than
250 publications (Albrecht 1904). Most of these consist of
a list of cases in which nephrectomy has usually been
performed.

This tumor should not be neglected just because it is
rare. Better methods of diagnosis should lead us to more
frequent preoperative recognition and thus to conservative
treatment.

Angiomyolipoma, or nemartoma, of the kidney is a benign
dysgenesis, which represents 3% of all renal tumours (5%
in our series). Our experience is based on 22 cases and
is reported in this paper.

CLINICAL ASPECTS

The difficulty of diagnosis varies according to the
circumstances in which the tumour is found:

(1) Tuberous sclerosis (Bourneville's disease)

In nearly 50% of cases angiomyolipomas are associated
with tuberous sclerosis (Bourneville 1880). This is a
hereditary disease transmitted as a dominant character.
It is associated with variable neurological and psychiatric
disorders, such as epileptic seizures and varying degrees
of mental deficiency, with cutaneous signs, such as
adenoma sebaceum of 'butterfly' distribution over the nose

and cheeks, pigmented spots, molluscum pendulum and the
periungual tumours of Koenen, and with visceral lesions
affecting the eyes, lungs, heart and especially the kidneys,
usually with renal angiomyolipomas as described by
Bourneville in his original article. In this condition the
angiomyolipomas are often multiple, frequently bilateral
and very variable in size.

(2) Complications leading to discovery

In 20 out of our 22 cases the angiomyolipoma was
brought to light by one of the following complications:

Haemorrhage: The abundance, complexity and fragility
of the blood supply to angiomyolipomas account for the
frequency of haemorrhagic complications (Keshin 1965;
Price, Mostofi 1965; Sairanen 1980). The most common
complication is bleeding within the tumour, and this accounts for most of the episodes of pain which occur in
nearly 90% of cases (Jardin et al. 1980; McCullough, 1974).
Sometimes the bleeding enters the urinary tract presenting
as haematuria. Finally, spontaneous retroperitoneal
bleeding occurs in 10% of cases and is the most serious
complication, leading all too often to nephrectomy (Jardin
et al. 1980; Louis 1980).

When the diagnosis of rupture of a hamartoma has been
made, selective embolization of the artery to the tumour
can stop the bleeding.

Infection: A picture of infection suggestive of acute
pyelonephritis was found in nearly one third of our cases -
rather more than in other series (Klapioth et al. 1959;
McCullough, 1974; Mazeman et al. 1977). There may be
several reasons for this. Bleeding within a tumor can
sometimes account for sustained fever (Huchon 1980) and
renal stone may rarely be associated, as in one of our
cases, but usually no obvious cause for this infective
picture can be found.

Hypertension: Like other renal tumours, hemartomas
may be accompanied by hypertension. The ischaemia produced by the tumour, or especially by a complicating intra-
or peri-renal haemorrhage, can perhaps explain it (Bagley
et al. 1981; Futter, Collins, 1974; Farrow et al. 1968).
Among our 3 hypertensive patients, one had associated

polycystic disease, another aortic insufficiency and the
third had no apparent renal cause for his hypertension, his
plasma renin being normal.

Renal insufficiency: This is not unusual with hemartomas
and occurs in 3-5% of cases (Anderson, Tannen 1969; Farrow
et al. 1968). Without doubt there are many different possible causes: destruction of renal tissue by invading
tumour (Farrow et al. 1968); associated polycystic disease
(Anderson, Tannen 1969); or associated interstitial
nephritis (Kleinkneicht et al. 1976), which was present
in one third of our cases.

(3) Tumour of the breast

Of the 27 hemartomas discovered at autopsy by Hajdu, 11
were found in women with breast cancer (Hajdu, Foote 1969).
Such a high incidence has not been found in other series.
In only one of our patients was the angiomyolipoma discovered during the course of investigation of a breast
nodule confirmed as breast carcinoma. Nevertheless, we
should search carefully for a breast tumour in all women
with hemartomas and we should not jump too hastily to the
conclusion that a tumour of the kidney in a woman with
breast cancer must be a secondary deposit.

DIAGNOSIS

The accuracy of diagnosis of angiomyolipomas has been
completely transformed by the CT scan. Intravenous urography (IVU) shows the presence of a space-occupying
lesion of the kidney, but rarely shows any translucent
zones within it (Barom et al. 1979; Brendler et al. 1971;
Seshanarayana, Keats, 1968). This was seen in only 2 of
our 22 cases. Arteriography demonstrates the hyper-
vascularity of these tumours. The blood vessels to the
tumours arise from the interlobular arteries and characteristically have a corkscrew appearance or end with
peripheral aneurysmal dilatations like bunches of grapes.
An onion skin effect can be seen in the nephrogram phase
(Brendler et al. 1971; McCallum 1975; Jardin et al. 1980).
These particular signs were found in 8 of the 12 patients
who had arteriography in our series.

In a patient with a space-occupying lesion of the kidney,
ultrasound can prove that it is solid. In our series it

has been used 6 times, but has not really allowed us to make a precise diagnosis of angiomyolipoma. However, with further refinement the diagnostic accuracy of ultrasound will probably improve (Pitts 1980; Bush et al. 1979), and it can already make the diagnosis of bleeding within or around a tumour. The CT scan is today the best method of diagnosis and it alone gives one an almost certain daignosis of angio-myolipoma, showing within a renal tumour areas of the same negative density as fatty tissue (Richard et al. 1979; Frija 1980; Bush et al. 1979; Marchal 1979). The correct pre-operative diagnosis of angiomyolipoma was made four times out of four in our series. Diagnostic pitfalls are tumours with severe bleeding which can easily be mistaken for necrotic carcinomas, especially if unilateral (Hansen et al. 1978).

HISTOLOGY

An absolute diagnosis of angiomyolipoma can only be made by histological examination. In most cases the clinical probability of angiomyolipoma is such that we believe biopsy and frozen section at the time of operation is justified. The histological characteristics of this tumour are sufficiently distinctive to allow an accurate diagnosis in all cases. There were no diagnostic errors in our series (Jardin et al. 1980). We did, however, carry out biopsy and frozen section in one patient with a carcinoma of the kidney. As such a procedure carries a possible risk, we now reserve it for cases in which the CT scan shows one or more areas of negative density within solid tumours.

TREATMENT

Various methods of management are described in the literature including radical nephrectomy, conservative surgery (enucleation of the tumour or partial nephrectomy) and observation.

Radical nephrectomy, in our opinion, can only be justified when the preoperative diagnosis is carcinoma of the kidney. As we have seen, the clinical, radiological and especially the CT findings usually allow us to make a preoperative diagnosis of angiomyolipoma and to confirm it histologically by frozen section at the time of opera-tion. Therefore, for these reasons, we believe that nephrectomy should be reserved for those rare cases in which the kidney has been completely destroyed by multiple tumours. In this context, measurement of the renal uptake of radioactive magnesium bichlorate may prove useful; one should not always rely on images when deciding whether to perform nephrectomy.

Observation has been advocated by some authors for the following reasons (Mazeman et al. 1977):

(1) Angiomyolipoma is a very slowly growing tumor.
(2) The life expectancy of patients with tuberous sclerosis is limited.
(3) Even large retroperitoneal haematomas may regress spontaneously.

In our opinion, this attitude is not safe. A large hemartoma is a serious condition and hemorrhagic complications often lead to nephrectomy or death (Cohen, Pearlman 1968; Jochimsen et al. 1969; Rao et al. 1981). Indeed, several cases have been published of bilateral nephrectomy (Renders, Defloor 1972) in patients who originally were 'observed' (Jochimsen et al. 1969).

Conservative surgery is, for us, the best solution. When the tumour is extrarenal it can generally be enucleated. 'Lumpectomy" of between 1 and 12 tumours from the same kidney has been carried out in our series. Partial nephrectomy may be needed to resect localized intrarenal tumours. In our series conservative surgery has been relatively safe; one patient died of biliary peritonitis shortly after the operation. One argument against conservative surgery is the possibility of leaving behind very small angiomyolipomas within the parenchyma. We do not think this argument is valid for the following reasons:

1) In all published series haemorrhagic complications were caused by tumours over 5 cm in diameter.
2) An 8-year follow-up of our first case using CT scanning suggests that small angiomyolipomas do not increase in size.

In fact, the only argument against conservative surgery is the risk of leaving behind a very small associated carcinoma. Five cases of such an association have been published; two were also associated with polycystic disease; in all five the carcinoma was over 5 cm in diameter (Guttierez et al. 1979; Jardin et al. 1980; Lynne et al. 1979). This association with carcinoma seems too rare to make us change our policy of conservative surgery.

SUMMARY

Angiomyolipoma of the kidney can often be diagnosed preoperatively. When this is possible, conservative surgery is the treatment of choice.

Albrecht E (1904). Uber Hamartome. Verh dt Path Ges 7:153.

Anderson D, Tannen RL (1969). Tuberour sclerosis and chronic renal failure. Potential confusion with polycystic kidney disease. Am J Med 47:163.

Bagley D, Appell R, Pingoud K, McGuire EJ (1981). Renal angiomyolipoma, diagnosis and management. Urology 1:1.

Barom M. Leiter E, Brendler H (1979). Preoperative diagnosis of renal angiomyolipoma. J Urol 117:701.

Bourneville DM (1880). Contribution à l'étude de l'idiotie. Sclérose tubéreuse des circonvolutions cérébrales; idiotie et épilepsie hémiplegique. Archs Neurol 1:81.

Brendler H, Maguire JW, Mitty HA (1971). Angiographic characteristics of renal hamartoma. Br J.Urp; 43:674.

Bush Jr WH, Freeny PC, Orme BM (1979). Characteristics images by ultrasonography and CT Scanning. Urology 14:531.

Cohen SG, Pearlman CK (1968). Spontaneous rupture of the kidney in pregnancy. J Urol 100:365.

Farrow GM, Harrison EG, Utz DC, Jones DR (1968). Renal angiomyolipoma. A clinicopathologic study of 32 cases. Cancer 22:564.

Fritz J (1980). Computed tomography diagnosis of renal angiomyolipoma. J Comput Assist Tomog :843.

Futter NG, Collins WE (1974). Renal angiomyolipoma causing hypertension. A case report. Br J Urol 46:485.

Guttierez OH, Burgener FA, Schwartz S (1979). Coincident renal cell carcinoma and renal angiomyolipoma in tuberous sclerosis. Amer J Roentgen 132:848.

Hadju SI, Foote FW (1969). Angiomyolipoma of the kidney. Report of 27 cases and review of the literature. J Urol 102:396.

Hansen GC, Hoffman RB, Sample WF, Becker R (1978). Computer tomography diagnosis of renal angiomyolipoma. Radiology 128:789.

Buchon A (1980). Angiomyolipome de rein révélé par une
fièvre prolongée. Nouv. Press med 1308:0.

Jardin A, Richard F, LeDuc A, Chatelain C, Le Guillou M,
Fourcade R, Camey M, Küss R (1980). Diagnosis and
treatment of renal angiomyolipoma (based on 15 cases).
Arguments in favor of conservative surgery (based on 8
cases). Eur Urol 6:69.

Jochimsen PR, Braunstein PM, Najardian JS (1969). Renal
allotransplantation for bilateral renal tumors. (1969).
J A M A 810:1721.

Keshin JG (1965). Three cases of renal hamartoma: two
cases presenting with spontaneous rupture and massive
retroperitoneal hemorrhage. J Urol 94:336.

Klaproth HJ, Putassse EF, Hazard JB (1959). Renal angiomyolipomas. Report of four cases. Arch Path 67:400.

Kleinkneicht D, Haiat R, Frija J, Mignon F (1976).
Sclérose tubéreuse de Bourneville avec bicuspidité
aortique et insuffisance rénale. Nouv Press Med 5:1196.

Louis JF (1980). Rupture d'angiomyolipomes (3 cas). J
Urol (Paris) 86:295.

Lynne CM, Carrion HM, Bakshandem K, Sadji M, Russel E,
Politano VA (1979). Renal angiomyolipoma polycystic
kidney and renal cell carcinoma in patient with tuberous
sclerosis. Urol 14:174.

McCallum RN (1975). The preoperative diagnosis of renal
hamartoma. Clin Radiol 26:257.

McCullough DL (1974). Renal hamartoma. Current concept
of diagnosis and surgical management. Urol 4:235.

Marchal G (1979). Etude ultrasonique et tomodensitomé-
trique dans l'angiomyolipome du rein (rapport de 4 cas).
J Belge Radiol 62:371.

Mazeman E, Wemeau L, Biserte J, Lemaitre G, Houcke M (1977).
Les angiomyolipomes rénaux. J Urol Nephrol 83:1.

Pitts WR (1980). Ultrasonography computerized transaxial
tomography and pathology of angiomyolipoma of the kidney.
Solution to a diagnostic dilemn. J Urol 907:124.

Price EB, Mostofi FK (1965). Symptomatic angiomyolipoma
of the kidney. Cancer 18:761.

Rao PN, Osborn DE, Barnard RJ, Best JJK (1981). Symptomatic renal angiomyolipoma. Br J Urol 53:212.

Randers G, Defloor E (1972). Hamartomes bilatéraux du
rein. Acta Urol Belg 40:537.

Richard F, Khoury S, Küss R, Parienti D, Dusselier R (1979).
Le rein en tomodensitométrie. Soc Fr Urol - J Urol
Néphrol

Sairanen H (1980). Renal angiomyolipoma. A cause of
 massive retroperitoneal hemorrhage. Ann Chir Gynecol
 69:3.
Seshanarayana KN, Keats TE (1968). Angiomyolipoma of the
 kidney. Diagnostic roentgenographic finding. Am J
 Roentg 104:334.

Renal Tumors: Proceedings of the First International Symposium on Kidney Tumors, pages 581–588
© 1982 Alan R. Liss, Inc., 150 Fifth Avenue, New York, NY 10011

THE TRANSPLANTED KIDNEY AS A VECTOR OF MALIGNANT CELLS

P. Frantz, C. Chatelain, J. Poisson, J. Luciani,
C. Jacobs, R. Küss
Hôpital de la Pitié
Paris, France

Organ transplantation opens the way to a new chapter
in oncology, with the possibility of grafting cancer cells
carried by the transplanted organ. It is difficult to
transplant human malignant cells under normal conditions
but this becomes possible in immuno-suppressed patients
(Southam et al, 1957). As a matter of fact, immunosup-
pression dramatically increases the general incidence of
cancer. This incidence varies from 2% (Hoover, Fraumeni,
1973) to 7% (Sheil, 1977). Penn reported that transplanted
patients were a hundred times more at risk to developing
cancer than age matched control groups (Penn, 1970). The
development of cancer in a transplanted kidney is a rare
event. Penn noted three cases out of 681 cancers in transplant recipients (Penn, 1979). In a cooperative study in
Europe involving 219 centers, we found 34 cancers which
developed (de novo) in 1978 transplant recipients. Two of
them were kidney tumors (one renal cell carcinoma and one
cancer of the pelvis). In addition, an apparently normal
transplanted kidney may act as a vector for malignant cells.
In the pioneering years of transplantation this possibility
was regarded as being without foundation. Thus, in the
three first years in the history of transplantation, donors
with cancer were accepted. A review of the literature
shows 25 cases of cancer transmitted by the graft in this
period (Table 1).

Table 1

CASE REPORT REVIEW OF THE LITERATURE

Author	Year case report	Year case	Donor source	Knolewdje of tumor	Site of primary tumor	Appearance of kidney
1) Martin	1965	1964	cadaver	+	bronchus	normal
2) MacIntosh	1965	1964	cadaver	+	larynx	normal
3) Maclean	1965	1964	cadaver	+	breast	normal
4) Wilson	1968	1964	cadaver	+	bronchus	normal
5) Tunner	1971	1964	living	+	kidney	carcinoma
6) Muiznieks	1968	1965	cadaver	+	Thyroīd	normal
7) Zukoski	1970	1966	cadaver	+	liver	normal
8) Lanary	1972	1965	cadaver	+	bronchus	normal
9) Lanary	1972	4/1966	cadaver	+	bronchus	normal
10) Lanary	1972	5/1966	cadaver	+	breast	normal
11) Lanary	1972	7/1966	cadaver	+	bronchus	normal
12) Jeremy	1972	1968 ?	cadaver	–	melanoma	normal
13) Cerilli	1972	1970	living	–	Kidney	abnormal
✱14) Poisson cited in Wilson		1970	cadaver	–	bronchus	normal
15) Traejer cited in Wilson		1971 ?	living	–	kidney	abnormal
16) Baird	1975	1973 ?	cadaver	–	Kidney	abnormal
17) Mocelin	1975	1974 ?	living	–	kidney	normal
18) Gokel	1977	1974	cadaver	–	choriocarcinoma	normal
19) Fairman 20)	1980	1975	cadaver	–	Malignant melanoma	{ normal normal
21) Peters	1978	1975	cadaver	–	Malignant melanoma	normal
22) Barnes	1976	1975 ?	cadaver	–	bronchus	normal
23) Forbes 24)	1981	1977	cadaver	–	bronchus	{ normal normal
✱25) Frantz	1981	1981	cadaver	–	kidney	normal

✱ 2 own case reports (14) cited by Wilson and Penn

Table 1 (continued)

Recipient diagnosis of renal carcinoma	Time elapsed between TR and diagnosis	Outcome
biopsy of allograft	4 months	Death 5 months after transplantation with metastases.
biopsy of liver	8 months	Death at 8 months widespread metastases.
histological examination of removed allograft	18 days	Death at 3 weeks from septicaemia.
biopsy of allograft	17 months	Allograft removed at 19 months. Alive and well on dialysis at 8 years after 3 grafts. Metastases rejected.
immediately	0	Death 15 weeks. Infection and renal carcinoma.
biopsy of allograft	7 days	Allograft removed at 7 days. Death at 13 months from natural renal carcinoma.
biopsy of allograft	35 months	Allograft removed. Metastases rejected. Died at 45 months after further transplant.
necropsy	10 months	Death from infection, carcinoma, metastases.
necropsy	16 months	Death from infection, carcinoma, without metastases.
necropsy	16 days	Death from infection, carcinoma, without metastases.
biopsy of allograft	12 months	Immunosuppression stopped. Allograft non removed. Carcinoma rejected. Death at 17 months without metastases.
histological examination of removed allograft	11 months	Death at 13 months with widespread metastases.
biopsy of allograft day 0	2 days	Allograft removed at 2 days. Alive and well at 2 years with a further transplant.
necropsy	7 months	Death with metastases at 7 months.
biopsy of allograft day 0	$<$ 7 days	Partial nephrectomy at 3 months. Alive and well at 3 years, with transplant.
biopsy of allograft day 0	$<$ 7 days	Tumor excise widely. Allograft removed at 44 days. No residual tumor. Well at 18 months after further transplant.
carcinoma in donor's nephrectomy scar	8 months	Death from metastases at 10 months (2 months after transplant nephrectomy.
Histological examination of controlateral kidney:metastases of choriocarcinoma	$<$ 7 days	Allograft removed at 7 days. Renal carcinoma and HCG high serum levels. Metastases rejected. Committed suicide at 7 months. No tumor at necropsy.
biopsy of skin nodule	3 1/2 years	Immunodepression stopped. Died at 46 months from brain metastases despite kidney removal.
histological examination of the removed allograft	45 months	Allograft rejected and removed. Outcome ?
biopsy of skin nodule donor necropsy	19 months	Died at 19 months from widespread metastases.
systematic allograft biopsy during transplantation	$<$ 7 days	Transplant nephrectomy refused by patient. Died at 6 months from metastases.
biopsy of allograft	13 months	Died at 15 months. Carcinoma and metastases.
nephrectomy of rejected transplant	18 months	Immunodepression stopped. Lung metastases rejected. Died at 20 months with abdominal metastases.
histological examination of removed rejected allograft	2 months	Alive and well at 8 months, on dialysis.

Transplantation of a kidney from a donor with a documented
cancer.

The first 11 cases in Table 1 were observed between
1964 and 1966. The donors were known as having a cancer
either before or after death (a cancerous kidney was even
transplanted to another patient ᴛ Case 5).

Death from widespread metastasis was the rule in these
cases (8 out of 11 cases). But in three cases (Cases 4,
7, 11) rejection of the primary cancer and its metastasis
was seen after administration of immunosuppressive drugs
retransplanted twice without the recrudescence of his
metastasis. Another case (Case 7) died in the aftermath of
the second transplantation 14 months after the first one
without any detectable cancer. The third (Case 11) died
after 17 months of bronchopneumonia and no cancer could be
detected on post-mortem.

Despite the possibility of cancer rejection after
stopping immunosuppressive drugs, the risks were considered
unacceptable and transplantations from cancerous donors
were stopped. However the problem of transmitting cancer
with the graft was not completely resolved. In the last
15 years, we could find in the literature 14 cases of cancer
transmitted by means of a graft from an apparently cancer
free donor.

Transplantation of a kidney from a donor with an unknown
cancer.

These are cases in which the cancer in the donor was
diagnosed early after transplantation. In 7 cases the
donors' cancers were diagnosed immediately after the
transplantation at post-mortem of donors as in Case 21,
histology of the donor's other kidney, biopsy of a suspicious zone on the graft (Cases 13, 15, 16), a routine
biopsy as in Case 22, or finally by histology of a transplanted kidney that was removed later (personal Case 25).

Case 25, a 27-year-old male was transplanted for the
first time in July 1979. The graft was removed in August
1979 after acute rejection. He had then 100% antibodies.
He was transplanted for the second time (7/1/81) and had
twin episodes of acute rejection and was put again on
hemodialysis (12/2/81). The second graft was removed

(8/3/81) and its histopathology showed to our surprise obvious lesions of acute rejection associated with a partly necrosed adenoma (4 cm in diameter) of the kidney. No visible metastasis occurred in the next 6 months. The donor was a 51-year-old man who died of head trauma without known history. No post-mortem was performed.

As soon as the diagnosis was made, the transplanted kidney was usually removed totally (Cases 17, 18, 25) or partially (Case 15, 16). These patients have survived or have died of unrelated causes without metastasis (Cases 16, 18) but in 2 cases (Cases 21, 22) the recipients refused removal of the graft and died from metastasis 19 and 5 months later.

Early removal of the graft does not always preclude the development of metastasis. For example, Case 18 is a man who developed coeliocarcinoma with a ligh level of HCG despite the fact that the kidney was removed on the 6th day following transplantation, i.e. as soon as the autopsy revealed that the donor died from a brain metastasis and not from brain hemorrhage. HCG levels were 10 times normal values at the 12th day and only came back to normal 8 weeks later.

Cancer in donors in other instances may be diagnosed late. For example, in 7 cases the cancer in donors remained unknown for long periods and became symptomatic in recipients as late as 45 months after the transplant, as demonstrated by Case 20. In this case the cancer could be mistaken for a "de novo" cancer and only analysis of the complete history of the donor and the conditions of death enabled us to find the primary tumor. In one of our patients (Case 14), a renal transplantation was done on 2/10/70 in a 70-year-old man. The donor was a 50-year-old man who died from a cerebral vascular accident. He had a horseshoe kidney, the left part of which was used for transplantation (the right part had too many arteries). Evolution was satisfactory for a period of 6 months. Then renal function started to fail. The general condition deteriorated quickly and the patient died suddenly on 8/5/71. Post-mortem revealed metastasis in the kidney and in the liver with no primary tumor found. Investigation revealed at post-mortem that the donor had a bronchial carcinoma with cerebellar necrosis responsible for his death. Histology was comparable in both donor and recipient.

In 2 other cases (Cases 11 and 20) the appearance of cancer in both kidneys collected from the same donor was related to the donor's primary tumor. At this stage it is usually too late for the patient, even if the graft is removed and immunosuppressive drugs stopped. The prognosis is very gloomy in such cases.

The final case (Case 17) involved development of a tumor at the site of the nephrectomy incision in a living donor. The recipient died from metastasis three months later.

DISCUSSION

Transmission of the donor's cancer by the means of a transplant graft is a real possibility. It was found 11 times in two years (1964 to 1966) in transplantations from donors with cancer. The same occurred 14 times in 15 years (1966 to 1981) from donors with no history of cancer. Does a graft from a cancer bearing donor lead inevitable to the development of cancer in the recipient? In 47 selected observations of patients who potentially could have trans- mitted cancer, out of a group of 12,389 kidney transplants (Renal Transplant Registry), only 15 did actually transmit cancer (Wilson, Penn, 1975). In 11 instances the cancer of the donor was known (patients transplanted before 1964) and in four cases it was unknown at the time of transplantation. In two cases of renal cancer the primary cancer could not be found in the donor and these were regarded as "de novo" cancers. In the 30 remaining cases there was no evidence of transmission of cancer; eleven of these patients died in the first three months of unrelated causes and might have developed cancer if they had lived long enough. It is known that cancer transmission may become manifest as late as 45 months after transplantation (Fairman et al, 1980).

The outcome of patients with a graft transmitted cancer is bad and no transplantation should be done from donors with known cancer, except perhaps in cases of primitive brain tumors. Eliminating cancer in donors is sometimes difficult especially when the cause of death was a coma following a vascular cerebral accident or following a presumed primitive brain tumor that might in fact be a secondary tumor. This happened in 4 cases (12, 14, 18, 21). Fortunately, CT scans of the brain now can provide a more precise diagnosis.

A small nodule in the lung may go unnoticed (Case 14) or may be mistaken for a tuberculous nodule (Cases 23, 24). In case of doubt it is better to biopsy such lung lesions and to quickly perform an histological examination of the specimen before transplanting the kidneys. This has become definitively possible since collected kidneys can be maintained in cold ischaemia for 48 hours. These precautions will decrease the risk of transplanting a graft from a cancer bearing donor. Also, in the event such a possibility occurs, the accident is quickly recognized and necessary steps can be taken.

REFERENCES

Baird RN, White HJO, Tribe CR (1975). Renal carcinoma in a cadaver kidney graft donor. Br Med J 2:371.
Barnes AD, Fox M (1976). Transplantation of tumour with a kidney graft. Br Med J 1:1442.
Cerilli GT, Nelsen C, Dorfmann L (1972). Renal homotransplantation in infants and children with the haemolytic uremic syndrome. Surgery 71:66.
Chatelain C, Frantz Ph, Luciani J, Jacobs C, Petit J, Gautier JP (1979). Tumeur et hémopathies malignes chez les insuffisants rénauz traités par transplantation rénale. Séminaires d'Uro-Néphrologie V, Masson Paris 184-196.
Fairman RM, Grossman RA, Barker CF, Perloff L (1980). Inadvertent transplantation of a melanoma. Transplantation 30:328.
Forbes GB, Goggin MJ, Dische FE, Saeed IT, Parsons V, Harding MJ, Bewick M, Pudge CT (1981). Accidental transplantation of bronchial carcinoma from a cadaver donor to two recipients of renal allograft. Clin Pathol 34:109.
Gokel JM, Rjosk HK, Meister P, Stelter WJ, Witte J (1977). Metastatic choriocarcinoma transplanted with cadaver kidney. Cancer 3:1317.
Hoover R, Fraumeni JF (1973). Risk of cancer in renal transplant recipients. Lancet 2:55.
Jeremy D, Farnsworth RH, Robertson MR, Annetts DL, Murnaghan GF (1972). Transplantation of malignant melanoma with cadaver kidney. Transplantation 13:619.
Lanari A, Rodo JE, Barcat JA 91972). Cuarto casos de desarrollo de un cancer del dador en el rinon injertado. Medecina (Buenos Aires) 32:79.

MacIntosh DA, McPhaul JJ, Peterson EW, Smith JR, Cook FE, Humphreys JW (1965). Homotransplantation of a cadaver neoplasm and a renal homograft. JAMA 192:1171.

MacLean CD, Dosseter JB, Gault MH, Oliver JA, Inglish FG, Mackinnon KJ (1965). Renal homotransplantation using cadaver donors. Arch Surg 91:288.

Martin DC, Rusini M, Rosen VJ (1965). Cadaveric renal homotransplantation with inadvertent transplantation of carcinoma. JAMA 192:82.

Mocelin AJ, Brandinal (1975). Inadvertent transplant of a malignancy. Transplantation 19:430.

Muiznieks HW, Berg JW, Lawrence W, Randall HT (1968). Suitability of donor kidneys from patients with cancer. Surgery 64:871.

Penn I (1970). Malignant tumors in organ transplant recipients. Springer Verlag, New York.

Penn I (1979). Malignant tumors in organ transplant recipients. in Seminaire d'Uro-Nephrologie V, Masson Paris 173.

Peters MS, Stuart ID (1978). Metastatic malignant melanoma transplanted via a renal homograft. Cancer 41:2426.

Sheil AGR (1977). Cancer in renal allograft recipients in Australia and New Zealand. Transplant Proc 9:1133.

Southam CM, Moore AE, Rhoads CP (1957). Homotransplantation of human cell lines. Science 125.

Tunner WS, Goldsmith EJ, Whitsell JC (1971). Human homotransplantation of normal and neoplastic tissue from the same organ. J Urol 105:18.

Wilson RE, Hager GB, Hampers CL, Corson JM, Merrill JP, Murray JE (1969). Immunologic rejection of human cancer transplanted with a renal allograft. N Eng J Med 278:479.

Wilson RE, Penn I (1975). Fate of tumors transplanted with a renal allograft. Transplant Proc 7:327.

Zukoski CF, Killen DA, Ginn E, Matter B, Lucas DO, Seigler HF (1970). Transplanted carcinoma in an immunosuppressed patient. Transplantation 9:71.

Renal Tumors: Proceedings of the First International Symposium on Kidney Tumors, pages 589–596
© **1982 Alan R. Liss, Inc., 150 Fifth Avenue, New York, NY 10011**

RENAL ONCOCYTOMA (PATHOLOGY, PREOPERATIVE DIAGNOSIS, THERAPY)

H.D. Lehmann and M.H. Blessing

Departments of Urology and Surgical Pathology
Hospitals of the city of Cologne
Cologne, R.F.A.

Renal oncocytes are epithelial cells which have lost the characteristic features of tubular cells and have attained a new differentiation. Functional alterations of the mitochondria seem to play an important role. The cells have a high concentration of ATP-ase and oxidative enzymes. Oncocytes and especially those of the kidney are not only found in elderly people but also in young adults (Cases 1 2). Synonyms for oncocytoma are proximal tubular eosinophilic adenoma, genuine hypernephroma, Riopelle-tumor, mitochondrioma and others. The fact that more renal oncocytomas are reported in recent literature does not prove an increase in incidence but merely indicates a better recognition of this growth.

Oncocytomas are usually a single growth of more than 3.5 cm in diameter and therefore larger than the more frequent ordinary tubular adenomas. They are not always situated strictly intrarenally. Frequently the cut-surface shows a slight striation and a characteristic mahogany-brown colour which is most likely due to a high concentration of cytochromes within the epithelial cells. There is no connective-tissue capsule and the consistency is somewhat softer than the surrounding renal parenchyma. Apparently only larger tumors reveal haemorrhages, necroses and scars.

O n c o z y t o m a   o f   k i d n e y

Nr.Name Age ♀ ♂	Symptoms BSR	preop.Diagnosis (Urography,SONO. CT,Angiography)	Operation-date preop.radiation Embolisation Approach	Specimen Weight Diameter Color	Histology Reclassification if any	p.op.course
1 K.H. 2o ♀	tumour 2 years, pain 4 weeks. 8/2o.	Cyst lower pole right kidney? Sono ∅,CT ∅ Angiogr.∅	retroperitoneal nephrectomy aft. frozen section 27.9.69	29o g 8 cm brown	Carcinoma. recl.Oncozyto-ma of kidney	normal healthy
2 M.B. 29 ♀	pain and haematuria 16/43	Tumour lower pole left kidney (Angiography)	3 x 5oo rad transperitoneal nephrectomy 21.4.74	3io g 6 cm brown	Carcinoma. recl.Oncozyto-ma of kidney	normal healthy
3 St.R. 49 ♂	colic r. kidney (stone)	Tumour left kidney,malignant in angiogr.	transperitoneal nephrectomy 15.11.71	22o g 9 cm brown	Carcinoma, recl.Oncozyto-ma of kidney	normal healthy
4 A.H. 6o ♂	none 6/17	Tumour lower pole r.kidney Angiogr.suspect	retroperitoneal nephrectomy 13.1o.76	2io g 4 cm brown	Oncozytoma of kidney,infil-tration of cap-sule ?	normal healthy
5 G.M. 6o ♂	pain left loin for 2 months 5/2o	Tumour upper pole left kid-ney.	retroperitoneal nephrectomy 17.5.76	32o g 5 cm brown-yellow	Oncozytoma of kidney	normal healthy
6 R.P. 64 ♂	Haematuria 21/64	2 tumours right kidney of diffe-rent vascular pattern.	Swan-Ganze cath. transperitoneal nephrectomy 15.6.77	3oo g 6 cm/6 cm brown/yellow	Oncozytoma and Carcinoma of kidney	normal healthy
7 St.T. 74 ♂	tumour since 3 years 23/59	great malignant tumour palpable Angiography!!	Swan-Ganze cath. retroperitoneal nephrectomy 31.1.77	92o g 16/12/11 brown-red yellow. grey.	Fibrosarcoma ex Oncozytoma	died on metasta-ses May 79
8 B.S. 49 ♂	pain for 3 years r.loin 1o/27	Sono + CT =malign. Angiogr.suspect	retroperitoneal nephrectomy 28.3.79	12oo g 22 cm brown-haemorrh.	Oncozytoma with necrosis	normal healthy
9 O.S. 65 ♂	Haematuria Varicocele right.2/7	hypervascul.Tu. lower pole r. kidney	Swan-Ganze cath. retroperitoneal nephrectomy 2.5.8o	brown 5 cm	Oncozytoma with haemorrhage	normal healthy
1o G.H. 74 ♂	none 53/87	Urogr.+Angiogr. hypervasc.Tumour right kidney	retroperitoneal nephrectomy aft. frozen section 31.3.81	19o g 5 cm brown	Oncozytoma of kidney with necrosis	normal died later on infarction

TABLE 1

It has been noted that oncocytoma is a benign tumor
which shows a different biological behavior than tubular
carcinoma. Occasionally, however, oncocytomas metastasize
and in one series of 90 renal tumors 2 had metastasized and
showed some cellular and nuclear atypia. In reclassifying
other cases 15% and 4.66% had oncocytic features in growth
between 3.5 and 13 cm in diameter.

Among our own 10 cases (Table 1) three were reclassi-
fied (Cases 1, 2, 3). Clinically and radiologically one
can only assume the existence of an oncocytoma, since the
final diagnosis can be made only histologically. Intraoperative frozen-sections can be helpful in determining
whether radical or conservative surgical management of the
patient is indicated.

MATERIALS AND METHODS

Between July 1963 and June 1981 we observed among 330
renal parenchymal tumors 10 oncocytomas (3.01%) with a
diameter between 4 and 22 cm. Eight patients were male
with a median age of 61.8 years and 2 were females, 20 and
29 years old. Six tumors were located in the right kidney,
five of which were in the lower pole, and one kidney was
almost completely replaced by a haemorrhagic growth (Case
8). Four oncocytomas were situated in the left kidney, one
in the upper and two in the lower pole, and one had replaced
the entire organ (Case 7).

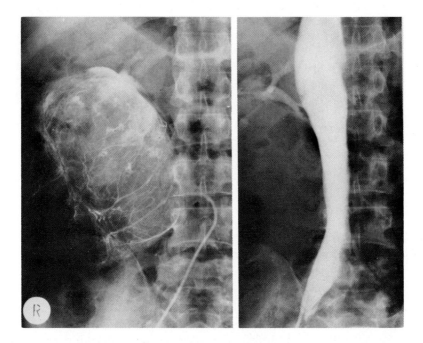

Fig. 1. (Case 8) Haemorrhagic oncocytoma.

In two cases the tumors were discovered accidentally.
Six patients had symptoms of pain, macro- or microhaematuria,
and had a right-side varicocele and in one patient the tumor
was known for three years (Case 7). Preoperatively we found
in two cases a second tumor with a different angiographic
pattern (Cases 6 and 7). One (Case 6) revealed histologically an independent tubular renal cell carcinoma (Fig. 2)
and the other showed a fibrosarcoma derived from scan and
granulation tissue within the oncocytoma (Fig. 3).

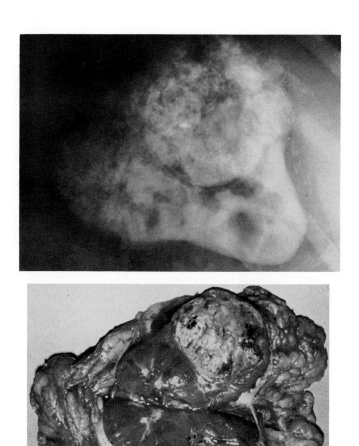

Fig. 2.   (Case 6) See text for comment.

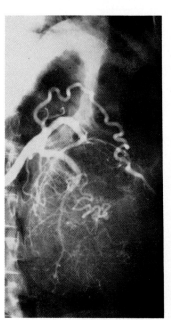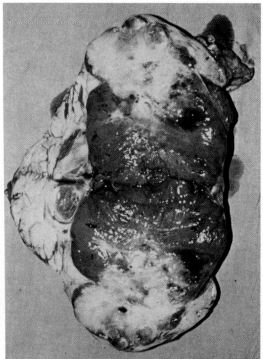

Fig. 3. (Case 7) Fibrosarcoma and granulation tissue within the oncocytoma.

Intravenous pyelogram usually shows an intraparenchymal or extending renal growth. An additional tomography reveals within the outlines of the kidney a tumor with a different density usually located in one of the poles. Sonography and computer tomography give indications as to necroses and the border to normal renal parenchyma. The density helps to differentiate between a solid tumor and a cyst: Angiography demonstrates the vascular component important for the therapeutic procedure. Sonography and CT are not indicative of the true nature of the tumor. In some of our cases (6, 8, 9, 10) quite different arteriographic patterns were demonstrated in spite of the subsequent histological diagnosis of oncocytoma. This is in accordance with other studies which revealed that with these procedures one can only suspect but not diagnose an oncocytoma.

TREATMENT

If selective angiography lets us suspect a malignant tumor, we usually embolize the renal artery with a Swan Ganze catheter. The preoperative angiography reveals whether radical nephrectomy, operative exposure of the kidney followed by a frozen section or enucleation of the tumor or partial resection of the kidney in cases with one kidney is indicated. In three of our 10 patients we performed a preoperative embolisation since there was indication for nephrectomy (Cases 6, 7, 9).

Preoperative laboratory data are not helpful in determining the malignancy of the tumor or the planned therapeutic procedure. We did not observe an excessive elevation of the sedimentation rate. In these cases where the type of the tumor cannot be ascertained before one or more frozen sections have been evaluated during the operation, it may be necessary to consider a second surgical intervention. This, however, under certain circumstances may be necessary. In cases with an oncocytic adenoma it is only occasionally possible e.g. when the tumor is very large and palpable or only a little parenchyma is left to decide on a primary nephrectomy. Special care should be taken when the frozen section reads "adenoma with oncocytic features" or when the tumor is grossly haemorrhagic and necrotic since in these cases one quite often faces a malignant growth. The question whether a radical tumor nephrectomy plus lymphadenectomy is too extensive a procedure in the case of an oncocytoma cannot be ascertained yet. Further histological investigations on multiple series from different sources as well as clinical behavior and survival rate have to be studied in the future.

It should be noted that cytofluorometry gives no relevant information as to the malignant potential of the oncocytoma of the kidney. Two of our cases were studied with this method. The tumor of Case 9 was hyperdiploid

with little tendency for proliferation and had a cytofluoro-
metric channel-value between 100 and 400.   Case 8 was
hypodiploid, the channel value was below 100, and there
was no sign of an elevated proliferation rate.

Renal Tumors: Proceedings of the First International Symposium on Kidney Tumors, pages 597-598
© **1982 Alan R. Liss, Inc., 150 Fifth Avenue, New York, NY 10011**

NEEDLE TRACT SEEDING FOLLOWING PUNCTURE OF RENAL ONCOCYTOMA

J. Auvert, C.C. Abbou, V. Lavarenne

Service d'Urologie

Hôpital Henri Mondor - 94010 - Creteil
Cedex, France

In 1973 a 59-year-old woman presented with asymptomatic
right lumbar mass which was evaluated by IVP and ultrasound
the conclusion from which was a right renal cyst. However,
percutaneous puncture failed to demonstrate a cyst and cytologic study after needle aspiration revealed renal carcinoma
cells.

The patient had a right radical nephrectomy and lymph
node dissection through a lumbo-abdominal approach.

The tumor specimen was a 9 X 6 cm-partly necrotic
lesion. On microscopy the tumor was comprised of plain
large eosinophilic cells, with few nuclear abnormalities,
in a trabecular and alveolar arrangement. The tumor did not
extend beyond the renal capsule and no tumor was found in
the regional lymph nodes. The diagnosis was Stage I renal
oncocytoma.

After a 7-year uneventful follow-up the patient at age
67 presented in October 1980 with a lumbar subcutaneous
1 X 2-cm mass located about 3 cm under the twelfth rib, that
is to say at the usual site for renal puncture. The patient
was in fair condition with no evidence of metastatic disease.
The removed lesion showed the same histologic features that
were found in the primary tumor. In our opinion that could
be a case of needle tract seeding of a tumor of intermediary
malignancy. Only one case of needle tract seeding after
renal cancer puncture seemed to be reported previously
(Gibbons et al, 1977).

References

Gibbons RP, Bush WH Jr, Burnett LL (1977). Needle tract
  seeding following aspiration of renal cell carcinoma.
  J Urol 118:865.

Renal Tumors: Proceedings of the First International Symposium on
Kidney Tumors, pages 599–600
© 1982 Alan R. Liss, Inc., 150 Fifth Avenue, New York, NY 10011

NATURAL HISTORY OF RENAL CELL CARCINOMA LEFT IN PLACE

G. Vallancien, Djedje Madi, F. Richard, R.
Kuss
Clinique Urologique, Hopital de la Pitié,
Paris

Surgical removal remains the only effective treatment
of renal cell carcinoma. The aim of this paper is to
evaluate the natural evolution of patients who were not
considered candidates for radical nephrectomy either because they had non-resectable tumors or because of poor
general physical condition. A total of 330 patients with
renal cell carcinoma treated at the Pitié Hospital in
Paris were reviewed. Of these, 33 (10%) did not have
nephrectomy. The diagnosis of unresectability of tumor
was made in 19 cases after exploratory laparotomy and in
14 cases based on clinical and/or CT scan evidence.

Table 1 summarizes the different cases who do not have
nephrectomy based on the diagnosis of unresectability
(laparotomy or CT scan). Two conclusions could be drawn:

(1) The use of CT scan rendered exploratory
laparotomy unnecessary in practice except in rare
cases where CT scan is unable to give exact tumor
extensions to renal hilus or to the liver.

(2) When patients have locally extensive disease
with no pain or hematuria the benefit of nephrectomy is
disputable. In our experience, the evolution without
surgery compares favorably with the expected evolution if
the tumor was resected.

TABLE 1A

CLINICAL FEATURES AND SURVIVAL OF PATIENTS WITH NO NEPHRECTOMY

	N°Patient	Mean Age	Stage	Metastasis	Scan
Exploratory laparotomy	19	57	IV 19	11	3
Not operated	14	70	IIIA 4		
			IIIC 4	6	11
			IVA 6		

TABLE 1B

	N°Patient	dead		living	
		<6 months	<1 year	+1 year	+ 2 years
Exploratory laparotomy	19	12	4	1	0
Not operated	14	5	4	3	2

In the group of patients not operated 3 patients were rehospitalized for edema of lower extremities or for hematuria.
In the group of patients operated (laparotomy) 2 died in post operative period and 9 were hospitalized 1 month.

Renal Tumors: Proceedings of the First International Symposium on Kidney Tumors, pages 601-602
© 1982 Alan R. Liss, Inc., 150 Fifth Avenue, New York, NY 10011

IMPROVEMENTS OF THE RENAL TUMOR EMBOLIZATION TECHNIQUE

Ph. Curet, M.D.

Department of Radiology, Hopital La Pitie
83 Bld de l'Hopital 75013 Paris

Since 1973, the vascular occlusive technique for kidney tumors has improved through prevention of ischemic renal pain and use of new embolization materials. An important limiting factor, ischemic pain due to abrupt occlusion of renal artery, is avoided and treated by upper peridural analgesia. This anesthesia begins prior to renal embolization. It is possible to prolong its action until nephrectomy or during the painful period. Analgesia begins with adrenalized bupivavaine, 0.5% given through a micro catheter positioned at L2-L3 level in peridural space, and can be continued through injection of the identical product or of morphine chlorydrate (Andrieu et al. 1981). Among recent vascular occlusive agents, we still retain the steel coil and fluid emboli. The advantages of this coil are its X-ray opacity and its easy employment. The level of obliteration is proximal but the distant result is not always definitive (Javeri et al. 1978). Moreover, the coil may cause a local aneurysm (Struthers et al. 1980). Therefore in our opinion its use is limited to preoperative embolization.

Butyl-cyanoacrylate is the most utilized fluid emboli. Its polymerization is induced by an ionic reaction (Dotter 1975). This reaction is exothermic and requires a few seconds. Mixing lipiodol and cyanoacrylate equally makes the emboli radiopaque and increases the polimerization time. This procedure provides an advantage that speeds up and modulates embolization. This material is not resorbable and the vascular obliteration is definitive (Fig. 1). Because its efficiency, its utilization must be in accordance with the radiologist ability and can be suggested for preoperative or palliative embolization.

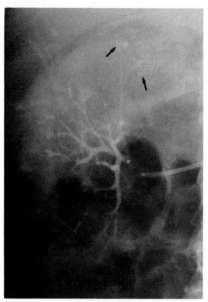

Fig. 1. Preoperative embolization realizes with butyl cyanoacrylate mixed with lipiodol. Note the existence of the contrast material and the arrows indicating the tumor localization.

Andrieu G, Harari A, Viars P, Samii K, Curet Ph, Richard F (1981). Analgésie péri-durale après embolisation artérielle viscérale. Nouv Presse Med 10:431.

Dotter CT, Goldman ML, Rosch J (1975). Instant selectiv arterial occlusion with isobutyl 2 cyano-acrylate. Radiology 114:227.

Jhaveri HS, Gerlock AJ, Ekelund L (1978). Failure of steel coil occlusion in a case of hypernephroma. Am J Roentgenol 130:556.

Struthers NW, Samu P, Chalvardjian A (1980). Renal artery aneurysm: complication of Gianturco Coil embolization of renal adenocarcinoma. J Urol 123:105.

Renal Tumors: Proceedings of the First International Symposium on
Kidney Tumors, pages 603–607
© 1982 Alan R. Liss, Inc., 150 Fifth Avenue, New York, NY 10011

THE INDICATIONS OF EMBOLISATION IN RENAL TUMOR: WHAT REMAINS
TO BE SAID?

M. LeGuillou, J.J. Merland

Bordeaux - Paris Lariboisiere

This purposely restricted title raises two thoughts.

1)   Each new technical innovation can be accomplished
by ill-considered enthusiasm. Without doubt, some
of the workers are caught up in the spirit of progress,
but without enough preparation especially in regard
to radiology. Precise aims must be defined, and new
techniques must be beyond reproach.

2)   In August, 1981, eight years after the indications
we suggested with René Kuss, it seemed essential to
state clearly the facts on methods employed, and
current perspectives evaluated. Four points are
worthy of discussion.

  a) Which technique should be suggested?
  b) What are the correct indications?
  c) What are the risks involved and how can
      they be avoided?
  d) What are the results from an analysis
      of 246 cases we have collected since
      the 17th Congress of the International
      Urology Congress?

TECHNIQUE

    High quality techniques are essential to achieve any
desired goal. For example, hyper-selective distal catheterisation of individual arterial pedicals, and not just of

arterial trunks, should be used to obtain distal obliteration, and also to avoid reflux of the embolus into the circulation. A very supple catheter should be used, which can be left in situ for long periods. Access should normally be via the femoral artery, and only exceptionally via the axillary.

The nature of the embolus is very variable, and, if spongel, with thrombin, is still the most frequently used material. The following material can also be used equally well: muscle, dura mater, granules of iron silicone directed electromagnetically, rapid polymerization solutions, and sclerosants, gold grains charged with a short half life isotope.

The following observations must be monitored cautiously: systematic control of renal insufficiency, monitoring of the limb distal to the puncture site, blood pressure and diuresis, and pain, which may herald the onset of infection.

Reasonable Indications

These indications have not altered since our presentation at the uro-nephrology seminar in the Pitié in 1976. A certain diagnosis, of course, must have been made. Pre-operative embolisation is preferentially found in voluminous and hyper-vascular tumors. This can pose subsequent technical problems if there is venous extension, particularly in the inferior vena cava. Embolisation allows one to control and ligate the venous axis without moving the tumor or ligating the renal artery. Such a check, with an immediate ligature of the vein does not involve any modification in the renal mass, and avoids the possibility of dislodging neoplastic emboli into the circulation. It also can simplify any operative intervention, by creating an actual edematous cleavage plane around the tumor. This is done after shutting down any collateral venous circulation. Finally, this procedure shortens the operating time and diminishes the blood loss.

Palliative embolisation may be indicated in certain cases of painful bony metastases, and in some renal tumors, where operation is contraindicated because of local or distal spread. Embolisation can reduce tumor volume and growth and can stop some catastrophic bleeding. It may slow down the development of the tumor, thus allowing any adjuvant anti-mitotic therapy time to achieve a greater effect on the

neoplastic cells. We cannot yet be sure that it improves
the immune status of the host and, while some metastases may
be slowed in their development, notably pulmonary metastases,
we have never observed their actual disappearance in contradistinction to other authors. In our opinion spongel-based
embolisation has no place in the treatment of small or
medium sized renal tumors. Its use may perhaps be justified
if an anti-mitotic is also used (especially Mitomycin C) in
the hope of diminishing the risk of metastatic disease.

The Risks of Embolisation: How They can be Avoided

The risk of embolisation, often undertaken under simple
analgesia, should not be ignored, but should be weighed
against the advantages in very ill patients, and in view of
the difficulty of performing surgery in a highly vascular
field.

Atheroma can be the cause of post-arteriography ischaemic
events, but the rigidity of the arterioles also raises the
possibility of haemorrhage in the target organ or at the
point of femoral puncture. This merely emphasizes the
necessity of an atraumatic catheterisation by an experienced
team, and constant surveillance of the limb subsequently.
There are four absolute contraindications:

1) Absence of certain diagnosis: not all tumors
should be embolised. Histology may indicate
that another more effective treatment should
be used.

2) The exact anatomical disposition should be
considered in great detail. The existence
of a direct arterio-venous fistula is a contraindication, even without an angioma. Similarly,
the presence of an abnormal pedicule of the
artery of Adamkiewicz, at the lumbar level,
would also constitute a contraindication.

3) Embolisation is contraindicated in purulent
tumors, for here one runs the risk of
establishing a septicaemia which can be
very difficult to treat.

4) Prior renal insufficiency is the 4th contra-

indication (creatinine level >20mg %).
During the procedure, there is an accumulation of contrast medium, which can produce
an undesirable exacerbation of this
insufficiency.

Results

The efficiency of embolisation is not in question, but
complete devascularisation can only be expected either
through the formation of thrombus inside the lesions, or by
the distal occulsion of all the afferent pedicules. The
whole problem revolves around subsequent revascularisation,
which throws the immediate benefit sustained as a result of
embolisation into doubt. It is difficult to be sure whether
this proces is secondary to incomplete embolisation, or if
it is due to the opening up on collateral circulation.
Presently, there is considerable doubt about lysis of the
embolus itself.

We carried out 203 pre-operative embolisations in
France in 1979. In all cases, the subsequent operations
were made easier and there was no mortality. No local
fibrinolysis or bacteraemia was observed. A number of
sequelae should be noted: 80% incidence of lumbar pain,
40% incidence of fever, 42% incidence of transitory elevation
of transaminases.

Three complications are worthy of mention.

1) Arterial disobstruction was required in
eight cases.

2) In 12 cases, emergency surgery was required
to stop bleeding.

3) Transient diminution in renal function for
15 days in 10% of cases, and prolonged
diminution with creatinine greater than 20 mg%
in eight cases. Two possibilities exist
here. Either there has been an inopportune
embolisation from the other side, or too
much medium had been injected.

In 44 cases of palliative embolisation, observed survival

ranged from several months to five years. This was similar
to the survival to be expected naturally.

Embolisation did seem to have a beneficial effect in
the majority of cases, especially with respect to severe
haematuria and diminution of pain. Some general improvement
was noted in 40% of cases, and in 16 patients there was a
definite stabilization of pulmonary metastases. Conversely,
infectious complications worsened the outlook in a number of
already inoperable patients. These have to be distinguished
from pneumatisation of the calyx, which was reversible within
three weeks (five cases).

In two cases of renal insufficiency, with creatinine
greater than 30mg%, no alteration in their short term
prognosis was noted.

Additional embolisations (66) carried out by our team
have confirmed the above findings.

Thus, after a total of 313 embolisations for renal
tumor, it can be said that this procedure is a useful tool
for the urologist, either on its own or in conjunction with
operative procedures. It appears especially useful where
there is metastasis.

The indications for using this technique should be
considered by a specialized team of radiologists. A refined
technique, exactly defined objectives, and constant
surveillance are essential for a satisfactory outcome.

Renal Tumors: Proceedings of the First International Symposium on Kidney Tumors, pages 609–616
© **1982 Alan R. Liss, Inc., 150 Fifth Avenue, New York, NY 10011**

PRE- AND POSTOPERATIVE RADIOTHERAPY, INFLUENCE ON PROGNOSIS

Lennart Andersson and Folke Edsmyr

Department of Urology and Radiuhemmet,
Karolinska sjukhuset, Stockholm, Sweden

Renal cell carcinoma is considered to be a radio-resistant tumour. Non-responsiveness like responsiveness to irradiation is a relative phenomenon. However, the dose necessary to sterilize renal cell carcinoma is of such magnitude that the surrounding normal tissues are destroyed. Radiotherapy therefore can never be an alternative to operation. On the other hand, irradiation has been rather widely used as an adjuvant therapy in association with surgery, both in the form of preoperative and postoperative irradiation.

In the USA preoperative irradiation in renal cell carcinoma was already in use in the early 1930's by Waters and co-workers (1934). In the 1950's Sir Eric Riches et al (1951) stimulated a new interest in preoperative ir-radiation in this form of cancer. He personally observed a number of patients over a long period and he collected a further large number of cases from various centers over the British Isles. In these series he noticed a better survival in those patients who had received preoperative irradiation. Based on his own and other authors' experience Riches et al (1951) recommended preoperative irradiation to all patients with renal cell carcinoma. Preoperative irradiation has a two-fold aim: to reduce tumour size, mainly the pericapsular spread, and thereby facilitate radical operation, and to reduce tumour cell viability and hopefully prevent tumour dissemination during the operation. A number of cases have been documented where the tumour size and vascularity diminished after irradiation and where tumours fixed to adjacent structures were rendered amenable to radical excision.

The irradiation presumably affects mainly the peripheral tumour cells and wide veins around the kidney are narrowed. If such a down-staging is aimed at, the operation should not be done in the hyperemic reactive phase immediately after irradiation but should be postponed until the fibrotic phase starts three to four weeks after cessation of irradiation.

It has also been presumed that preoperative irradiation by reduction of tumour cell viability would diminish the risk of intraoperative tumour spread due to manipulation of the kidney. If distant metastases are already present preoperative irradiation is, of course, useless in this respect.

Saksela and co-workers (1973) studied in vitro the effect of preoperative irradiation on renal cell carcinoma. In a randomized series the patients were either nephrectomized immediately or given irradiation from a linear accelerator in a dose of 30-35 Gy to the kidney and operated upon three weeks later. In the operative specimen cells both from the tumour and from normal renal tissue were taken and grown in tissue culture. As is seen in Table 1, there was growth of tumour cells from 71% of the non-irradiated kidneys but only from 18% of those kidneys exposed to irradiation. There was a similar difference between the growth from the non-affected part of the kidneys, but this difference was much less conspicuous.

Since metastases are slowly growing colonies of disseminated tumour cells or cell clusters, the findings of Saksela et al (1973) would support the hypothesis that preoperative irradiation might prevent, to some extent, tumour spread. However, the reports on the value of preoperative irradiation are contradictory. There are many investigations on record. This review will be confined to reporting briefly on two relatively recent investigations where the tumours were characterized in a reproducible way.

Van der Wert-Messing (1973) reported on a randomized trial where patients with renal cell carcinoma were either treated by immediate nephrectomy or given preoperative irradiation, 30 Gy, to the kidney area and regional nodes over three weeks, and operated on immediately after. One

TABLE 1

GROWTH IN RENAL CULTURE OF CELLS FROM KIDNEYS

REMOVED FOR RENAL CELL CARCINOMA (SAKSELA ET AL, 1973)

	Preoperative irradiation		No irradiation	
	17		21	
Tumour	3	18%	15	71%
Normal tissue	12	71%	18	86%

TABLE 2

INCOMPLETE REMOVAL IN 52 P_3 CASES OF

RENAL CELL CARCINOMA (VAN DER WERF MESSING, 1973)

Preop	X	8/30	27%
No preop	X	11/22	50%

hundred twenty-six patients could be evaluated. A difference occurred mainly in the P_3 category which comprised 52 cases. Removal of the tumour was incomplete in 27% of the 30 patients given preoperative irradiation, but in 50% of those 22 operated on without previous irradiation (Table 2). During the observation period, distant metastases occurred in 45% of the P_3 patients who had a locally complete tumour removal, but in 79% of those cases where the removal was locally incomplete. A non-radical operation carries a higher risk of subsequent metastases.

Fig. 1 reports postoperative survival of the P_3 patients. In the first 18 months the patients given irradiation did better than the controls, but after two years the survival was the same in both groups. In the other P categories no difference in survival was observed. Preoperative irradiation was recommended in such cases where it is suspected that the local tumour can not be removed completely.

In our departments preoperative irradiation has been given on a non-randomized basis, mainly in those cases where the preoperative fine needle biopsy, which is done routinely, indicated poorly differentiated renal cell carcinoma. Irradiation, 35 Gy, was given by linear accelerator to the kidney and regional glands over 35 days and nephrectomy was done 3-4 weeks after cessation of irradiation. In a series of 24 irradiated patients with poorly differentiated carcinoma, 5-year survival was 54%. In a previous series of 103 patients with poorly differentiated carcinoma and given no irradiation, 5-year survival was 31%. In the categories of well or moderately well differentiated carcinoma, there was no difference in survival whether preoperative irradiation was given or not. Analysis of an extended series is under way to evaluate whether preoperative irradiation secures signifantly improved survival in those cases of high grade malignancy.

The rationale for postoperative irradiation is to eradicate or reduce recurrence of the tumour following surgery, either in the tumour bed, scar or local lymph node areas.

There are on record three large and several smaller series comparing survival following nephrectomy for renal

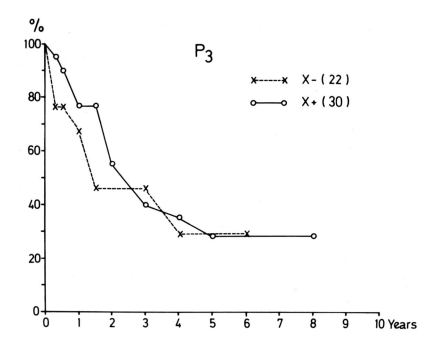

Legend to figure

Fig. 1.   Survival in 52 P_3 cases of renal cell
carcinoma.   In 30 cases preoperative
radiation was given (van der Werf-
Messing, 1973).

cell carcinoma with and without postoperative irradiation.
In Table 3 are reported the 5-year survival in a series
of over 800 cases from various British hospitals and reported by Riches (1964) and in two other large series
reported by Flocks & Kadesky (1958) and by Bratherton
(1964). In these studies, which were all retrospective
and non-randomized, survival was somewhat more favorable
in the groups given irradiation.

Finney (1973) reported on a controlled study of 100
cases of renal cell carcinoma and randomly allocated to
postoperative irradiation by a standard treatment regime
or no irradiation. Five-year survival was 36% in the
patients given irradiation and 44% in the controls.
Cancer deaths, both from local recurrence and from
distant metastases, were about equal in both groups, but
there occurred significantly more deaths from other causes
in the irradiated patients. Four died of liver damage.
These four patients had right-sided tumours. Finney
(1973) concluded that postoperative irradiation fails to
control local tumour recurrence and has no place in the
routine management of renal cell carcinoma.

Today, postoperative irradiation is only given in
those cases where the removal of the local tumour was
incomplete or suspected to be incomplete. This is a
generally accepted indication as an attempt at palliation.

Our own series of postoperative irradiation is non-
randomized and comprises 41 cases where the tumour invaded the renal vein, the renal pelvis or the perirenal
tissue, all factors of unfavourable influence on the
prognosis. These patients were individually planned for
irradiation and given a mean dose of 50 Gy to the renal
bed and regional nodes in 6-7 weeks with a three-field
technique and linear accelerator. The irradiation was
started 3-4 weeks after surgery. The 5-year survival
in this series was 45% in grade 2 tumours and 33% in
grade 3 tumours. Some patients with right-sided carcinoma had a temporary alteration of liver function tests
but there was no case of irreversible liver disturbance
and no case of renal failure. Our experience is in accordance with that of some other authors that postoperative irradiation in a suitable dose and with
adequate technique can be given without undue risk to the

TABLE 3

FIVE YEAR SURVIVAL IN PERCENT IN PATIENT WITH RENAL
CELL CARCINOMA WITH AND WITHOUT POSTOPERATIVE IRRADIATION.

	N	Surgery	Surgery + X
Flocks & Kadesky (1958)	353	48	53
Riches (1964)	816	30	49
Bratherton (1964)	125	29	43

patient, even in tumours of the right kidney.

In summary, irradiation is too little effective against renal cell carcinoma to be an alternative to surgery. In tumours with large pericapsular spread preoperative irradiation is useful to facilitate the operation and favours radical excision. There is preliminary evidence that preoperative irradiation improves survival rate in high grade carcinoma. Postoperative irradiation is given as an adjunctive measure in cases where tumour tissue had to be left behind in the renal bed or regional nodes. The opinions on the value of irradiation in renal cell carcinoma have often been based on inadequately controlled studies. The problem deserves further investigation under controlled conditions where the tumours are properly categorized with respect to local extension, regional and distant metastases and malignancy grade.

Bratherton DG (1974). The place of radiotherapy in the treatment of hypernephroma. Brit J Radiol 37:141.

Edsmyr F, Schreeb T von, Johansson B, Esposti PL (1977). Radiation therapy of malignant renal tumours. Pathologie und Radiologie von Hochdruck und Nierenkrankheiten, p. 270. Ed. T. Kröpelin, Thieme, Stuttgart.

Finney R (1973). The value of radiotherapy in the treatment of hypernephroma - a clinical trial. Brit J Urol 45:258.

Flocks RH, Kadesky, MC (1958). Malignant neoplasms of the kidney: An analysis of 353 patients followed five years or more. J Urol 79:196.

Riches, Sir EW (1964). Surgery of renal tumours. In "Neoplastic Disease at Various Sites. Tumours of the kidney and Ureter," Vol. 5, Edinburgh: Livingstone, p. 275.

Riches, Sir EW, Griffiths, IH, Thackray AC (1951). New growths of the kidney and ureter. Brit J Urol 23:297.

Saksela E, Alfthan O, Malmio K (1973). Effect of preoperative radiotherapy on the growth of human renal carcinoma tissue in vitro. Scand J Urol Nephrol 7:181.

Waters CA, Lewis LG, Frontz, WA (1934). Radiation therapy of renal cortical neoplasms with special reference to preoperative irradiation. Southern Med J 27:290.

Werf-Messing B, van der (1973). Carcinoma of the kidney. Cancer 32:1056.

Renal Tumors: Proceedings of the First International Symposium on Kidney Tumors, pages 617–622
© 1982 Alan R. Liss, Inc., 150 Fifth Avenue, New York, NY 10011

KIDNEY CARCINOMA: IS PREOPERATIVE RADIOTHERAPY OF ANY VALUE?

L. Boccon Gibod, G. Benoit, F. Eschwege, A. Steg
Clinique Urologique de l'Hopital Cochin 75014
Department de Radiation, Service de Telecobal-
therapie - Institut G. Roussy 94800 Villejuig
FRANCE

Is adjunctive preoperative radiotherapy of any value in
the management of kidney carcinoma? We report here on its
use and effects on a series of 70 consecutive patients.
From 1972 to 1978, 55 men and 15 women aged 58.7±10.9 years,
suffering from renal adenocarcinoma (36 right side, 34 left)
were treated by nephrectomy preceded by irradiation (3000R)
of the kidney. Irradiation was given in 300R increments
over a period of three weeks, and delivered through two
anterior and posterior portals limited superiorly by the
diaphragm, inferiorly by the iliac crest and medially by the
prevertebral vessels so as to comprise the median lymph nodes.

Radical nephrectomy without lymphadenectomy was performed three weeks after completion of radiotherapy and was
effectively realized in 69 cases, 59 of which were through
an 11th or 12th rib flank incision, and 10 cases were through
a thoracoabdominal incision opening the diaphragm in cases
of large upper pole tumors.

RESULTS

The surgical procedure was usually easy: the postradiotherapy oedema facilitated the development of anatomical
cleavage planes. Hemorrhage was moderate and the mean blood
replacement volume was 2.4 units. Mean operating time
(residents and staff surgeons) was three and one-half hours.

Two patients died in the first month. Postoperative
complications were minimal and the usual postoperative duration

of hospital stay was 20 days.   The pathology report showed,
using Robson's classification, that there were 15 Stage I,
10 Stage II, 20 Stage III and 12 Stage IV tumors.   Fifty-
seven patients having been followed for a minimum of eight
months were eligible for estimation of actuarial survival.
Thus the five-year survival for all stages is 34%, and for
Stages I, II, III it is 50% (Figures 1 and 2).   Among the
24 surviving patients seven are alive with metastasis.

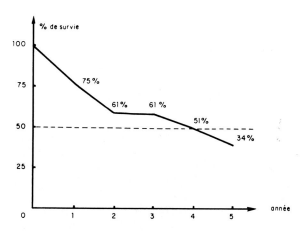

4. Survie actuarielle des stades I, II, III, IV.

Fig. 1.   Actuarial survival, Stages I, II, III, IV.

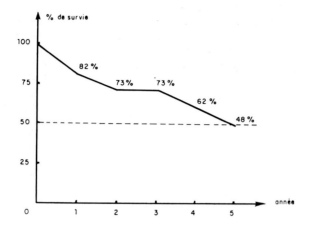

5. Survie actuarielle des stades I, II, III.

Fig. 2. Actuarial survival, Stages I, II, III.

DISCUSSION

There are four purposes for preoperative radiotherapy. The first is to sterilize tumor cells mobilized by surgical manipulation and presumed to be the source of local recurrence and/or distant metastases. The other purposes are to sterilize the lymph nodes draining the kidney, facilitate surgical extirpation, and expand survival figures. Although Saksela showed that radiotherapy significantly diminished the possibility of cultivating cells of kidney carcinoma, there is no demonstrated efficiency of preoperative irradiation in the prevention of metastasis (Saksela et al, 1973). Positive lymph nodes which occur in 22% of the cases can only be effectively treated in cases of microscopic metastases (Angerval, Wahlquist 1978; Robson et al, 1969). Preoperative radiotherapy undoubtedly facilitates the surgical procedure, owing to reduction of tumor volume (Cox et al, 1969) and

mainly to postradiotherapy oedoma, which allows a radical
nephrectomy through a flank incision. This is far less
aggressive than the thoracoabdominal incision opening the
diaphragm, the necessity of which is limited to large upper
pole tumors and cases of caval thrombosis. Although well
tolerated, preoperative radiotherapy has little or no effect
on the survival of the patients. Our five-year survival
rate of 48% (Figure 3) compares well with those of other
authors using the same protocol (Juusela et al, 1977; Rost,
Brosig 1977; Van der werf 1973, 1975) of simple radical
nephrectomy, but seems lower compared to those obtained by
radical nephrectomy with lymphadenectomy (Figure 4).

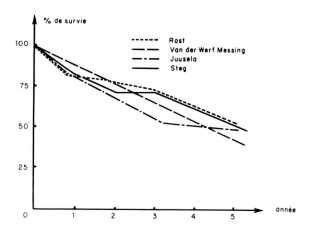

6. Survie actuarielle, comparée, de la radiothérapie préopératoire suivie de néphrectomie élargie.

Fig. 3. Comparative acturial survival of patients receiving
preoperative radiotherapy before radical nephrectomy.

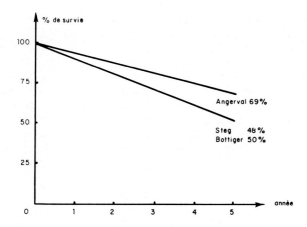

7. Comparaison de la survie à cinq ans suivant le type d'intervention.

Fig. 4. Comparative five-year survival in different types of surgical procedures.

CONCLUSION

The adjunction to radical nephrectomy of preoperative radiotherapy using a dose of 3000R over three weeks does not have any demonstrable effect on survival. On the other hand, facilitation of the surgical procedure is unquestionable. Therefore although we have abandoned routine preoperative irradiation in favor of the adjunction of lymphadenectomy to radical nephrectomy, a procedure the efficiency of which has yet to be clearly demonstrated, we still recommend it in cases of very large (>10 cm in diameter) upper pole kidney adeno-carcinoma, which can thus be extirpated through a flank incision using a subtotal 11th rib resection, avoiding opening of the diaphragm.

REFERENCES

Angerval L, Whalquist L (1978). Follow up and prognosis of
  renal carcinoma in a serie operated by perifascial
  nephrectomy with adrenalectomy and retroperitoneal lymphadenectomy. Eur Urol 4:13.
Cox C, Lacy S, Montgomery W, Boyce W (1979). Renal adenocarcinoma 28 years review with emphasis on national and
  feasibility of preoperative radiotherapy. J Urol 104:53.
Juusela H, Malmio K, Alfthan O, Oravisto K (1977). Preoperative irradiation in the treatment of renal adenocarcinoma. Scand J Urol Nephrol 11:277.
Robson C, Churchill B, Anderson W (1969). The result of
  radical nephrectomy for renal cell carcinoma. J Urol
  101:297.
Rost A, Brosig W (1977). Preoperative irradiation of renal
  cell carcinoma. Urology 10:414.
Van der werf messing B (1975). Carcinome du rein: un essai
  therapeutique. J Radiol 55:785.
Van der werf messing B (1973). Carcinoma of the kidney.
  Cancer 32:1056.

Renal Tumors: Proceedings of the First International Symposium on Kidney Tumors, pages 623–640

HORMONAL THERAPY OF RENAL CELL CARCINOMA (RCC)

Ulrico Bracci, Franco DiSilverio and Giuseppe Concolino
University of Rome
00161 Rome, Italy

INTRODUCTION

Hormonal therapy of human renal cell carcinoma (RCC) is based on the effects of additive or ablative endocrine treatment in experimental animals. The relationship between hormone agonists and antagonists on kidney tissue has been extensively documented in animals, particularly in the Syrian hamster which provides the best experimental model of hormone-induced RCC (Bloom 1973; Bloom et al, 1963a,b; Horning 1956a,b; Letourneau et al, 1975; Li, Li 1975; Kirkman 1959; Matthews et al, 1947). Following clinical observations in man, attempts have been made to prove that human RCC can be considered hormone-dependent tumor. Recent studies on steroid receptors both in animal and human RCC have provided the biochemical basis for the hormonal treatment of RCC (Bojar et al, 1975; Concolino et al, 1975; Concolino et al, 1979; Fanestil et al, 1974; Li, Li 1975; Li, Li 1977; Li et al, 1974; Li et al, 1976). It is worthwhile to point out that control of tumor growth with hormones can be obtained with a selective modification of some physiological processes and therefore without serious side effects for the patients.

Hypothesis of Hormone-Dependence of RCC

Statistical and epidemiological data as well as clinical findings have led to the conclusion that human RCC has some analogy with experimental RCC. RCC, in fact, occurs twice as frequently in men as in women with a decrease in the male/female ratio from 4:1 to 2:1 at the age of 40-44 years i.e., at end of gonadal activity (Bennington 1973).

The higher incidence of RCC during the child-bearing period of the human female suggests a protective action of progesterone in women.

Racial differences have also been reported, the frequency being higher in white races than in negro and yellow races (Bennington 1973; Kantor et al, 1976). There are no data available on the effects of hormonal status on these racial differences.

The possibility that adrenal corticoids could inhibit human RCC was suggested by the report of renal cancer regression in the presence of developing adrenal tumor (Bartley, Hulquist 1950). We have unpublished data on this phenomenon.

Furthermore, implants of testosterone, or administration of testosterone plus progestins and cortisone led to the regression of lung metastasis from human RCC (Bloom 1971; Bloom, Wallace 1964; Bracci et al, 1973; Paine et al, 1970). Some authors consider the regression of lung metastases following hormonal therapy as a spontaneous regression of lung metastases. Spontaneous regression, however, was found to occur in 474 (0.8%) patients with RCC (Montie et al, 1977), while in another series there were 67 such patients from 1928-1980 (Fairlamb 1981).

Trials of Hormonal Therapy of Human RCC

In 1964 Bloom reported the possible effect of testosterone upon the regression of metastases of human RCC (Bloom, Wallace 1964). Bloom extended hormonal treatment with medroxy-progesterone acetate (MPA) to patients with advanced metastatic disease. The overall percent response reported by Bloom is 15-16% (Bloom 1971) which is comparable with that of 16-17% reported by Wagle and Murphy (1971) in advanced RCC. Progestins generally have no effect on lymph nodes or bone metastases. Talley reported a response of 11.4% with androgen treatment in patients failing to respond to progestin treatment (Talley 1973).

Between 1967 and 1976 Bracci and Di Silverio (1976) used

progestational compounds as post-operative adjuvent treatment
in a group of patients submitted to nephrectomy for RCC and
reported a lower incidence of metastases in patients given
adjuvant treatment than in those submitted only to nephrectomy.

Antiestrogens have been used in the attempt to treat
patients with advanced metastatic RCC; a 9-16% response rate
as stable disease has been reported. It should be mentioned,
however, that the response to endocrine therapy was estimated
in absence of studies on estrogen receptors (Al Sarraf et al,
1981; Glick et al, 1979).

A low response rate to chemotherapy both with single
and combined agents has been reported in the literature.
Even recent attempts to treat human RCC with cis-platinum
(Rodriquez, Johnson 1978) or methyl-GAG (Todd et al, 1981)
or estracyt (Swanson, Johnson 1981) have been disappointing
although a higher response rate (36%) has been reported by
some authors using MPA associated with chemo-immunotherapy
or with vinblastine (Bartley, Hulquist 1950; Glick et al, 1979;
Hahn et al, 1977, Stolbach et al, 1981).

Biochemical Basis

On the basis of the effects of hormonal treatment and
taking into consideration the recent findings on the mechanism
of action of steroid hormones, it appeared reasonable to
study steroid receptors in RCC.

Estradiol receptors (ER), progesterone receptors (PR)
and androgen receptors (AR) have been studied in many experimentally induced RCC. Particular attention has been paid to
the study of ER, PR and AR in the estrogen-induced RCC of
Syrian hamster (Li, Li 1975a,b; Li, Li et al, 1974a,b, 1976).
The PR concentration which in response to estrogen treatment
showed a 17-27 fold increase in renal tissue with respect to
treated control levels, became 620 times higher in RCC than
in control animals. In order to establish whether human RCC
showed some analogy with the estrogen induced tumor in
experimental animals, steroid receptors have been investigated
in normal human renal tissue and in the cytoplasmic and
nuclear fractions of human RCC (Bojar et al, 1976; Concolino
et al, 1975, 1976, 1978, 1979a, b, 1980). Steroid receptors
in fact, appear to support the hypothesis of human RCC
suggested on the basis of previous clinical data. Renal

tissue, the tissues of the female genital tract, mammary gland and prostate may be considered target organs of sex hormones. Estrogen and androgen act upon human renal cells and induce opposite morphological and biochemical changes. Therefore, ER, PR, and AR have been studied both in the cytosol and nuclear RCC. Our investigations have recently focused on the meaning of the nuclear AR as a marker of hormone responsiveness of human RCC to pharmacological doses of MPA. Furthermore, we have preliminary data showing an increase in PR concentration in RCC of patients treated with Tamoxifen (TAM) seven days before nephrectomy (Table 1), which would support the concept that estradiol acts on RCC through a receptor mechanism.

TABLE 1

EFFECT OF TAMOXIFEN* ON PROGESTERONE RECEPTOR IN NORMAL
HUMAN KIDNEY AND IN HUMAN RENAL CELL CARCINOMA

	Progesterone Receptor (fmol/mg protein)	
	No Treatment	Tamoxifen
Normal Kidney Tissue	2.96	66.13
Renal Cell Carcinoma	4.09±2.81	16.43±4.05

*Patients treated with Tamoxifen (20mg/p.d. for seven days)before surgery.

Current Status of Hormonal Treatment of Human RCC

The first approach to the treatment of human RCC by our group began in 1967, following the preliminary report of Bloom. At that time, our investigations did not, of course, include receptor studies. Following favorable results in 82 patients on hormonal therapy in that first ten-year period, a second study was performed in which ER, PR and AR were examined in 50 patients with no metastatic disease, and survival was also taken into consideration. At present, hormonal therapy as adjuvant treatment to radical nephrectomy is performed only on the basis of the result of receptor studies. The next approach in the study of the effectiveness of endocrine treatment will be based on the randomization of the patients with hormonal treatment in those patients with RCC containing steroid receptors. Results of a preliminary study of this type have recently been reported (Concolino et al, 1979, 1980).

Therefore the study programs carried out so far address survival in patients with and without adjuvant hormonal therapy, and survival in patients submitted to nephrectomy plus hormonal therapy with regard to the presence of steroid receptors.

The first series of 82 patients examined between 1967 and 1976 were divided into a group of 40 who underwent only nephrectomy (mean age 57.3 years male/female ratio 3:1) and a second group of 42 who received adjuvant therapy with MPA at pharmacological doses (mean age 51.5 years, male/female ratio 3:1). The TNM classification in both groups was $pT_{2-3} N_{0-1} M_0$. The percent survival in these two groups is comparable in the first two years but at the end of a six-year follow-up period a significant difference ($p < 0.05$) is observed in the survival rate between the two groups (29% vs. 61%) (Figure 1).

The second study was carried out on 50 patients (out of 67 patients on whom tumor receptor studies had been performed). The mean age was 61.4 years, the male/female ratio 2.3:1, and each submitted to radical nephrectomy and MPA therapy at pharmacological doses. According to the TNM classification the histological stage was pT_2 in 34 patients and pT_3 in 16; lymph node involvement (N_1) was found in 35% of patients in both groups. Since no evidence of metastases was detected (M_0), death rate, survival and life expectancy were studied. A slight increase in the percentage of positive tumors was found in the pT_2 and pT_3 groups (Table 2).

Preliminary analysis of the data emerging from the present study (Figure 2) reveals that the death rate is higher in the patients with receptor negative cancers regardless of the type of receptors and histological stage considered.

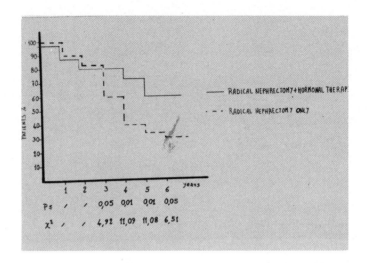

Fig. 1. Actuarial survival of 82 patients with tumor stage pT_{2-3} N_{0-1} M_0.

TABLE 2

DISTRIBUTION OF STEROID RECEPTORS (ER, PR AND AR) IN pT_2 AND pT_3 PATIENTS

Receptors	pT_2		pT_3	
	Number	Percent	Number	Percent
ER+	20	58.9	9	56.2
ER-	14	41.1	7	43.8
PR+	20	58.9	10	62.5
PR-	14	41.1	6	37.5
AR+	9	64.3	7	70.0
AR-	5	35.7	3	10.0

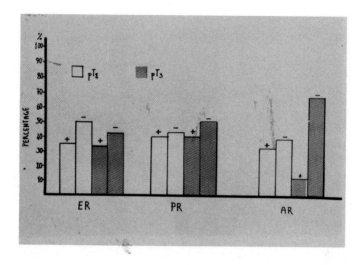

Fig. 2. Steroid receptors and death rate in pT$_2$ and pT$_3$ patients.

Within 36 months, in fact, 50% of the ER- patients died, while only 35% of the ER+ patients died. Note that the death rate is lower in patients with receptor positive cancers. This observation is more clearly demonstrated when the combined ER and PR are considered. In fact, as shown in Figure 3, the highest death rate (66%) occurs in the group of pT$_2$ patients with ER- PR- RCC, while in the ER+ PR-, ER- PR+, and ER+ PR+ groups, the mean death rate is 37%. This correlation could not be demonstrated in the pT$_3$ group on account of the limited number of patients.

In these 50 patients, observed between 1975 and 1980 with a follow-up period ranging between 6 months and 6 years, death occurred in 20 (40%) regardless of the presence of steroid receptors. It is not possible, on the basis of the data obtained, to prepare an actuarial curve of survival, inasmuch as the latter, to be sufficiently reliable, should refer to a larger number of observations, a homogeneous follow-up period and a larger number of patients. Nevertheless, calculations were made on the life expectancy per period and overall life expectancy. It should be pointed out, however, that even if standard errors were assumed in these calculations,

the results cannot be considered reliable on account of the
limited number of patients studied.

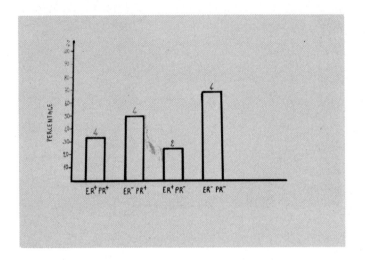

Fig. 3. Combined steroid receptors (ER and PR) and death
rate in pT$_2$ patients.

A comparison was made between ER+ patients, PR+ patients
and the respective negative groups. Positive estradiol
receptors and probability of the survival are reported in
Figure 4 which also shows the number of patients still alive
in each period under consideration as well as the probability
of survival for that period. The latter is calculated by
dividing the number of patients alive at the end of the
period by the number alive at the beginning minus the number
of cases no longer in the follow-up study. Death occurs
within the first 30 months and the life expectancy in that
period is about 85%. In the case of the ER- patients, most
deaths occur within the first 24 months with a life expectancy
ranging between 80% and 90%, whereas at 42 months life
expectancy drops to 65% (Figure 5).

The prognostic value of ER is confirmed by the results
reported in Figure 6 which shows the overall life expectancy
in the groups with and without ER. It can be seen that the

presence of ER shows a favorable prognostic significance for life expectancy beyond the third year.

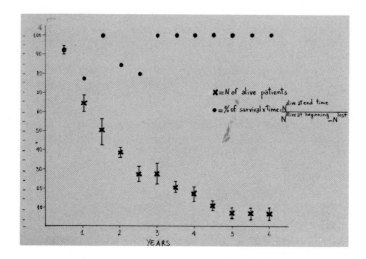

Fig. 4. Life expectancy per period in ER+ patients.

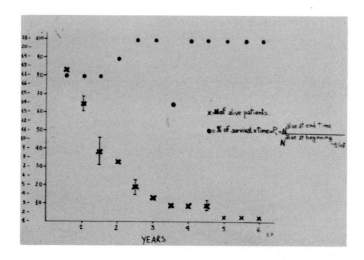

Fig. 5. Life expectancy per period in ER- patients.

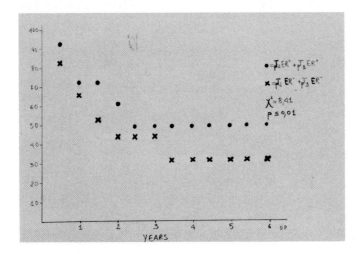

Fig. 6. Overall life expectancy in the groups with and without ER.

Considering the wide margin of error of our statistics, we also calculated the number of deaths per period out of the number of patients present at beginning of the follow-up period and the confidence level. The latter expresses the casual life expectancy, i.e. the probability that two samples belong to completely different populations and not to the same populations. A difference exists between the two groups both in terms of the absolute number of deaths per period and the overall number (Table 3). However, the confidence level suggests caution in the interpretation of these data.

Data from the group of patients with PR+ tumors are given in Figure 7. Deaths are fairly uniformly distributed in the first 36 months, with a life expectancy per period of about 90%. From data obtained in the PR- patients (Figure 8), it has been demonstrated that all deaths occur within the first 12 months, with a mean life expectancy per period of about 70%. When the overall life expectancy is taken into consideration (Figure 9), the prognostic importance of the progesterone receptors within the first two years appears evident, whereas in the next phase values coincide. Also in this instance calculations were made on the number of

TABLE 3

FOLLOW-UP PERIOD DEATHS OF PATIENTS WITH ER+ AND ER- TUMORS

Months	ER+	ER-	Confidence Level
12	7/29	7/21	≈ 40%
18	7/29	9/21	≈ 25%
24	9/29	10/21	≈ 30%
30	10/29	10/21	≈ 35%

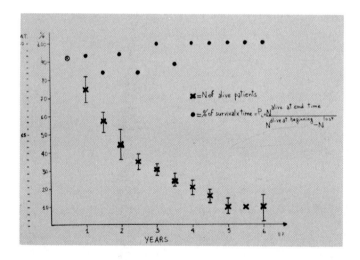

Fig. 7.   Life expectancy per period in PR+ patients.

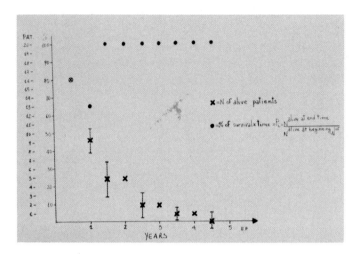

Fig. 8. Life expectancy per period in PR- patients.

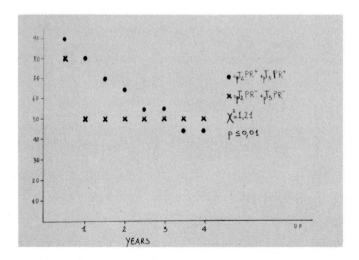

Fig. 9. Overall life expectancy in the groups with and without PR.

deaths per period out of the number of patients at the beginning of the follow-up observation, extrapolating the statistical significance with the relative confidence level (Table 4). Statistical differences were observed particularly at 12 and 18 months. The very low confidence level provides an excellent safety margin on the statistical reliability of data from the first two periods under examination.

TABLE 4

FOLLOW-UP PERIOD DEATHS OF PATIENTS WITH PR+ AND PR- RENAL TUMORS

Months	PR+	PR-	Confidence Level
12	5/30	9/20	≃ 3.5%
18	8/30	9/20	≃ 17.0%
24	9/30	9/20	≃ 30.0%
30	11/30	9/20	≃ 50.0%

DISCUSSION AND CONCLUSIONS

Results reported on experimental models and those obtained in man with hormonal treatments based on receptor analyses (which represents the biochemical support of hormone-dependence of renal cancer) led to the conclusion that the hormone responsiveness of RCC may be related to the different proportion of tumor cells with and without receptors. It is clear, in fact, that only receptor positive cells will respond to hormonal manipulation. The presence of two different cell lines, one hormone-dependent, the other hormone-independent, is demonstrated by the higher response rate obtained with the combination of chemo and hormonal agents. When we approached the problem of treating RCC, a tumor with low radiosensitivity and scarcely affected by chemotherapy, in the pre-receptor era, we decided to treat all the patients with MPA on the basis of a few preliminary favorable results. The encouraging data obtained with a combination of radical nephrectomy plus hormonal therapy particularly on survival, but also on stabilization of the disease, led us to investigate whether this tumor might be considered a hormone-responsive tumor.

Based on the above mentioned animal models and taking into consideration that normal human kidney as well as RCC possess steroid receptors (as does RCC in experimental animals), we started adjuvant hormonal treatment following receptor studies in patients submitted to radical nephrectomy for RCC. The good results obtained on stabilization of the disease, tumor-free interval and death rate in receptor positive RCC patients, as well as survival, further support the hormone-dependence hypothesized on the basis of clinical findings and sustained by biochemical data.

For these reasons we therefore propose the use of hormonal treatment as an adjuvant form of therapy for the rest of the life of such patients. Progestational treatment could act as "prophylaxis of metastatic disease" (Di Silverio et al, 1977) and furthermore could even have a blocking effect on those agents considered to play an active role in the etiology of the disease. Although these agents are not yet known, it is reasonable to believe that they act on the remaining kidney or are involved in the onset of silent metastatic foci.

Further trials on a larger series of randomized patients will shed further light on the hormonal responsiveness of human RCC and the usefulness of endocrine treatment in this neoplasia.

ACKNOWLEDGEMENT

The collaboration of Drs. Raffaele Tenaglia, Ermanno Pannunzio and Fabio Ferrarotto in the elaboration of the data and preparation of this report is gratefully acknowledged.

This work was supported in part by a grant of C.N.R. (Italy) Special Project "Control of Neoplastic Growth".

REFERENCES

Al Sarraf M, Eyre H, Bonnet S, Saiki S, Gagliano R, Pugh R, Lehane D, Dixon D, Bottomley R (1981). Study of tamoxifen metastatic renal cell carcinoma and the influence of certain prognostic factors: a South West Oncology Group Study. Cancer Treat Rep 65:447.

Bartley O, Hulquist GT (1950). Spontaneous regression of hypernephromas. Acta Path Microbiol Scand 27:448.

Bennington JL (1973). Cancer of the kidney. Etiology, epidemiology and pathology. Cancer 32:1017.

Bloom HJG (1971). Medroxyprogesterone acetate (Provera) in the treatment of metastatic renal cancer. Br J Cancer 25:205.

Bloom HJG (1973). Hormone induced and spontaneous regression of metastatic renal cancer. Cancer 32:1066.

Bloom HJG, Baker WH, Dukes CE, Mitchley BCV (1963a). Hormone-dependent tumours in the kidney: II Effect of endocrine ablation procedures on the transplanted oestrogen-induced renal tumour of the Syrian hamster. Br J Cancer 17:646.

Bloom HJG, Dukes CE, Mitchley BCV (1963b). Hormone-dependent tumours of the kidney: I The oestrogen-induced renal tumours of the Syrian hamster; hormone treatment and possible relationship to carcinoma of the kidney in man. Br J Cancer 17:611.

Bloom HJG, Wallace DM (1964). Hormones and the kidney: possible therapeutic role of testosterone in a patient with regression of metastasis from renal adenocarcinoma. Br Med J 2:476.

Bojar H, Wittliff JL, Balser K, Dreyfurst R, Boeninghans F, Staib W (1975). Properties of specific estrogen binding components in human kidney and renal carcinoma. Acta Endocrinol (Kbh) Suppl 193:51.

Bojar H, Dreyfurst R, Baller K, Staib W, Wittliff JL (1976). Oestrogen binding components in human renal cell carcinoma. J Clin Chem and Clin Biochem 14:521.

Bracci U, Gagliardi V, Di Silverio F (1973). Les progestatifs dans les tumeurs du rein. In "Proc XVI Congres of Inter Soc Urol", Doin Paris, vol 2, p 569.

Bracci U, Di Silverio F (1976). Attuali orientamenti nella diagnosi e terapia dei carcinomi del rene: l'ormonodipen-denza. Atti del XLIX Congresso SIU, Vol I p 167. Ferrara Italy.

Concolino G, Di Silverio F, Marocchi A, Conti C, Tenaglia R, Bracci U (1978). Human renal cell carcinoma as a hormone-dependent tumor. Cancer Res 34:4340.

Concolino G, Di Silverio F, Marocchi A, Bracci U (1979a).
Renal cancer steroid receptors: biochemical basis for
endocrine therapy. Eur Urol 5:319.

Concolino G, Marocchi A, Martelli ML, Gagliardi V, Di Silverio
F (1975). Human renal carcinoma and steroid hormone
receptors. J Steroid Biochem 6:15.

Concolino G, Marocchi A, Di Silverio F, Conti C (1976).
Progestational therapy in human renal carcinoma and steroid
receptors. J Steroid Biochem 7:923.

Concolino G, Di Silverio F., Marocchi A, Tenaglia R, Bracci U
(1979b). Steroid receptors in normal kidney and in human
renal adenocarcinoma. In "Proc X Congres of the European
Federation of the International College of Surgeons",
Turin, Italy: Minerva Medica, p 383.

Concolino G, Marocchi A, Conti C, Liberti M, Tenaglia R,
DiSilverio F (1980). Endocrine treatment and steroid
receptors in urological malignancies. In Iacobilli S
"Hormones and Cancer", New York: Alan R. Liss.

Di Silverio F, Concolino G, Marocchi A, Tenaglia R, Bracci U
(1977). Le basi biochimiche della ormono-terapia sugli
adenocarcinomi renali. Urologia ed ormoni. Volume unico:
65 Reggio Emilia, Italy.

Fairlamb DS (1981). Spontaneous regression of metastases of
renal cancer. Cancer 47:2102.

Fanestil DD, Vaughn DA, Ludens JH (1974). Steroid hormone
receptors in human renal cell carcinoma. J Steroid Biochem
5:338.

Glick J et al (1979). Tamoxifen in metastatic prostate and
renal cancer. Proc AACR/ASCO 20:311.

Hahn DM, Schimpff SC, Ruckdeschel JC, Wiernik PH (1977).
Single agent therapy for renal cell carcinoma: CCNU,
vinblastine, thiotepa, or bleomycin. Cancer Treat Rep
61:1585.

Hahn RG, Temkin NR, Savlov ED, Perlia C, Wampler GL, Horton J,
Marsh J, Carbone PP (1978). Phase II study of vinblastine,
methyl-CCNU, and medroxyprogesterone in advanced renal cell
carcinoma. Cancer Treat Rep 62:1093.

Horning ES (1956a). Observations on hormone-dependent renal
tumours in the golden hamster. Br J Cancer 10:678.

Horning ES (1956b). Endocrine factors involved in the
induction, prevention and transplantation of kidney tumours
in the male golden hamster. Z Krebsforschung 61:1.

Letourneau RJ, Li JJ, Rosen S, Villee CA (1975). Junctional
specialization in estrogen induced renal adenocarcinoma of
the golden hamster. Cancer Res 35:6.

Li JJ, Li SA (1975). Cell free cytosol-nuclear oestrogen

receptor translocation in the hamster oestrogen-dependent renal tumour and uterus. (Abstract) Am Assoc Cancer Res Inc Annual Meeting, San Diego.

Li JJ, Li SA (1977). Translocation of specific steroid hor hormone receptors into purified nuclei in Syrian hamster tissues and oestrogen dependent renal tumours. In Vermeulen et al: "Research on Steroids", Amsterdam: North Holland Publ. Co., Vol VII.

Li SA, Li JJ (1975). Specific progesterone binding in the estrogen dependence renal adenocarcinoma of the golden hamster. (Abstract). The Endocrine Society

Li JJ, Li SA, Merry BJ, Villee CA (1974). Lack of induced protein in the hamster uterus and in the oestrogen dependent renal adenocarcinoma. J Steroid Biochem 5:340.

Li JJ, Talley DJ, Li SA, Villee CA (1974). An oestrogen binding protein in the renal cytosol of intact, castrated and estrogenized golden hamsters. Endocrinology 95:1134.

Li JJ, Talley DJ, Li SA, Villee CA (1976). Receptor characteristics of specific oestrogen binding in the renal adenocarcinoma of the dolden hamster. Cancer Res 36:1127.

Kantor ALF, Meigs JM, Heston JF, Flannery JT (1976). Epidemiology of renal cell carcinoma in Connecticut, 1935-1973. J Natl Cancer Inst 57:495.

Kirkman H (1959). Estrogen-induced tumours of the kidney in the Syrian hamster. J Natl Cancer Inst Monogr 1:1.

Matthews VS, Kirkman H, Bacon RL (1947). Kidney damage in the golden hamster following chronic administration of diethylstilbestrol and sesame oil. Proc Soc Exp Biol Med 66:195.

Matulich DT, Spindler BJ, Schambelan M, Baxter JD (1976). Mineral-corticoid receptors in human kidney. J Clin Endocrinol Metab 43:1170.

Montie IE, Stewart BH, Straffon RA, Bonowsky LH, Hevitt CB, Montagne DK (1977). The role of adjuntive nephrectomy in patients with metastatic renal cell carcinoma. J Urol 117:272.

Paine CH, Wright FW, Ellis F (1970). The use of progesterone in the treatment of metastatic carcinoma of the kidney and uterine body. Br J Cancer 24:277.

Rodriguez LH, Johnson DE (1978). Clinical trial of cis-platinum (NSC 119875) in metastatic renal cell carcinoma. Urology 11:344.

Stolbach LL, Begg CB, Hall T, Horton J (1981). Treatment of renal carcinoma: a phase III randomized trial of oral medroxyprogesterone (Provera), hydroxyurea and nafoxidine. Cancer Treat Rep 65:7.

Swanson DA, Johnson DE (1981). Estramustine phosphate (Emcyt) as treatment for metastatic renal carcinoma. Urology 17: 344.

Talley RW (1973). Chemotherapy of adenocarcinoma of the ki kidney. Cancer 32:10.

Todd RF, III, Garnick MB, Cannellos GP, Richie SP, Gittes RF, Mayer RS, Skarin AT (1981). Phase I-II trial of Methyl-GAG in the treatment of patients with metastatic renal adenocarcinoma. Cancer Treat Rep 65:1.

Wagle DG, Murphy GP (1971). Hormonal therapy in advanced renal cell carcinoma. Cancer 28:318.

Renal Tumors: Proceedings of the First International Symposium on Kidney Tumors, pages 641–659
© **1982 Alan R. Liss, Inc., 150 Fifth Avenue, New York, NY 10011**

TREATMENT OF ADVANCED RENAL CELL CARCINOMA

Jean B. deKernion, M.D.* & Arie Lindner, M.D.**

Chief Urologic Oncology*   Clinical Fellow**
UCLA School of Medicine
Los Angeles, California 90024

INTRODUCTION

Renal cell carcinoma is not a common tumor, but accounts for approximately 7,000 to 8,000 new cases annually in the United States. Because of the anatomic relationships of the kidney, renal carcinoma is often not identified until it has become far advanced. The relative inefficacy of management modalities for advanced renal carcinoma have prompted extension of surgical management to include excision of tumor in the solitary kidney, excision of locally invasive tumors, and removal of vena caval thromboses. The results of such extensive surgery have been satisfactory in most reported series.

Little progress has been realized in three categories of patients with renal cell carcinoma. First, patients with incomplete excision or with extension into the regional lymph nodes have a poor prognosis, and thus far no modality of adjuvant therapy has proven to improve survival. Secondly, patients who develop metastatic disease following nephrectomy have little prospect for even two year survival. Finally, patients who initially present with metastases at the time of diagnosis have a uniformly poor prognosis in spite of traditional treatment methods. Since approximately one-half of patients who undergo radical nephrectomy with curative intent will at some time develop metastases, and since approximately one-third of patients present with metastases at the time of diagnosis, the need for systemic therapy is clear. Chemotherapy, hormonal therapy, immunotherapy and surgery have been proposed as appropriate methods of treatment of such patients with advanced renal carcinoma.

CHEMOTHERAPY

The traditional management of advanced solid tumors is with cytotoxic agents, either as single agents or in combination. However, renal cell carcinoma has remained one of the few solid tumors which appears to be almost totally refractory to standard cytotoxic drugs, and numerous individual and collected series have demonstrated the paucity of response of this tumor to any form of chemotherapeutic agent. An occasional report has suggested a beneficial effect of single agent therapy, but followup studies invariably fail to support the original optimism.

A large number of single agents have been utilized against renal carcinoma. Table 1 is a summary of the existing literature relating results of single agent chemotherapy. Although response criteria are not uniform, and drug dosage schedules varied, the lack of therapeutic efficacy is nonetheless obvious. Furthermore, in view of the occasional stabilization of growth of metastatic renal carcinoma for extended periods and the variability of growth of pulmonary metastases, the validity of some partial responses may be questioned. The rare complete response might also simply be a manifestation of the natural history of the tumor, since complete regression of this tumor occasionally occurs even with no therapy (Freed, et.al., 1977).

The agent most commonly used in the United States is vinblastine. Hrushesky (1977) recently retrospectively reviewed the activity of thirty-five chemotherapeutic agents. He reported a 25% objective response rate following therapy with vinblastine sulfate. This surpassed the activity of any other single agent or any combination of agents. As noted in Table 1, several partial responses have been attributed to vinblastine sulfate. Anecdotal reports of responses to vinblastine therapy are often mentioned although seldom documented. We have treated sixteen patients with vinblastine sulfate and noted arrest of growth of metastases in three patients for three or more months, and partial regression in one patient. Another patient had disappearance of obvious tumor for three years, followed by rapid progression and death. No patient had complete regression of metastases. The other agent often recommended is CCNU (see Table 1). Occasional responses have been reported, but the general experience, after an initial optimism, has been disappointing. Recently,

TABLE 1

Drug		No. Pts.	CR	PR
AMSA	(Schneider, Van Echo 1980)	37	0	1
Baker's Antifol	(Bukowski 1980)	17	1	0
MTX	(Baumgartner 1980)	20	0	2
IFOSFAMIDE	(Fossa 1980)	15	0	1
CTX (High dose)	(Wajsman 1980)	12	0	0
Methyl-GAG	(Todd Callahan 1981)	76	1	6
CCNU	(Merrin 1975)	23	0	4
5-FU	(Talley 1973)	12	0	0
Hydroxy urea	(Stolbach 1981, Talley 1973)	24	0	1
Velban	(Talley 1973)	15	0	2
Actinomycin D	(Hahn 1981, Talley 1973)	65	0	1
Triazimate	(Hahn 1981)	59	1	2
cis-Platinum	(Rodriguez 1978)	32	0	0

CR = Complete response
PR = Partial response
MTX = Methotrexate

an early study utilizing methyl-GAG reported several impressive partial regression (Knight, et.al., 1979). The toxicity was severe, however, and a subsequent report indicated three partial responses and three mixed responses out of fifty-one evaluable patients (Callahan, et. al., 1980).

Therefore, the maximum objective regressive rate one can expect from single agent chemotherapy is approximately 15%. In light of the natural history of the tumor, the significance of this low level of activity must be questioned. However, faced with the patient who has diffuse metastases, and who wishes the full extent of therapeutic options, even the small level of activity warrants a trial of chemotherapy. Vinblastine sulfate, CCNU, or methyl-GAG appear to be the most appropriate choices.

Traditionally, combination chemotherapy is structured from single agents which have shown some level of activity. In view of the poor response rate of renal carcinoma to single agents, selection of agents for combination therapy has often been based on criteria of toxicity and patient tolerance rather than antitumor effect.

The reported experience with combination chemotherapy is reviewed in Table 2. The response rate is somewhat better than that of single agents alone, especially with combinations of vinblastine and other agents. The numbers reported are often small and the toxicity of these combinations is usually significant. Complete responses are rare and the duration of responses is often short.

Treatment of patients with combination chemotherapeutic agents therefore seems to be of questionable benefit. The increased toxicity imposed by such combinations must be carefully balanced against the projected response rate. Little benefit can reasonably be expected from combinations of agents which show little or no activity when used singly. However, few options are available to the physician treating metastatic renal carcinoma and any well-structured, well-executed chemotherapeutic trial in properly informed patients seems appropriate. For the moment, however, our preference is for established single agents or new Phase I trial agents.

The inability to identify effective chemotherapeutic agents has prompted the utilization of new in vitro chemotherapeutic tests to determine sensitivity of renal carcinoma

TABLE 2

Drug	No. Pts.	CR	PR
VLB + CCNU (Davis 1978, Hahn 1981, Merrin 1978, Tirelli 1980)	95	3	9
VLB + methyl CCNU (Merrin 1975)	15	0	1
VLB + MTX + Bleomycin (Levi 1980)	14	0	5
VLB + MTX + Bleomycin + Tamoxifen (Levi 1980)	14	0	5
VLB + CTX + 5-FU (Halpern 1981)	10	0	0
VLB + CTX + hydroxy urea + MPA + prednisone (Talley 1979)	45	1	6
CTX + 5-FU + vincristin + MTX (van der Werf-Messing 1974)	18	0	0
VLB + CTX + Adriamycin + Bleomycin + BCG (Dana 1981)	14	0	3

VLB = Vinblastine
CTX = Cyclophosphamide
MTX = Methotrexate
MPA = Medroxyprogesterone acetate

to single agents. Day, et.al., (1981) determined response
of both explanted renal carcinomas and tumor implanted into
athymic mice. The renal carcinomas maintained in the athymic
mice demonstrated identical chemotherapeutic sensitivity
patterns as demonstrated in vitro. Salmon, et.al. (1978)
described a method for growth of human tumor stem cells on
soft agar in vitro. This clonogenic assay has been applied
to a number of tumors, and recently has been utilized in assessing cytotoxic drugs against renal carcinoma. Lieber and
Kovach (1980) established clonogenic growth in soft agar in
seven of thirty-one human renal carcinomas. In vitro chemotherapy sensitivity testing was successfully achieved in
five of the seven tumors. Rare response to single agents
was observed, but the authors concluded that further study
of the soft agar assay as a means of identifying effective
single agents for individual patients was feasible. The
clonogenic assay is currently undergoing extensive trials
in a number of centers in the United States. Its role in
accurately predicting clinical response to human tumors has
yet to be established and, in view of the lack of activity
of cytotoxic agents against renal carcinoma, its role in
this tumor is very uncertain.

HORMONAL THERAPY

The observation that progestational agents inhibit the
growth of the diethyl-stilbestrol-induced kidney tumor of the
Syrian hamster provided a basis for clinical trials of progestational agents in humans (Bloom, 1971). After the encouraging initial report, isolated reports of regressions of
tumors after progestational therapy appeared. Bloom (1973)
reviewed the literature and reported an objective response
rate of approximately 15% in patients with metastatic renal
carcinoma. This represented a collection of the published
literature of non-randomized studies, and therefore suffered
from the same shortcomings as the Phase II trials of single
agent chemotherapy. In recent years, the enthusiasm for progestational therapy has faded greatly in most centers. In a
review of 110 patients at UCLA, no patient was found to have
an objective response to progestational agents (deKernion,
1978). In a prospective randomized study, no objective benefit was noted with progesterone or testosterone as compared
to placebo (Claire Cox, M.D., personal communication.) The
major impetus for continued use of progestational agents is
the lack of effective chemotherapeutic agents, and the relative

paucity of side effects from hormonal therapy. Patients occasionally experience nausea, vomiting, edema, breast tenderness and uterine bleeding, but these symptoms are seldom severe.

The poor response to progesterones has occasionally been attributed to inefficient dosage schedules. The dosage ranges used in various reports are quite variable as is the type of progestational agent employed. At the present time, orally administered divided doses of 160 milligrams per day are well tolerated and seem to be appropriate. Others have utilized twice weekly injections of medroxyprogesterone acetate with little toxicity. However, no good study has been reported to compare the relative advantages of various dosages and routes of administration.

Other hormonal agents have occasionally been tested against metastatic renal carcinoma. Table 3 represents a summary of recent reports of hormonal therapy in renal carcinoma. Progesterone was the only agent which showed any antitumor effect. Four of the six complete responses and two of the partial responses were reported by Tally (1973). As indicated in Table 3, the overall response to progesterone is less impressive.

If a true antitumor effect can be ascribed to progestational agents, it seems reasonable to measure hormone receptors in renal carcinoma. Concolino, et.al. (1978) attempted to identify patients who are likely to respond to progesterone on the basis of the presence or absence of hormone receptors. A few patients with progesterone receptors responded to therapy while those with no receptors did not. This interesting approach deserves further study. However, the major question as to whether hormonal agents truly exert any antitumor effect against renal carcinoma has not been answered, and the wealth of reported experience would suggest that the activity, if present, is minimal.

IMMUNOTHERAPY

The unusual clinical behavior of renal cell carcinoma, especially the variability of growth of metastases, the prolonged dormancy of some metastases, and the occasional spontaneous regression, suggest that innate host factors play an important role in the natural history of this tumor. Although

TABLE 3

Drug		No. Pts.	CR	PR
MPA	(Pizzocaro, Tirelli 1980 Stolbach 1981, Talley 1973)	116	7	4
Testosterone	(Talley 1973, Tirelli 1980)	48	0	0
Tamoxifen	(Al-Sarraf, Glick, Mulder 1979, Ferrazzi 1980, Weiselberg 1981)	106	0	2
Nafoxidine	(Feun 1979, Stolbach 1981)	39	2	2
Estramustin P.	(Swanson 1981)	16	0	0

MPA = Medroxyprogesterone acetate

no firm evidence has yet been presented to implicate host
immunity as the regulating factor, alterations in cellular and
circulating immune functions in patients with renal cell carcinoma have been demonstrated (deKernion, 1980). It is therefore not surprising that a number of immunotherapeutic modalities have been proposed.

The most commonly used agents have been non-specific
immunostimulants, especially BCG. Brosman, et. al. (1977)
treated twelve patients with advanced renal carcinoma and
compared survival to ten patients who received no immunotherapy. Survival of the treated patients was somewhat increased, although the difference was not significant. Morales and Eidinger (1976) treated eight patients with metastatic renal carcinoma with systemic BCG. Objective improvement was noted in five of the eight patients, although the
criteria for improvement included stabilization of growth
of metastatic foci in one patient. These responses were
transitory and the mean duration of the followup was brief.
Drs. Paul Lange and Elwin Fraley (personal communication)
at the University of Minnesota treated patients with cutan-
eously administered BCG after removing the bulk of the tumor.
Stabilization or regression occurred in a few patients, but
the investigators concluded that survival did not seem to be
increased by this approach of surgery plus immunotherapy.
Minton, et. al. (1976) noted clinical responses in four of
nine patients with pulmonary metastases from renal carcinoma
treated with intradermal BCG.

A number of other methods of active immunotherapy have
been utilized, although only a few patients have been treated
and followup series are seldom conducted. Allogeneic lymphocytes (Humphrey, et. al., 1971) and microsomal renal cell
carcinoma fractions (Nairn, et. al., 1971) were earlier
approaches to active immunotherapy which have not been expanded into decisive clinical trials. Recently, however,
other approaches to active immunotherapy have been reported
in Phase II trials.

Tykkä, et. al., (1978) treated thirty-one patients with
active specific immunotherapy after palliative nephrectomy.
A soluble fraction of autologous tumor prepared by hypotonic
cell lysis was polymerized to small particles by addition of
ethylchlorformiate. The polymerized tumor was injected intradermally along with PPD tuberculin or Candida antigen as
adjuvant. The survival of treated patients was improved over

controls although only 20% of treated patients were alive at
five years. The only objective responses noted were those in
patients with pulmonary metastases, which disappeared in six
of sixteen treated patients. Selection of controls and heterogeneity of the treated patients may present some problem in
interpretation, although this method of immunotherapy appears
to have a role in the management of this tumor. Other centers
are currently investigating this approach.

A somewhat similar approach which was used by Prager,
et.al. (1981). Irradiated autologous tumor cells were polymerized with DDA and injected intracutaneously. Twenty-seven
patients with metastatic renal carcinoma were treated. Survival of treated patients was significantly improved over
controls.

A recent report by Schapira, et.al. (1979) in which
irradiated autologous tumor cells were mixed with C.parvum
as an adjuvant and injected intradermally suggested some
activity against a number of solid tumors. Regression of
pulmonary metastases occurred in two patients with renal
carcinoma and a third patient with extensive metastases had
symptomatic improvement with stabilization of tumor for more
than twelve months. A subsequent report by McCune, et.al.
(1981) indicated a partial response in four of fourteen
patients with metastatic renal cell carcinoma. Based on
these data, we have instituted a Phase III trial of this
approach in patients who present with metastases at the
time of the diagnosis. Following adjunctive nephrectomy,
patients are randomized to receive either progestational
agents or the autologous tumor-C.parvum vaccine. This is one
of the first Phase III trials of immunotherapy of renal carcinoma, comparing standard therapy to a new immunotherapeutic
modality.

Juillard, et.al. (1979) recently demonstrated successful
intralymphatic injection of irradiated tumor cells in patients
with several types of metastatic cancer. We have collaborated
with Dr. Juillard and associates in the treatment of five
patients with metastatic renal carcinoma by this approach and
temporary regression was noted in one patient. This Phase II
trial is being expanded.

Interferons have shown some effect against a number of
human tumors, but no trial of interferon therapy of renal
carcinoma has been reported. We are currently instituting a

Phase II trial of alpha-interferon in renal carcinoma, which
may be extended to other interferon types if a significant
response rate is achieved.

Some of the earliest clinical experiments in the treatment of renal carcinoma were in the form of serotherapy.
Horn, et.al. (1971) infused plasma from a patient previously
cured of renal carcinoma into a family member with diffuse
metastases. The patient remained clinically free of tumor
for twenty months but subsequently died of cerebral metastases. Another patient with pulmonary metastases received
plasma infusions from a family member who had undertone
curative nephrectomy for renal carcinoma. One pulmonary
metastasis resolved but others remained stable and the
patient succumbed to CNS metastases (Hellström, et.al., 1972).
Other anecdotal cases have been reported or verbally noted,
but no formal trial of this form of therapy has been initiated.

Adoptive immunotherapy in the form of transfer factor
and immune-RNA have been used more extensively than other
forms of therapy for this tumor. Montie, et.al. (1977)
reported some objective response in a few patients with metastatic renal cell carcinoma treated with transfer factor. In
a subsequent report from the same institution, Bukowski, et.
al. (1979) combined transfer factor with other modalities.
Nine patients received transfer factor alone of which one had
a complete response. Another small group received transfer
factor plus TICE strain BCG by scarification. Two of eight
had partial regression of measurable metastases. The third
group received transfer factor plus CCNU plus progesterone.
One of the fourteen patients had a complete response and four
had partial regressions. The incidence of tumor response
seen in this study is higher than one would expect from the
inherent natural history characteristics of the tumor. It is
also interesting that in this study as in most other immunotherapeutic studies reported, patients who responded were
usually those with pulmonary metastases.

Based on experiments on animal tumors, a clinical trial
of xenogeneic immune-RNA was instituted in patients with
advanced renal cell carcinoma. The RNA was extracted from
the lymphoid organs of sheep which had been immunized with
human renal cell carcinoma. Patients were treated with
weekly intradermal injections of four milligrams of the RNA.
Toxicity was minimal over a very wide dosage range. No
patient had a complete regression of tumor. Seven patients

had a partial response defined as any measurable regression
or stability of measurable previously growing tumors for over
three months (Ramming and deKernion, 1977). In view of these
findings it was felt that RNA given by this method had no
value in treatment of widely disseminated carcinoma. In
addition, survival was not significantly increased over com-
puter-matched controls. However, patients with pulmonary
metastases initially had an improved survival over patients
with pulmonary metastases who were not treated with RNA. By
four years, however, most patients with metastases had died,
whether or not RNA therapy had been given (deKernion, 1980).

Recently, other approaches to immune-RNA therapy have
attempted to circumvent the problem of degradation by ribo-
nucleases in human tissue. In vitro incubation of separated
leucocytes with xenogeneic RNA and subsequent re-infusion
successfully avoids this problem and initial reports show a
suggestion of therapeutic efficacy (Richie, et.al., 1981).
However, the role of immune-RNA administered by any route for
the treatment of renal cell carcinoma is still unclear.

NEPHRECTOMY FOR METASTATIC RENAL CARCINOMA

The management of metastatic renal cell carcinoma has
been markedly influenced by the lack of any effective systemic
therapeutic agent. Approximately 30% of patients have metastases at the time they are first seen, and approximately
another half of those treated for "cure" develop metastases
at some future date. For decades, the treatment of choice
for patients who present with renal carcinoma with concomitant metastases has been palliative nephrectomy. This was
based on the observation that some patients had regression of
metastatic tumor after the primary was removed, and upon the
palliative effect of removal of a large primary tumor which
was causing significant symptoms.

Palliative nephrectomy for control of severe symptoms
seems justified in a patient who otherwise has a reasonable
life expectancy of six months or greater. However, in view
of the current therapeutic modalities including angiographic
infarction for symptom management, a major surgical procedure
for symptomatic relief is seldom indicated. When considering
palliation in such patients, one must be cognizant that the
mean survival of these patients is approximately four months,
and only 10% of such patients survive one year (deKernion, et.

al., 1978). Nonetheless, nephrectomy for palliation is sometimes warranted.

Nephrectomy for the patient with concomitant metastases who does not have symptoms has been a common practice. The purpose of the surgery is either to induce regression of metastases or to prolong survival. Literature reports are not unified in their opinion, and some authors still advocate so-called adjunctive nephrectomy. In view of the lack of effectiveness of systemic agents, it is easy to understand the desire for the urologist to attempt even the most remotely effective method of therapy.

As discussed above, spontaneous regression of metastatic renal carcinoma does occur. However, regression may occur even in the patient who has not undergone a nephrectomy. Furthermore, the incidence in which regression occurs is very small, approximately 0.4% or one in two hundred fifty patients (Montie, et.al., 1977). This figure in itself may be optimistic, since in 533 patients reviewed at the Mayo Clinic, no incidence of metastases was noted (Myers, et.al., 1968). The incidence with which regression of metastases occurs after adjunctive nephrectomy is less than 1% (deKernion and Berry, 1980). Furthermore, many of these regressions were short lived and the mortality rate from surgery ranges somewhere from 2-15%, depending upon patient selection. Therefore, it seems impossible to support the routine practice of adjunctive nephrectomy in patients with concomitant metastases.

The contention of some advocates of adjunctive nephrectomy is that survival is increased following surgery. The effect on survival will, of course, depend to a great extent on patient selection. However, little evidence suggests that patient survival is improved unless only the patients with the best performance status and least amount of disease are selected for nephrectomy. In a study from this institution (deKernion, et.al., 1978), survival of patients who underwent adjunctive nephrectomy was the same as for the general population of patients with metastatic renal cell carcinoma.

It therefore has not been our practice to advise routine adjunctive nephrectomy. However, adjunctive nephrectomy may be reasonable in certain instances. Due to the significant five year survival in patients with solitary lesions (Middleton, 1967), excision or radiation of the solitary lesion along with nephrectomy may be reasonable in such patients. Another indication may be in the patient who is willing to undergo experimental therapy, part of which involves removal of the primary tumor. Such studies can only be justified under the proper environment of careful experimental protocols and patient consent. Finally, the recent reports suggesting regression of metastases in patients who undergo percutaneous infarction of the tumor followed by nephrectomy may justify this approach.

The rationale for renal infarction has not been firmly established although the enhancement of the host immune response is postulated. In a recent report, forty-nine patients were treated by percutaneous renal artery occlusion followed in three to five days with nephrectomy and hormonal therapy (Wallace, et.al, 1979). Six of thirty-six evaluable patients had complete regression of tumor for six to eighteen months, five had a partial regression and nine had some form of stabilization for prolonged periods. Median survival was increased over the expected survival in such patients. This, therefore, seems to be a fruitful field of further clinical research. However, certain specific aspects of the study must be examined. First, thirteen patients were excluded as non-evaluable and one wonders if perhaps this did not provide an unintentional bias in the results. Secondly, most or all patients had pulmonary metastases which are those lesions most commonly affected by any form of therapy, and which most commonly undergo temporary or permanent regression. This is, therefore, a particularly good group of patients who would be expected to do well in a number of therapeutic trials.

This author has treated nine patients with concomitant metastases by infarction followed by nephrectomy. One patient with liver metastases and a large tumor mass and retroperitoneal lymph nodes has survived two years with no evidence of persistent tumor. No other patients seemed to be benefited.

The complications of infarction may be significant. Almost all patients undergo stigmata of the postinfarction syndrome including severe abdominal pain, nausea, vomiting, diarrhea, fever and paralytic ileus. Some patients also have hypertension and severe sepsis. One patient treated by this author developed a renal abscess followed by gram negative septicemia, pancreatitis and death. Unintentional embolization of peripheral vessels may also occur.

CONCLUSIONS

Chemotherapy of advanced renal carcinoma seldom produces regression or prolongs survival. The best single agents seem to be vinblastine, CCNU, and methyl-GAG. In view of the poor results and severe toxicity of these drugs, we first offer the patient some form of experimental immunotherapy. For patients who do not wish to have experimental immunotherapy, we usually reserve chemotherapy for those who are symptomatic.

Hormonal therapy produces little toxicity, but also has little demonstrated antitumor activity. Patients who do not wish to have immunotherapy or chemotherapy may experience at least a subjective response to hormones.

Patients who present with metastases at the time of initial diagnosis should be aggressively treated if they are in good general health. While we do not advocate routine palliative or adjunctive nephrectomy, we do feel that nephrectomy or part of a planned experimental approach (immunotherapy or infarction-nephrectomy) is warranted. If the metastases progress after immunotherapy with C. parvum-autologous cell vaccine or after infarction-nephrectomy, other forms of therapy such as intralymphatic immunotherapy or interferon should be considered. Established or new chemotherapeutic agents can also be offered to the patient at various times during the course of the disease.

Patients with advanced renal carcinoma are often young and in good physical condition, and multiple therapeutic options should be presented to them. The relative ineffectiveness of current standard drug and hormonal treatment is no reason for therapeutic nihilism.

Al-Sarraf M (1979). The clinical trial of tamoxifen in patients with advanced renal cell cancer. A Southwest Oncology Group study. Proc Am Soc Clin Oncol 20:378.

Baumgartner G, Heinz R, Arbes H, Lenzhofer R, Pridun N, Schuller J (1980). Methotrexate-citrovorum factor used alone and in combination chemotherapy for advanced hypernephromas. Cancer Treat Rep 64(1):41.

Bloom HJC (1971). Medroxy progesterone acetate (provera) in the treatment of metastatic renal cancer. Br J Cancer 25:205.

Bloom HJG (1973). Hormone-induced and spontaneous regression of metastatic renal cancer. Cancer 32;1006.

Brosman S (1977). Non-specific immunotherapy in GU cancer. Proc Chic Symp Publ Franklin Inst Press Chic 97.

Bukowski RM, Groppe C, Reimer R, Weick J, Hewlett JS (1979). Immunotherapy of metastatic renal cell carcinoma. Am Soc Clin Oncol 20:402.

Bukowski RM, LoBuglio A, McCracken J, Pugh R (1980). Phase II trial of Baker's antifol in metastatic renal cell carcinoma: a Southwest Oncology Group study. Cancer Treat Rep 64(12):1387.

Callahan SK, Knight III WA (1981). A Phase II trial of methyl-glyoxal bisguanybydrazone (MGBC, methyl-GAG) in renal carcinoma. Proc Am Soc Clin Oncol 22:164.

Concolino G, Marrachi A, Conti C, Tenaglia R, DiSilverio F, Bracci U (1978). Human renal cell carcinoma as a hormone dependent tumor. Cancer Res 38:4340.

Dana BW, Alberts DS (1981). Combination chemoimmunotherapy for advanced renal carcinoma with adriamycin, bleomycin, vincristine, cyclophosphamide plus BCG. Cancer Clin Trials 4:205.

Davis TE, Munalo FB (1978). Combination chemotherapy of advanced renal cell cancer with CCNU and vinblastine. Proceedings Am Assoc Cancer Res 19:316.

Day JW, Sharivastav S, Lin G, Bonar RA, Paulson DF (1981). In vitro chemotherapeutic testing of urologic tumors. J Urol 125:490.

deKernion JB, Ramming KP, Smith RB (1978). Natural history of metastatic renal cell carcinoma: computer analysis. J Urol 120:148.

deKernion JB, Ramming KP (1980). The therapy of renal adenocarcinoma with immune RNA. Invest Urol 17:378.

deKernion JB, Berry D (1980). The diagnosis and treatment of renal cell carcinoma. Cancer 45(8):1947.

Ferrazzi E, Salvango L, Fornasiero A, Gartei G, Fiorentino M (1980). Tamoxifen treatment for advanced renal cell cancer. Tumori 66:601.

Feun LG, Drelichman A, Singhalow A, Vaitkevicius VK (1979). Phase II study of nafoxidine in the therapy for advanced renal carcinoma. Cancer Treat Rep 63:149.

Fossa SD, Table K (1980). Treatment of metastatic renal cancer with ifosfamide and mesnum with and without irradiation. Cancer Treat Rep 64(10-11):1103.

Freed SZ, Halperin JP, Gordon M (1977). Idiopathic regression of metastases from renal cell carcinoma. J Urol 118:538.

Glick J, Wein A, Nesendank W, Harris D, Brodovsky H, Padavic K, Torri S (1979). Tamoxifen in metastatic prostate and renal cancer. Proc Am Assoc Cancer Res 20:311.

Hahn RG, Begg CB, Davis T (1981). Phase II study of vin-blastin-ccnu, triazinate and dactinomycin in advanced renal cell cancer. Cancer Treat Rep 65(7-8):711.

Halpern J, Brufman G, Shnider B, Biran S (1981). Vinblastin, cyclophosphamide and 5 fluorouracil combination chemotherapy for metastatic hypernephroma. Oncology 38(4):193.

Hellström I, Hellström KE (1972). Some aspects of human tumor immunity and their possible implications for tumor prevention and therapy. Front Radiation Ther Onc 7:3.

Horn L, Horn HL (1971). An immunological approach to the therapy of cancer. Lancet 2:466.

Hrushesky WJ, Murphy GP (1977). Current status of the therapy of advanced renal carcinoma. J Surg Oncol 9:277.

Humphrey LJ, Murray DR, Boehm OK (1971). Effect of tumor vaccines in immunizing patients with lung cancer. Surg Gynecol Obstet 132:437.

Juillard GJF, Boyer PJJ, Yamashiro CH (1979). A Phase I study of active specific intralymphatic immunotherapy. Yearbook of Cancer, p 289.

Knight III WA, Livingston RB, Fabian C, Costanzi J (1979). Methyl-glyoxal bis-guanylhydrazone (methyl GAG, MGBG) in advanced human malignancy. Proc Am Soc Clin Oncol 20:319.

Levi JA, Dalley D, Aroney R (1980). A comparative trial of the combination vinblastine methotrexate and bleomycin with and without tamoxifen for metastatic renal cell carcinoma. Proc Am Assoc Cancer Res (21:426).

Lieber MM Kovach JS (1981). A soft agar clonogenic assay for primary human renal carcinoma: in vitro chemotherapeutic drug sensitivity testing. Abstract annual AUA meeting Boston.

McCune CS, Schapira DV, Henshaw EL (1981). Specific immuno-therapy of advanced renal carcinoma: evidence for the polyclonality of metastases. Cancer 47:1984.

Merrin C, Mittelman A, Famous N, Wajsman Z, Murphy GP (1975). Chemotherapy of advanced renal cell carcinoma with vin-blastine and ccnu. J Urol 113:21.

Middleton RG (1967). Surgery for metastatic renal carcinoma. J Urol 97:973.

Minton JP, Pennline K, Nowrocki JF (1976). Immunotherapy of human kidney cancer. Proc Am Soc Clin Oncol 17:301.

Montie JE, Bukowski R, Deodhar S, Hewlett JS, Stewart BH, Straffon RA. Immunotherapy of disseminated renal cell carcinoma with transfer factor. J Urol 117:553.

Montie JE, Stewart BH, Straffon RA, Bunowsky LHW, Hewitt CB, Montague OK (1977). The role of adjunctive nephrectomy in patients with metastatic renal cell carcinoma. J Urol 117:272.

Morales A, Eidinger D (1976). Bacille Calmette-Guerin in the treatment of adenocarcinoma of the kidney. J Urol 115:377.

Mulder JH, Alexieva-Figusch I (1979). Tamoxifen in metastatic renal cell carcinoma. Cancer Treat Rep 63:1222.

Myers GH, Fehrenbaker LG, Kelalis PP (1968). Prognostic significance of renal vein invasion by hypernephroma. J Urol 100:420.

Nairn RC, Ghose PH (1963). Production of a precipitin against renal cancer. Br Med J 1:1702.

Pizzocaro G, Valente M, Cataldo I, Vezzoni P, DiFronzo G (1980). Estrogen receptors and MPA treatment in metastatic renal carcinoma. A preliminary report. Tumori 66:739.

Prager MD, Baechtel FS, Peters PC, Brown GL, Greene CL (1981). Specific immunotherapy of human metastatic renal cell carcinoma. Proc Am Soc Clin Oncol 22:163.

Ramming KP, deKernion JB (1977). Immune RNA therapy for renal cell carcinoma: survival and immunologic monitoring. Ann Surg 186:459.

Richie JP, Wang BS, Steele Jr GD, Wilson RE, Mannick JA (1981). In vivo and in vitro effects of xenogeneic immune RNA in patients with advanced renal cell carcinoma: a phase I study. J Urol 126:24.

Rodriguez LH, Johnson DE (1978). Clinical trial of cis-platinum (NSC 119875) in metastatic renal cell carcinoma. Urology 11:344.

Salmon SE, Hamburger AW, Soehnlen B, Durie BGM, Alberts DS, Moon TE (1978). Quantitation of differential sensitivity of human-tumor stem cells to anticancer drugs. New Engl J Med 298:1321.

Schapira DV, McCune CS, Henshaw EL (1979). Treatment of advanced renal cell carcinoma with specific immunotherapy consisting of autologous tumor cells and c.parvum. Proc Am Soc Clin Oncol 20:348.

Schneider RJ, Woodcock TM, Yagoda A (1980). Phase II trial of 4'-(g-acridinylamino) methanesulfon-m-anisidide (AMSA) in patients with metastatic hypernephroma. Cancer Treat Rep 64(1):183.

Stolbach LL, Begg CB, Hall T, Horton J (1981). Treatment of renal carcinoma: a Phase III randomized trial of oral medroxyprogesteron (Provera), hydroxyurea and nafoxidine. Cancer Treat Rep 65)7-8):689.

Swanson DA, Johnson DE (1981). Estramustine phosphate (Emcyt) as treatment for metastatic renal carcinoma. Urology 17(4):344.

Talley RW (1973). Chemotherapy of adenocarcinoma of the kidney. Cancer 32:1062.

Talley RW, Oberhauser NA, Brownlee RW, O'Bryan RM (1979). Chemotherapy of metastatic renal adenocarcinoma with five drug regimen. Henry Ford Hosp Med J 27(2):110.

Tirelli S, Frustaci S, Galligioni E, Veronesi A, Trovo' MG Magri DM, Crivellari D, Roncadin M, Tumolo S, Grigoletto E (1980). Medical treatment of metastatic renal cell carcinoma. Tumori 66:235.

Todd RF, Garnick MB, Canellos GP, Richie JP, Gittes RF, Mayer RJ, Skarin AT (1981). Phase I-II trial of methyl-GAG in the treatment of patients with metastatic renal adenocarcinoma. Cancer Treat Rep 65(1-2):17.

Tykkä H, Oravisto KJ, Lehtonen T (1978). Active specific immunotherapy of advanced renal cell carcinoma. Eur Urol 4:250.

van der Werf-Messing, B, Mulder J (1974). Metastatic kidney cancer treated with multiple drug therapy at the Rotterdam Radiotherapy Institute. Br J Cancer 29:491.

Van Echo DA, Markus S, Aisner J, Wiernik PH (1980). Phase II trial of 4'(g-acridinylamino) methanesulfon-m-anisidide AMSA) in patients with metastatic renal cell carcinoma. Cancer Treat Rep 64(8-9):1009.

Wajsman Z, Beckley S, Madajewicz S, Dragone N (1980). High dose cyclophosphamide in metastatic renal cell carcinoma. Proc Am Assoc Cancer Res 21:423.

Wallace S, Chuang V, Green B, Swanson CA, Bracken RB, Johnson EE (1979). Diagnostic radiology in renal carcinoma in: cancer of the genitourinary tract, Johnson DE and Samuels ML (eds) Raven Press NY.

Weiselberg L, Budman D, Vinciguerra V, Schulman P, Degnan TJ (1981). Tamosifen in unresectable hupernephroma. Cancer Clin Trials 4:195.

Renal Tumors: Proceedings of the First International Symposium on Kidney Tumors, pages 661–662
© **1982 Alan R. Liss, Inc., 150 Fifth Avenue, New York, NY 10011**

COMBINED CHEMOTHERAPY AND RADIOTHERAPY IN METASTATIC RENAL
CARCINOMA

Lennart Andersson and Folke Edsmyr

Department of Urology and Radiumhemmet,
Karolinska Sjukhuset, Stockholm, Sweden

Since there is no effective therapeutic alternative
available in disseminated renal cell carcinoma and since
chemotherapy alone is rather unsatisfactory we have evaluated combined chemotherapy and irradiation in cases of
multiple pulmonary metastases. In a pilot study we have
used a technique proposed by Terashima and co-workers
(1968) and based on tissue culture studies of tumour cells.

The treatment was given to patients previously subjected to nephrectomy and who had developed bilateral
pulmonary metastases. The diagnosis was verified by at
least two chest X-ray examinations and by aspiration
biopsy from a pulmonary lesion using fine neddle technique.

The treatment was given over 4 weeks with irradiation
5 days/week. Two days every week chemotherapy was given
as Vincristine 0.5 mg i.v., followed 6 hours later by
Bleomycin 15 mg i.m. The irradiation was given 1/2 hour
later. In the remaining three days only irradiation was
given. The irradiation was given by a conventional X-ray
equipment, alternatively from in front and behind, and to
a total central dose of 10 Gy.

In a pilot study 20 patients were treated. One of
these 20 patients had a complete disappearance of the
pulmonary lesions. Twenty-four months later pulmonary
lesions recurred. The patient has been observed for a
further 3 years with a slow progression of his pulmonary
metastases. A reduction of the lesions was observed in a
further 11 cases, whereas no change or progression occurred

in 8 cases.   The average duration of remission was 5 months.

There was no respiratory or other untoward reactions.
On the other hand, those patients with respiratory distress
reported a relief; whether this was from organic cause or a
psychological reaction is not known.

The results were apparently not very encouraging.
Still, until a more effective treatment is available, this
kind of combination therapy can be tried in cases of progressive disease with multiple pulmonary metastases.

Terashima K (1968).   Personal Communication.

Renal Tumors: Proceedings of the First International Symposium on Kidney Tumors, pages 663–667
© **1982 Alan R. Liss, Inc., 150 Fifth Avenue, New York, NY 10011**

METHYL-GAG IN ADVANCED RENAL CELL CARCINOMA

J.A.Child, M.D., F.R.C.P.
and the EORTC Urological Group

The General Infirmary at Leeds
Leeds LS1 3EX, England, U.K.

Methyl-GAG (methyl-glyoxal bis-guanylhydrazone) was first synthesised in 1958 and was used in the treatment of the leukaemias in the early 1960's. Toxicity with daily administration was considerable but recently, weekly administration schedules have been shown to cause much less toxicity and to produce responses in a variety of solid tumours, including kidney cancer (Knight,Livingston, Fabian, Costanzi 1979). The drug has an antiproliferative effect on cancer cells which probably reflects two principal properties: selective binding to mitochondria with resulting structural and functional damage; and inhibition of polyamine synthesis, notably the inhibition and depletion of spermidine (Porter, Mikles-Robertson, Kramer, Dave 1979; Oliverio, Adamson, Henderson, Davidson 1963).

It was against this background that the EORTC Urological Group formulated a protocol for a phase II study of the anti-tumour effect of methyl-GAG in patients with renal cell carcinoma with measurable metastases not amenable to surgery. A secondary objective was to assess the morbidity of the treatment.

MATERIAL AND METHODS

It was required that the patients should be under 75 years of age with a Karnofsky index > 60%. Concurrent, but not previous, treatment excluded, as did the existence of brain metastases and evidence of significant bone marrow depression or renal failure. Measurable metastases

of histologically or cytologically proven renal cell
carcinoma were necessary.

Methyl-GAG(supplied to the EORTC for the study by Riom
Laboratories, France) was administered weekly in a dose of
500mg/m^2 by intravenous infusion over 30 minutes. Dose
modifications were not allowed but delay of up to 3 weeks
was permissable in the event of bone marrow depression
(wbc < 3000/mm^3) or renal dysfunction (serum creatinine
> 1.5 mg/100ml.).

Physical examination, whole blood count, biochemistry
profile and roentgenographic examinations were done before
the start of therapy and at regular intervals during
treatment. Full description and measurement of indicator
lesions were recorded. Investigations necessary for the
assessment of indicator lesions were repeated as appropriate
but were required in all cases after seven treatment cycles.

Strict criteria (WHO Handbook, 1979) were applied with
complete remission necessitating disappearance of all lesions
and partial remission a 50% or more decrease in the product
of the two largest perpendicular diameters of all measurable
lesions. Complete and partial remissions had to be
maintained for no less than four weeks with no new lesions
appearing. Stable disease and progression were the other
two recognised categories. Arbitrarily, patients were
considered evaluable for response if they had received a
minimum of four treatment cycles with methyl-GAG.

RESULTS

Forty-five patients were entered into the study. Only
3 of these were completely non-evaluable because of lack
of data or protocol violation. Thirty patients received
4 or more treatment cycles and were evaluable for response.
Twelve patients were only partially evaluable, i.e. for
assessment of toxicity.

Of the 30 fully evaluable patients, 3 achieved partial
remission, 11 showed no significant change and in 16 the
disease progressed. No complete remissions were observed.
The duration of the partial remissions in no case exceeded
8 weeks.

Patients Evaluable/ Patients entered	Partial Remission	Stable Disease	Progression
30/45	3	11	16

Table 1. Results of Methyl-GAG in Metastatic Renal Cell Cancer

The commonest side-effects were anorexia, nausea and vomiting (43%), moderate or severe in 19% of all patients. Neuropathy, myopathy and myalgia also proved troublesome in some patients and was encountered in 21% overall (moderate or severe in 14% of all patients). Mucositis was moderate or severe in 7%. Six patients had to be taken off treatment because of the severity of side-effects. Evidence of bone marrow depression was unusual and leucopenia necessitated delay in treatment in only 3 patients.

Side-effects	Number of Patients		
	Mild	Moderate	Severe
Anorexia, nausea, vomiting	10	5	3
Neuropathy, myopathy myalgia	3	4	2
Mucositis	3	2	1
Skin reactions	2	2	1
Leucopenia	2	2	0
Diarrhoea	2	1	1

Table 2. Toxicity of Methyl-GAG 500 $mg/m^2/wk$ (42 patients)

DISCUSSION

The results of this EORTC study add to information which is accumulating as to the effects of methyl-GAG in advanced renal cancer. The data from SWOG (Knight, Livingston, Fabian, Costanzi 1980) indicated significant responses to methyl-GAG in a weekly dose of 500 mg/m^2 with 100 mg/m^2 dose escalation per treatment cycle, occuring both within four and after four treatment cycles. One complete and two partial remissions were seen in 23 patients. Todd, Garnick,

Canellos (1980), who also gave 500 mg/m^2 weekly but with
50 mg/m^2 escalation, reported one complete and three partial
remissions among 18 patients. All these remissions occurred
within four weeks. However, in a more recent study (Zeffren,
Yagoda, Watson, Natale, Blumenreich, Howard 1981) no remissions were seen in 30 patients, in whom toxicity was
apparently severe - including muscle weakness, lethary,
myalgia, mucositis and skin rashes. In the study reported
here, where a fixed dose was adopted, three partial
remissions have been recorded among the 30 patients
receiving at least four treatment cycles. The toxicity
observed was moderate to severe in some patients, necessitating cessation of treatment in six patients.

There is good evidence that methyl-GAG has limited
activity of short-term duration in renal cell cancer.
However, the degree of toxicity encountered with the use
of this drug may well preclude further study.

Killin J, Hoth D, Smith F, Schein P, Woolley P (1980).
  Methyl-glyoxal bis-guanylhydrazone (NSC 32946) (methyl-GAG)
  Phase II experience and clinical pharmacology. Proc Am
  Assoc Cancer Res 21:368.
Knight WA III, Livingston RB, Fabian C, Costanzi J (1979).
  Phase I-II trial of methyl-GAG: a southwest oncology
  group pilot study. Cancer Treat Rep 63:1933.
Knight WA III, Livingston RB, Fabian C, Costanzi J (1980).
  Methyl-glyoxal bis-guanylhydrazone (methyl-GAG, MGBG) in
  advanced renal carcinoma. Proc Am Assoc Cancer Res 21:367.
Oliverio VT, Adamson RH, Henderson ES, Davidson JD (1963).
  The distribution, excretion and metabolism of methylglyoxal
  bis (guanylhydrazone C^{14}). J Pharmacol & Exper Therap
  141:149 .
Porter CW, Mikles-Robertson D, Kramer D, Dave C (1979).
  Correlation of ultrastructural and functional damage to
  mitochondria of ascites L1210 cells treated in vivo with
  methylglyoxal bis (guanylhydrazone) or ethidium bromide.
  Cancer Res 39:2414 .
Todd RF, Garnick MD, Canellos GP (1980). Chemotherapy of
  advanced renal adenocarcinoma with methyl-glyoxal bis-
  guanylhydrazone (methyl-GAG). Proc Am Assoc Cancer
  Res 21:340.

WHO Handbook for Reporting Results of Cancer Treatment (1979).
  Definitions of objective response. WHO Offset
  Publication 48:23.
Zeffrin J, Yagoda A, Watson RC, Natale RB, Blumenreich MS,
Howard J (1981).
  Phase II trial of methyl-glyoxal bis-guanylhydrazone in
  advanced renal cancer. Cancer Treat Rep 65:525.

PRINCIPAL PARTICIPANTS

1. Bono AV, Ospedale Di Circolo E Fondazione E.e S. Macchi,
    Varese
2. Fossa SD, The Norwegian Radium Hospital, Oslo
3. Bokkel Huinink WW ten, Antoni van Leeuwenholkhuis,
    Amsterdam
4. Stoter G, Ac: 'emisch Ziekenhuis der Vrije Universiteit,
    Amsterdam

Renal Tumors: Proceedings of the First International Symposium on Kidney Tumors, pages 669–671
© **1982 Alan R. Liss, Inc., 150 Fifth Avenue, New York, NY 10011**

CHEMOTHERAPY OF RENAL TUMOURS.   PERSONAL EXPERIENCE

C. Jacquillat, G. Auclerc, M.F. Auclerc, N. Chamsedine, J. Mara, M. Weil
Medical Oncology Service
Hôpital de la Salpétrierè
47 Blvd de l'hôpital, Paris

Kidney tumours account for 2% of all malignancies, and over a quarter of them, when first diagnosed, have metastases. Nephrectomy can reduce the incidence of metastases by 1%: thus because of possible operative or postoperative mortality (2, 3, 10%), one hesitates to propose nephrectomy in advanced cases, even if the prognosis is grave. Numerous studies have indicated a 5-year survival rate between 0 and 8%. Some have suggested strongly the presence of an interval between diagnosis and the appearance of metastases: if metastases present more than 2 years after onset, one can perhaps hope for a 20% 5-year survival rate. In addition, the nature of the metastases can alter the prognosis. In a case of a solitary bony metastasis, the median survival was reported to be 21 months, falling to 10 months if the bony metastases were diffuse.

Because this pathology has such a disastrous prognosis, numerous therapeutic agents have been proposed, ranging from hormonal therapy to chemotherapy. During the 1970's, the progestogens were said to have a 10-17% response rate. Since then, however, the results have been disappointing, with a 0-2% response rate after 10 years. Hopes were raised with the appearance of anti-oestrogens and results showing a 16% response rate to tamoxifen. Other reports indicated a lower response (8.1%) to tamoxifen based on literature values, and a 3% response to androgens. Mono-chemotherapy was often used in phase II of the disease. Here, at least 22 drugs have been tested, though few have been found to be of any use. Vincaleucoblastine (VLB) appears to be the least inefficient since a 25% response rate was found in a study of 200 patients. If, however, one takes into account only regressions greater than 50%, this response rate falls to 15%. Other products have shown some activity: Mitomycin C (11% in 26 cases), 5-fluoro-uracil (8% in 90 cases), CCNU, methyl-CCNU (7% in 116 cases) and hydroxyurea (5% in 45 cases). More recently, quite interesting results have been noted with Methyl-GAG, PALA, Triazinate, (Baker antifolate) and 20_H-9 methyl-ellepticinium. Conversely, no response was shown to Adriamycin on cis-Platinum.

In addition to the product selected, the dose used is also relevant. For example, with VLB, in particular, the response rate rises from 15% to 31% depending on whether the dose used is 0.1-0.2 mg/kg or 0.2-0.3 mg kg.

With such mediocre results, the association of several products was tried, but the results here were either less than or just equal to VLB on its own. A combination of VLB and CCNU gave a 24% response; other combinations were less effective, except for the combination of acetate and medroxyprogesterone, MPA. A protocol involving MPA and Vincristine and Adriamycin and BCG gave a 33% response rate in a series of 31 cases, and a 19% rate with VLB and CCNU and cyclophasphamide and MPA was reported in another study. The median survival was 52 weeks in those showing a response and 12 weeks in those with no response. Some randomized trials have been undertaken with fairly mediocre results. One study reported a 16% response rate with nafoxidine.

If there exists a problem of the efficiency of the medication, there exists an equal problem of evaluation of response, because some workers take into account even very minor responses, thus giving rise to differences in observed response rate. It would be better if everyone agreed not to describe a "response" unless there was at least a 50% regression. Furthermore, the benefit of progestagens is not always demonstrable, and similary one wonders if antioestrogens have an action. Again, all the drug combination studies have failed to demonstrate any clear superiority over VLB on its own in large doses.

Despite all, we continue to use a drug combination for metastatic disease following primary renal tumor:

VLB (8 mg/m^2/weekly i.v.) and MPA (1,000 mg 2 times per week i.m.) and Tomoscifen in large doses (60 mg/daily).

However, the future will bring new active preparations (Methyl-GAG, 20H-9 methyl-ellepticinium), different techniques, potentration of methyl-GAG by diffuro-methyl-ornithine (DFMO), for example, or continuous infusion of VLB. Finally, the future might bring better drug screening either by evaluating drug sensitivity in vitro or neoplastic cell cultures or by using allografts on mice. Only cooperative studies can provide the means necessary for progress in this direction.

Renal Tumors: Proceedings of the First International Symposium on Kidney Tumors, pages 673–685
© 1982 Alan R. Liss, Inc., 150 Fifth Avenue, New York, NY 10011

THERMOMAGNETIC SURGERY FOR RENAL CANCER

Robert W. Rand, Ph.D., M.D.*, Harold D. Snow,
D.V.M.**, W. Jann Brown, M.D.***
*Department of Surgery, UCLA School of Medicine,
Los Angeles CA, **The Leo G. Rigler Center for
Radiological Sciences, UCLA Center for the
Health Sciences, Los Angeles, CA, ***Depart-
ment of Pathology, UCLA School of Medicine,
Los Angeles, CA

Supported in part by grants from UCLA Medical
Center Auxiliary and Max and Victoria Dreyfus
Foundation.

ABSTRACT

   Thermomagnetic surgery is a technique that uses
hysteresis heating of ferromagnetic materials to produce
focally controlled temperatures within solid organs or
tumors to cause coagulation necrosis. The degree of
heating of a neoplasm is controlled by manipulating the
power of the electromagnetic coil system through
temperature monitoring. This effectively limits the
region of destruction to the disease process and thereby
avoids damage to surrounding structures. If the ferromagnetic material is delivered by an arterial route
to the tumor or organ additional beneficial effect of
ischemic necrosis of tissue may be achieved. This new
technique is applicable to selected cases of human cancer.
Exposure in the electromagnetic fields or use of the
ferromagnetic material in experimental animals has
produced no ill effects.

INTRODUCTION

   Thermomagnetic surgery is a technique which was
developed to effect destruction of cancerous tissue by
focally controlled hyperthermia. It uses the physical

phenomenon of hysteresis heat loss of microferromagnetic materials to produce cancer cell destruction. These materials are placed directly within the cancer by implantation or by arterial embolization in anesthetized animals. Animals are positioned in a specially designed low frequency alternating current Litz tank coil system (Fig. 1). The ferromagnetic particles change their polarity to produce hysteresis heat loss in the low frequency alternating current magnetic field. The intense focal heat thus generated is conveyed by convection and contact to the surrounding neoplastic tissue. As the temperature rises the cancer is destroyed by coagulation necrosis and denaturation (Fig. 2).

The ferromagnetic particles ($0.1 - 1\mu$) and the carrier fluid combine to cause occlusion at the pre-capillary and capillary levels of the selected vascular system of the cancer when the transarterial route is employed. Residual neoplastic cells may remain at the interface between cancer and the normal tissue where the blood and lymphatic supply exist. This neoplastic tissue that may have escaped the initial ischemic necrosis may be destroyed subsequently by coagulation necrosis. Thermo-magnetic surgery constitutes an attempt to totally destroy the primary origin of the renal cancer so that any subsequent surgical maneuver would be advantaged by minimal risk of spreading the cancer by metastasis (Fig. 3).

Thermomagnetic surgery though still in an investigative stage, has been proven to be effective in totally destroying whole normal solid organs such as kidney within experimental dog and rabbit models. The surgery has been performed without producing acute or chronic ill effects from the exposure to the powerful alternating current low frequency magnetic field of the micro-ferromagnetic material. These magnetic fields do, however, produce muscle spasm of varying degrees, depending on the orientation of the animal relative to the magnetic field during treatment. Such spasm can be controlled effectively by appropriate drugs.

METHODS AND MATERIALS

Twenty-four New Zealand white rabbits were injected selectively, into the renal artery of one kidney with rabbit (VX_2) carcinoma. Active cancer in recipient rabbits, confirmed both by histological examination for cell viability and by the capacity for transplanted cells to grow in other rabbits, was evident in 5 days.

The VX_2 neoplasm appears on the surface of the kidney and develops within 10 days. Metastasis to the peritoneum and a generalized spread to other organs occurs. Control rabbits with this anaplastic VX_2 type of cancer have invariably died.

A transfermoral catheter is passed into the renal artery of a rabbit under general anesthesia. An aliquot of 10^7 malignant VX_2 cells in 0.5 - 1.0 mL of carrier liquid is made under fluoroscopy. An abdominal laparotomy under general Pentothal anesthesia is done five days later and the diseased kidney exposed. Ligation of the renal artery and vein is performed and 2-3 ml of micro-ferromagnetic material suspended in 50% concentrations in sterile saline is injected into the pelvis and renal calcyes of the kidney. A radiograph establishes the location and distribution of this radio-opaque ferromagnetic material. Fine thermocouples are placed on the surface and within the cancerous kidney and held by a biologic adhesive. The wire leads are brought out through the abdominal incision (Fig. 4).

An alternating current low-frequency 2-KH_z coil in a strong, alternating magnetic field of 0.1 Tesla rms amplitude is produced by a tank circuit. The ferro-magnetic particles oscillate and hysteresis heat is produced to which the VX_2 renal cancer model rabbits are then exposed.

In 12 rabbits with VX_2 renal carcinoma the temperature of the kidney surface was raised in 1 to 2 minutes to 55^OC. The power activating the coil system was then switched off resulting in a cooling of the kidney for a period of 5 min. Power was resupplied when the temperature fell to 43^OC causing a second sudden rise in temperature within the kidney. The cancer was exposed to several of these periods of hysteresis heating.

The rabbits recovered from anesthesia, and the exposure to the magnetic field produced no acute ill effects. Later autopsy examinations demonstrated that although the majority of the cancer within the kidney was destroyed some islands of carcinoma had remained in arteries and within the parenchyma (Fig. 5).

In six experiments the increases of kidney surface temperature was raised more gradually. When the temperature reached the level of 50°C the power to the coil was reduced slowly in order to maintain a steady renal surface temperature of 50°C for 5, 10 or 15 minutes. In these rabbits total destruction of the cancer was achieved. The successful results were due to the longer exposure of the cancer cells to intense controlled focal heat. All animals survived the thermomagnetic surgery and showed no evidence of metastases when sacrificed after 7 to 10 days and tissues were compared to control animals (Fig. 6, 7).

This microferromagnetic material has been placed in the lungs and kidneys of dogs for a period of over 3 years without any clinically evident ill effects. Liver, kidney and bone marrow function have remained unimpaired. Dogs and rabbits have been exposed to the magnetic field and have not shown ill effects after 3 and 1 years respectively.

DISCUSSION

Gilchrist (Gilchrist et al. 1957; Gilchrist 1960) reported on the potential use of hysteresis heating in cancer. The studies revealed not only the potential value of hysteresis hyperthermia in destroying cancerous tissue but also that the magnetic fields had no apparent adverse effects on normal adult tissue or embryonic tissue. The experimental work was not given a clinical trial and was discontinued.

Prior research using ferrosilicone embolization to produce ischemic necrosis of organs and human neoplasms lead to the current development of the technique of thermomagnetic surgery. Ferrites, which show strong hysteresis heating characteristics were substituted for the spherical carbonyl iron that has poor ferromagnetic properties. Many ferromagnetic materials were tested to determine which ferromagnetic needle-shaped particles would not interfere with vulcanization of the medical liquid silicone (Mosso, Rand 1973; Rand, Mosso 1972; Rand et al. 1976). These electromagnetic and silicone experiments were successful so that it was possible to inject these compounds into the vascular tree of normal tissue and organs. The combination of ischemia and coagulation necrosis secondary to hysteresis heating effects total necrosis of the desired tissue, wuch as a kidney (Fig. 8; Rand et al. 1976; Turner et al. 1975).

The poorly differentiated VX_2 rabbit carcinoma was employed to develop a renal tumor model. The VX_2 rabbit carcinoma has rarely undergone spontaneous remission. This cancer uniformly causes death of the rabbit within several months by metastasis.

These experiments have demonstrated that a sustained constant surface heating of $50^{\circ}C$ for longer periods of time, induced by adjusting the power to the coil was more effective in destroying renal cancer than earlier periodic on-off surface heating to $55^{\circ}C$. The temperature within the kidney was higher by at least $15^{\circ}C$. Histologic examination by both light and electron microscopy of these later model tumor specimens made the nature of the necrosis in kidney and of the cancer within it unquestioned (Fig. 6, 7).

The animals survived the various operative procedures and exposure in the magnetic field without evidence of ill effects including chronic dogs which have been followed for up to 3 years after exposure to the magnetic fields with the ferromagnetic material in the lungs and kidneys.

The authors suggest that thermomagnetic surgery is ready for limited clinical application in selected patients with proven accessible cancer using the ferro-magnetic material suspended in medical grade silicone. A patient with hypernephroma could benefit first by the ischemic necrosis of the cancerous kidney followed by hysteresis hyperthermia to assure complete destruction of any residual cancer in the kidney prior to any surgical manipulation.

CONCLUSIONS

Thermomagnetic surgery is an effective method of producing intense controlled focal heating resulting in total necrosis and destruction of the renal cancer VX_2 in rabbit models. This technique of thermomagnetic surgery is a feasible and a reasonable procedure for clinical trials with selected human cancer patients.

Gilchrist RK, Medal R, Shorey WD, Hanselman RC, Parrot, JC, Taylor CB (1957). Selective Inductive Heating of Lymph Nodes. Ann Surg 146:596.

Gilchrist RK (1960). Potential Treatment of Cancer by Electromagnetic Heating. Surg Gynecol & Obstet 110:449.

Mosso. JA, Rand RW (1973). Ferromagnetic Silicone Vascular Occlusion: A technique for selective infarction of tumors and organs. Ann Surg 178:663.

Rand RW, Mosso JA (1972). Ferromagnic silicone vascular occlusion in superconducting magnetic field: Preliminary Report. Bull LA Neurol Soc 37:67.

Rand RW, Snyder M, Elliott D, Snow H (1976). Selective radiofrequency heating of ferrosilicone occulded tissue: Preliminary Report. Bull LA Neurol Soc 41:154.

Turner RD, Rand RW, Bentson, JR, Mosso JA (1975). Ferromagnetic silicone necrosis of hypernephromas by selective vascular occlusion to the tumor: A new technique. J Urol 113:455.

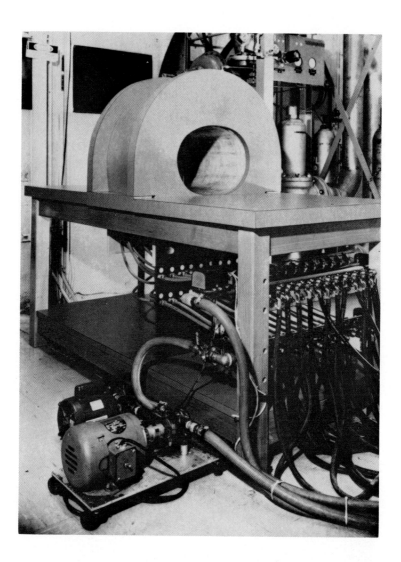

Fig. 1 A specially designed low frequency alternating
current system which produces the physical
phenomena of hysteresis heat loss of ferromagnetic
particles to produce cancer cell destruction.

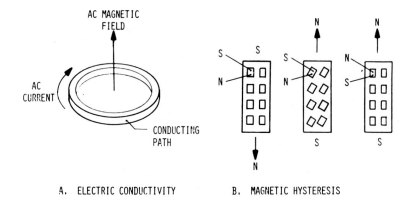

A. ELECTRIC CONDUCTIVITY   B. MAGNETIC HYSTERESIS

Fig. 2. Diagram of mechanism of magnetic hysteresis heat loss. The alternating position of the ferrosilicone particles produces heat by friction.

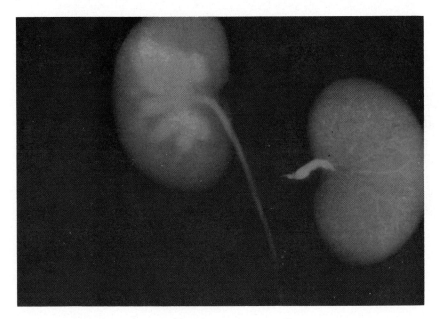

Fig. 3. Radiograph of ferromagnetic particles placed in the renal pelvis of the dog kidney (left), and within the arterial tree of the kidney of another dog (right).

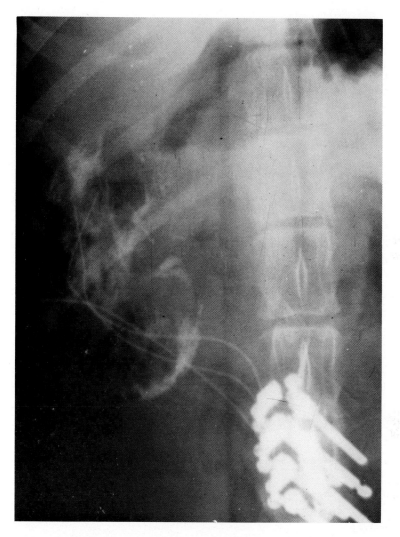

Fig. 4   Fine thermocouples placed on surface and within
kidney containing ferromagnetic particles.   The
thermocouples monitor the temperature to control
the hysteresis heating of the cancerous kidney.

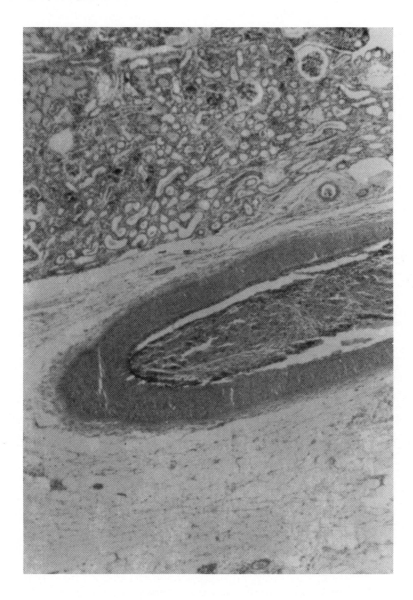

Fig. 5 Microphotograph of residual VX$_2$ carcinoma in an
arterial of rabbit kidney after on-off hysteresis
heating technique.

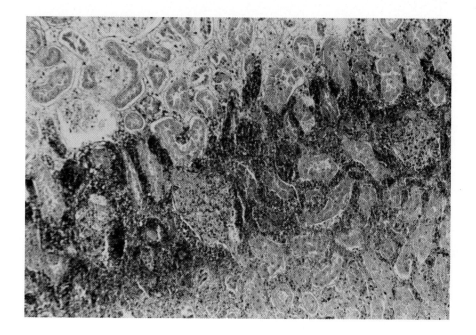

Fig. 6   Photomicrograph of rabbit kidney showing total
          destruction of kidney parrenchyma and VX_2
          carcinoma after continuous controlled hysteresis
          heating.

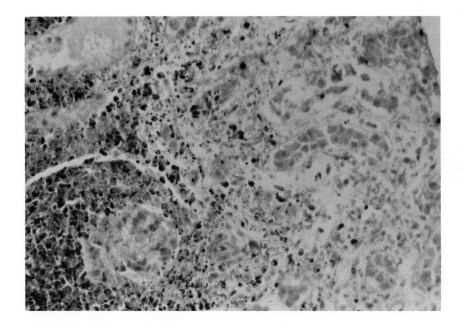

Fig. 7 Similar results of total coagulation necrosis in
        another rabbit kidney containing VX$_2$ carcinoma
        seen at higher magnification.

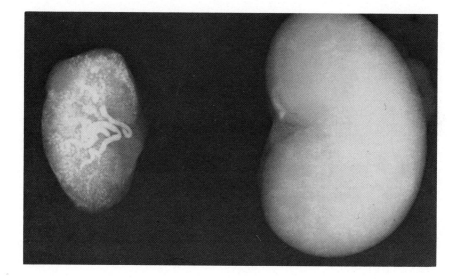

Fig. 8   Roentgenogram of canine kidneys showing gross
total necrosis of left kidney by ischemic
necrosis and hysteresis heating.   The total
necrosis was confirmed by subsequent microscopic
examination.

Index

Abdomen irradiation, 102–103
ACTH, 281
Actinomycin D
    and renal cancer, 199–200
    and Wilms' tumor, 111–116, 119,
        131–132, 134, 169–170
Adenomatous hyperplasia, 323
Adriamycin, 115, 141
Alkylating agents, 264–265
Amyloidosis, 449
Anaplasia, 2–5, 12
Androgen receptors, 231–232, 248–249,
    252, 625–627
Anemia, 449
Angiomyolipomata, 385
Aniridia, 44
Anticancer agents, 265
Aromatic amines, 264
Arteriography and
    nephroblastoma, 65–66, 77
    renal angiomyolipoma, 575
    renal cancer, 349–368, 498

Benzpyrene, 267
Biochemical syndromes, 278
Bladder surgery, 561–566, 569
Bone metastasis, renal cancer, 9–11,
    331, 544–546
Bourneville's disease, 573–574
Bowel, 497, 501–504
Brain metastasis, renal cancer, 541,
    545–546, 651
Breast tumor, 575

Cadmium, 266–267
Calcification, tumor, 386
Calcitonin, 298, 308
cAMP, 296

Chemical carcinogens, 256, 262–263,
    268
Chemotherapy, 50
    and bladder tumor, 565
    preoperative, for Wilms' tumor,
        131–143
    and renal cancer, 198–201, 545, 642–
        646, 655, 661–666, 669–671
    side effects of, 112–116, 119–120
    and Wilms' tumor, 26–36, 111–116,
        119–120, 125–128, 131–143,
        169–170
Children, 1–13
Chloroform, 267–268
Computerized tomography, 51, 54
    and inferior vena cava obstruction,
        399–408
    and nephroblastoma, 67–70, 77–80,
        83
    and renal angiomyolipoma, 576
    and renal cancer, 377–394, 497
    and renal cancer recurrence, 409–415
    and renal tumor, 418, 422–423, 438–
        439, 442
Congenital mesoblastic nephroma. See
    Mesoblastic nephroma
Cycas circinalis, 267
Cycasin, 201, 267
Cystic lesions, kidney, 49, 268
Cystic nephroblastoma, 8–9, 13
Cysts, renal, 8–9, 13, 84, 377, 382, 385,
    417–423, 433–434
Cytology, 425–432

DNA, 198

Echotomography, 61–65, 76–77
Endocrine syndromes, 279–281
Enteropathy, 450

Enzymes and
    renal tumor, 281
    Wilms' tumor, 21–22
Epidemiology, 258–259, 268
Epithelioma, clear cell, 84
Erythropoietin, 25–26, 280, 308
Estradiol receptors, 233–237, 625–627,
    629–631
Estrogen, 261–262, 625–626
Estrogen receptor, 249–253
Extrarenal tumor, 76

Fetal. *See* Foetal
Fever, 279, 283–289, 449
Foetal lobulation hypertrophy, 385

Gastrointestinal tract, 106
Genetics and
    renal cell carcinoma, 259–260, 268
    Wilms' tumor, 43
Genito-urinary anomalies, 44
Gerota's fascia, 390, 458, 487
Gonadotrophins, 280–281, 450

Haematologic. *See* Hematologic
Haematuria. *See* Hematuria
Haemorrhage. *See* Hemorrhage
Hemangioblastoma, 331–332
Hemartoma, 574–575, 577
Hematologic syndromes, 278
Hematologic toxicity, 107
Hematuria, 338–340, 448–449
Hemihypertrophy, 43
Hemorrhage, 574
Hepatic
    dysfunction, 301–312, 449
    toxicity, 105–106
    see also Liver
Herpes simplex virus, 260, 268
Histologic grading, 145–153
Histology and
    angiomyolipoma, 576
    renal cell carcinoma, 426
Histopathology, 1–13
Hormones and
    renal cancer, 211–238, 261–262, 268
    renal tumor, 279–281, 310

Hormone therapy, 175–176, 189–193,
    623–636, 646–647, 655
Hydrazine, 264
Hydronephrosis, 84
Hypercalcemia, 293–298, 307–308, 450
Hypernephroma. *See* Renal cancer
Hypertension, 279, 308, 450, 574–575

Immune system and
    renal cancer, 310–311
    Wilms' tumor, 26, 39
Immunological syndromes, 279
Immunotherapy, 647–652, 655
Indomethacin, 298
Infection, 574
Inflammatory syndromes, 287–288
Interferon, 650–651
International Society of Paediatric On-
    cology, 131–143
Irradiation. *See* Radiation

Kidney. *See* Renal
Kupffer cells, 309

Lead, 266
Levamisole, 26
Lipomatosis, 373
Liposomes, 200–201
Liver
    and renal cancer, 497–499, 503–504,
        546
    see also Hepatic
Lung, 330, 333
    irradiation, 103–104, 134
    metastasis, 543–544, 640–651
    toxicity, 107–108
Lymph node
    lymphadenectomy, 486–487, 491,
        493–495
    and renal cancer, 393–394, 448,
        471–473
    retroperitoneal dissection, 489–492

Malignant cells, transplanted, 581–587
Malignant rhabdoid tumor, kidney,
    11–12

Mesoblastic nephroma
  diagnosis, 84
  histopathologic aspects of, 7–8,
    12–13
  and Wilms' tumor, 45, 49
Metabolic syndromes, 279
Metastasis
  renal cancer, 195–198, 274–275,
    317–333, 393–394, 448, 450,
    533–547, 610–611, 641,
    647–655
  spontaneous regression, 333, 535,
    653–654
  Wilms' tumor, 22–23, 33, 47–48,
    91–94, 134, 137, 141
Methyl-GAG, 663–666
Mice, 207–209; see also Murine
Mithramycin, 298
Murine renal cell carcinoma, 175–202
Murine Wilms' tumor, 26–33

Nephroblastomas
  bilateral, 73–74
  computerized tomography in, 67–70
  differential diagnosis of, 71–80
  evaluation of, 59–66
  see also Wilms' tumor
Nephroblastomatosis
  diagnosis, 74, 84
  histopathologic aspects of, 5–6, 12
  and Wilms' tumor, 45
Nephrotomography, 345–347
Neuroblastoma, 76
Neurofibromatosis, 45
Nitrosamines, 46, 263–264
NMRI Nu/Nu mouse tumor, 207–208
Nu/Nu mice, 207–209

Oestrogen. See Estrogen
Ovary, 332

Paraneoplastic syndromes, 277–281,
    307–308, 339–340
Parathormone, 280, 294–296
Pelvic tumor surgery, 569–570
Perinephric space, 388–390
Polycythemia, 449–450

Progesterone, 646–647
Progesterone receptors, 625–627,
    629–630
Progestin, 624
Progestin receptors, 222–231
Prostaglandins, 280, 294–295, 308
Pseudo-hyperparathyroidism, 294
Pulmonary. See Lung
Pyrexia. See Fever
Pyrogens, 288–289

Radiation
  abdomen, 102–103
  lung, 103–104, 134
  renal bed, 99–102
  and renal cancer, 260, 268
Radioactive isotope scans, 51–53
Radiology, 59–61
Radiotherapy
  and bladder tumor, 565
  complications of, 104–108, 120–121
  preoperative, and renal cancer,
    609–621
  and renal cancer, 661–662
  and Wilms' tumor, 97–108, 120–121,
    125, 131–132, 134–135, 139,
    142–143, 169–170
Rats, Wilms' tumor in, 15–25
Receptor profiles, 211–238
Renal abscess, 386, 388
Renal adenocarcinoma. See Renal
  cancer
Renal adenoma, 256–257
Renal angiomyolipoma, 573–578
  clinical aspects of, 573–575
  diagnosis of, 575–576
  histology, 576
  treatment, 576–578
Renal arteriography. See Arteriography
Renal autotransplantation with
    pyelovesical anastomosis, 563,
    566, 569–570
Renal bed irradiation, 99–102
Renal cancer
  arteriography, 349–368, 498
  associated with other conditions,
    257–258

and chemotherapy, 198–201, 545,
    642–646, 655, 661–666,
    669–671
clear cell adenocarcinoma, 324–325,
    327–328
clear cell sarcoma, 9–11, 13, 45–46,
    53
clinically unrecognized, 273–275
clinical signs of, 337–340
combined chemotherapy and
    radiotherapy, 661–662
computed tomography, 377–394,
    399–415, 497
cytologic diagnosis, 425–432
diagnosis, 79–80, 341–342, 349–352,
    378
differential diagnosis, 342–343
etiology, 194–198, 255–268
fever, 279, 283–289
genitourinary spread, 327
hematogenous spread, 326–327
and hepatic dysfunction syndrome,
    301–312
hormonal studies of, 189–193
and hormone therapy, 623–636,
    646–647, 655
and hypercalcemia, 293–298
immunotherapy for, 647–652, 655
and inferior vena cava obstruction,
    399–408
invasion, 497–505, 529–531
kinetics, 179–183
local signs of, 448–449
lumbar flank approach, 457–459
lymphatic metastasis, 325–326
metabolic studies, 183–189
metastasis, 195–198, 274–275,
    317–333, 393–394, 448, 450,
    533–547, 610–611, 641,
    647–655
methyl-GAG for, 663–666
natural history of, 447–450, 599–600
nephrotomography in, 345–347
preoperative radiotherapy in,
    609–621
prognosis of, 483, 486–487, 545–546

radiotherapy in, 661–662
receptor profiles in, 211–238
recurrence of, 487
recurrence of, in renal fossa and/or
    abdominal wall, 549–559
sonography in, 369–375
spontaneous, 257
spontaneous regression in, 450
staging in, 321, 378, 439–445,
    483–486, 557
surgery, 453–505, 509–526, 533–542,
    641, 652–655
survival, 324, 480, 485–492, 526,
    534–535
systemic signs, 449–450
thermomagnetic surgery in, 673–684
in transitional cells, 256
treatment of advanced, 641–655
tumor grade, 487, 557
tumor size, 322–333
urologic signs of, 338–339
and vinblastine sulfate, 209
weight loss, 339
see also Renal tumor
Renal cell carcinoma. See Renal cancer
Renal infarction, 654–655
Renal insufficiency, 575
Renal oncocytoma, 589–596
    needle tract seeding after puncture,
        597
    treatment, 595–596
Renal pelvis, 256, 385
Renal sinus, 53
Renal toxicity, 107
Renal transplantation, 581–587
Renal tumor
    calcification, 386
    in children, 1–13
    and computerized tomography,
        438–439, 442
    diagnosis, 417–418, 433–434
    embolization, 601–607
    explorative lumbotomy, 435–436
    investigation, 431–438
    pelvis, 385
    percutaneous puncture, 417–423

sonography, 437–438
steroid receptors in, 245–253
see also Renal cancer
Renal vein, 390–393, 443–444
Renin, 279–280, 308, 450
Rhabdoid tumor, 11–13, 45–46, 53
RNA therapy, 651–652

Sarcoma, clear cell, 9–11, 13, 45–46, 53
Serotherapy, 651
Serum alkaline phosphatase, 309–310
Skin, 106–107, 332
Sonography, 51, 54
    and nephroblastoma, 74, 77, 79, 83,
        84
    and renal cancer, 369–375
    and renal tumor, 418, 422–423,
        437–438
Squamous cell carcinoma, 256
Stauffer's syndrome, 301–312
Steroid hormones, 625–627, 636
Steroid receptors, 216–222, 238,
    245–253
Surgery
    abdominal approach, 461–464,
        530–531
    anterior transabdominal transversal
        sub-costal approach, 465–469
    bench, 509–516
    extracorporeal, 509–516
    incision choice, 471–473
    lumbar flank approach, 457–459
    nephrectomy, 652–655
    nephrectomy, partial, 519–526
    nephrectomy, radical, 481–495,
        533–540
    nephrectomy, radical without
        lymphadenectomy, 475–480,
        491
    nephroureterectomy, 561–562, 564,
        569
    renal angiomyolipoma, 576–578
    renal cancer, 453–505, 509–526,
        533–542, 641, 652–655
    thermomagnetic, 673–684

thoraco-abdominal nephrectomy,
    radical, 481–488
thoracophrenolaparotomy, 453–455
urinary tract, 561–566
Wilms' tumor, 85–89, 124–125,
    155–164

Tomodensitometry, 394
Transfer factor, 651
Transitional cells, 256, 561–566
Tuberous sclerosis, 573–574, 577
Tumor
    bladder, 565
    breast, 575
    calcification, 386
    cell kinetics, 179–183
    extrarenal, 76
    mouse, 207–208
    pelvic, surgery, 569–570
    rhabdoid, 11–13, 45–46, 53
    ureter, surgery, 569–570
    see also Renal cancer; Renal tumor;
        Wilms' tumor

Ultrasound. *See* Sonography
Ureter tumor surgery, 569–570
Urinary tract
    anomalies, 44
    and renal cancer, 338–339
    transitional cell tumors, 561–566

Vena cava, 393
    obstruction of inferior, 399–408
    and renal cancer, 497–501, 503,
        529–531
Vinblastine sulfate, 209, 642, 644
Vincristine, 113–116, 119, 131, 134,
    169–170
Virus, 260–261, 268

Wilms' tumor
    adjuvant therapy for, 26–36
    anaplasia in, 2–5, 12
    bilateral, 36, 47, 103, 155–164
    cell studies, 23–25

chemotherapy for, 26–36, 111–116,
    119–120, 125–128, 131–143,
    169–170
clinical signs and symptoms, 48–49
cystic lesions, 49
diagnosis, 50–53
differential diagnosis, 49–50
etiology, 46, 54
experimental, 15–39
familial, 44
genetics, 43, 54
histologic grading, 145–153
histopathology of, 2–3, 12, 46
immunologic factor in, 26, 39
late-recurring, 165–166
metabolic effects of, 25–26
metastasis, 22–23, 33, 47–48, 91–94,
    134, 137, 141

natural history of, 47
preoperative chemotherapy for,
    131–143
preoperative diagnosis of, 83–84
prognosis, 94, 128–129
radiotherapy for, 97–108, 120–121,
    125, 131–132, 134–135, 139,
    142–143, 169–170
staging, 48, 53, 91–94, 131–133
surgery, 85–89, 124–125, 155–164
survival, 134–137, 141, 151–153,
    167–168
TNM, 91–94
treatment side effects, 119–121,
    167–171
understanding of, 123–124
see also Nephroblastomas

PROGRESS IN CLINICAL AND BIOLOGICAL RESEARCH

Vol 1: **Erythrocyte Structure and Function,** George J. Brewer, *Editor*

Vol 2: **Preventability of Perinatal Injury,** Karlis Adamsons and Howard A. Fox, *Editors*

Vol 3: **Infections of the Fetus and the Newborn Infant,** Saul Krugman and Anne A. Gershon, *Editors*

Vol 4: **Conflicts in Childhood Cancer: An Evaluation of Current Management,** Lucius F. Sinks and John O. Godden, *Editors*

Vol 5: **Trace Components of Plasma: Isolation and Clinical Significance,** G.A. Jamieson and T.J. Greenwalt, *Editors*

Vol 6: **Prostatic Disease,** H. Marberger, H. Haschek, H.K.A. Schirmer, J.A.C. Colston, and E. Witkin, *Editors*

Vol 7: **Blood Pressure, Edema and Proteinuria in Pregnancy,** Emanuel A. Friedman, *Editor*

Vol 8: **Cell Surface Receptors,** Garth L. Nicolson, Michael A. Raftery, Martin Rodbell, and C. Fred Fox, *Editors*

Vol 9: **Membranes and Neoplasia: New Approaches and Strategies,** Vincent T. Marchesi, *Editor*

Vol 10: **Diabetes and Other Endocrine Disorders During Pregnancy and in the Newborn,** Maria I. New and Robert H. Fiser, *Editors*

Vol 11: **Clinical Uses of Frozen-Thawed Red Blood Cells,** John A. Griep, *Editor*

Vol 12: **Breast Cancer,** Albert C.W. Montague, Geary L. Stonesifer, Jr., and Edward F. Lewison, *Editors*

Vol 13: **The Granulocyte: Function and Clinical Utilization,** Tibor J. Greenwalt and G.A. Jamieson, *Editors*

Vol 14: **Zinc Metabolism: Current Aspects in Health and Disease,** George J. Brewer and Ananda S. Prasad, *Editors*

Vol 15: **Cellular Neurobiology,** Zach Hall, Regis Kelly, and C. Fred Fox, *Editors*

Vol 16: **HLA and Malignancy,** Gerald P. Murphy, *Editor*

Vol 17: **Cell Shape and Surface Architecture,** Jean Paul Revel, Ulf Henning, and C. Fred Fox, *Editors*

Vol 18: **Tay-Sachs Disease: Screening and Prevention,** Michael M. Kaback, *Editor*

Vol 19: **Blood Substitutes and Plasma Expanders,** G.A. Jamieson and T.J. Greenwalt, *Editors*

Vol 20: **Erythrocyte Membranes: Recent Clinical and Experimental Advances,** Walter C. Kruckeberg, John W. Eaton, and George J. Brewer, *Editors*

Vol 21: **The Red Cell,** George J. Brewer, *Editor*

Vol 22: **Molecular Aspects of Membrane Transport,** Dale Oxender and C. Fred Fox, *Editors*

Vol 23: **Cell Surface Carbohydrates and Biological Recognition,** Vincent T. Marchesi, Victor Ginsburg, Phillips W. Robbins, and C. Fred Fox, *Editors*

Vol 24: **Twin Research, Proceedings of the Second International Congress on Twin Studies,** Walter E. Nance, *Editor* Published in 3 Volumes: Part A: **Psychology and Methodology** Part B: **Biology and Epidemiology** Part C: **Clinical Studies**

Vol 25: **Recent Advances in Clinical Oncology,** Tapan A. Hazra and Michael C. Beachley, *Editors*

Vol 26: **Origin and Natural History of Cell Lines,** Claudio Barigozzi, *Editor*

Vol 27: **Membrane Mechanisms of Drugs of Abuse,** Charles W. Sharp and Leo G. Abood, *Editors*

Vol 28: **The Blood Platelet in Transfusion**

Therapy, G.A. Jamieson and Tibor J. Greenwalt, *Editors*

Vol 29: **Biomedical Applications of the Horseshoe Crab (Limulidae),** Elias Cohen, *Editor-in-Chief*

Vol 30: **Normal and Abnormal Red Cell Membranes,** Samuel E. Lux, Vincent T. Marchesi, and C. Fred Fox, *Editors*

Vol 31: **Transmembrane Signaling,** Mark Bitensky, R. John Collier, Donald F. Steiner, and C. Fred Fox, *Editors*

Vol 32: **Genetic Analysis of Common Diseases: Applications to Predictive Factors in Coronary Disease,** Charles F. Sing and Mark Skolnick, *Editors*

Vol 33: **Prostate Cancer and Hormone Receptors,** Gerald P. Murphy and Avery A. Sandberg, *Editors*

Vol 34: **The Management of Genetic Disorders,** Constantine J. Papadatos and Christos S. Bartsocas, *Editors*

Vol 35: **Antibiotics and Hospitals,** Carlo Grassi and Giuseppe Ostino, *Editors*

Vol 36: **Drug and Chemical Risks to the Fetus and Newborn,** Richard H. Schwarz and Sumner J. Yaffe, *Editors*

Vol 37: **Models for Prostate Cancer,** Gerald P. Murphy, *Editor*

Vol 38: **Ethics, Humanism, and Medicine,** Marc D. Basson, *Editor*

Vol 39: **Neurochemistry and Clinical Neurology,** Leontino Battistin, George Hashim, and Abel Lajtha, *Editors*

Vol 40: **Biological Recognition and Assembly,** David S. Eisenberg, James A. Lake, and C. Fred Fox, *Editors*

Vol 41: **Tumor Cell Surfaces and Malignancy,** Richard O. Hynes and C. Fred Fox, *Editors*

Vol 42: **Membranes, Receptors, and the Immune Response: 80 Years After Ehrlich's Side Chain Theory,** Edward P. Cohen and Heinz Köhler, *Editors*

Vol 43: **Immunobiology of the Erythrocyte,** S. Gerald Sandler, Jacob Nusbacher, and Moses S. Schanfield, *Editors*

Vol 44: **Perinatal Medicine Today,** Bruce K. Young, *Editor*

Vol 45: **Mammalian Genetics and Cancer: The Jackson Laboratory Fiftieth Anniversary Symposium,** Elizabeth S. Russell, *Editor*

Vol 46: **Etiology of Cleft Lip and Cleft Palate,** Michael Melnick, David Bixler, and Edward D. Shields, *Editors*

Vol 47: **New Developments With Human and Veterinary Vaccines,** A. Mizrahi, I. Hertman, M.A. Klingberg, and A. Kohn, *Editors*

Vol 48: **Cloning of Human Tumor Stem Cells,** Sydney E. Salmon, *Editor*

Vol 49: **Myelin: Chemistry and Biology,** George A. Hashim, *Editor*